Clinical Guide to
Sunscreens and
Photoprotection

BASIC AND CLINICAL DERMATOLOGY

Series Editors

Alan R. Shalita, M.D.
Distinguished Teaching Professor and Chairman
Department of Dermatology
SUNY Downstate Medical Center
Brooklyn, New York

David A. Norris, M.D.
Director of Research
Professor of Dermatology
The University of Colorado
Health Sciences Center
Denver, Colorado

Clinical Guide to Sunscreens and Photoprotection

Edited by

Henry W. Lim
Henry Ford Hospital
Detroit, Michigan, USA

Zoe Diana Draelos
Dermatology Consulting Services
High Point, North Carolina, USA

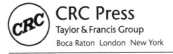

CRC Press
Taylor & Francis Group
Boca Raton London New York

CRC Press is an imprint of the
Taylor & Francis Group, an **informa** business

CRC Press
Taylor & Francis Group
6000 Broken Sound Parkway NW, Suite 300
Boca Raton, FL 33487-2742

First issued in paperback 2019

© 2009 by Taylor & Francis Group, LLC
CRC Press is an imprint of Taylor & Francis Group, an Informa business

No claim to original U.S. Government works

ISBN-13: 978-1-4200-8084-1 (hbk)
ISBN-13: 978-0-367-38615-3 (pbk)

Library of Congress Cataloging-in-Publication Data

Clinical guide to sunscreens and photoprotection / edited by Henry W. Lim, Zoe Diana Draelos.

      p. ; cm. — (Basic and clinical dermatology ; 43)

    Includes bibliographical references and index.

    ISBN-13: 978-1-4200-8084-1 (hardcover : alk. paper)

    ISBN-10: 1-4200-8084-9 (hardcover : alk. paper) 1. Sunscreens (Cosmetics) 2. Photosensitivity disorders—Treatment. I. Lim, Henry W., 1949- II. Draelos, Zoe Kececioglu. III. Series.

    [DNLM: 1. Sunscreening Agents—therapeutic use. 2. Photosensitivity Disorders—prevention & control. 3. Skin—radiation effects. 4. Sunlight—adverse effects. 5. Ultraviolet Rays—adverse effects. W1 CL69L v.43 2008 / QV 63 C641 2008]

      RS431.S94C55 2008

      616.5'1505—dc22

                               2008037841

Visit the Taylor & Francis Web site at
http://www.taylorandfrancis.com

and the CRC Press Web site at
http://www.crcpress.com

Series Introduction

In the last 30 years, there has been a vast explosion in new information relating to the art and science of dermatology as well as fundamental cutaneous biology. Furthermore, this information is no longer of interest only to the small but growing specialty of dermatology. Clinicians and scientists from a wide variety of disciplines have come to recognize both the importance of skin in fundamental biologic processes and the broad implications of understanding the pathogenesis of skin disease. As a result, there is now a multidisciplinary and worldwide interest in the progress of dermatology.

With these factors in mind, we have undertaken this series of books specifically oriented to dermatology. The scope of the series is purposely broad, with books ranging from pure basic science to practical, applied clinical dermatology. Thus, while there is something for everyone, all volumes in the series will ultimately prove to be valuable additions to the dermatologist's library.

Dermatology has played a vital role in informing the public about skin cancer and its prevention. In this regard, sunscreens and photoprotection have proved essential tools in skin cancer prevention. Drs. Lim and Draelos have produced a definitive book on this subject which is both informative and comprehensive. They have assembled an exceptional group of international thought leaders in the field of photobiology and photomedicine to contribute to our understanding of this important subject and have produced a volume that should prove to be a valuable addition to the libraries of dermatologists, skin biologists, and cutaneous oncologists.

Alan R. Shalita, M.D.
SUNY Downstate Medical Center
Brooklyn, New York, U.S.A.

Preface

Over the last 20 years, significant advances have been made in the understanding of the biologic and clinical effects of ultraviolet (UV) radiation, including erythema, delayed tanning, photoimmunosuppression, photoaging, and photocarcinogenesis. Furthermore, better appreciation of the biologic and clinical effects of different spectra of UV radiation has also been achieved.

Together with the increased knowledge about the effects of UV, advances in photoprotection have occurred. While sunscreen has been in use since the late 1920s, new filters and formulations that provide final products with excellent cosmesis and broad-spectrum photostable UVB/UVA protection are now available. Protective effects of sunscreens are better understood, and active research on new and more effective UV filters and on oral photoprotective agents is ongoing. This has prompted worldwide regulatory activity covering the use of novel sun protective chemicals and appropriate labeling of products for increased consumer awareness. It is now recognized that clothing, window glass, contact lenses, and sunglasses are an integral part of photoprotection, affording physical protection to supplement the use of topical sunscreens. Current areas of research in photoprotection include novel delivery systems, topical antioxidants, and technology to simulate a tan without sunlight. General public understanding of the many novel photoprotection alternatives is indispensable to communicating a positive educational message to patients.

This book is designed for practicing dermatologists, dermatology trainees, physicians, and scientists interested in photoprotection. It covers the history of photoprotection, UV filters and other photoprotective agents, physical photoprotection, and public education in photoprotection. Each chapter, which starts with a synopsis, is written by authors who have made significant contributions to the topic. We hope that the readers will find this book an informative and practical reference on this important subject.

Henry W. Lim
Zoe Diana Draelos

Acknowledgments

Henry W. Lim, M.D., would like to thank his wife, Mamie, for her unending patience and support.

Zoe Diana Draelos, M.D., appreciates the encouragement of her two sons, Mark and Matthew, who provided challenging insights into sun protection during the preparation of this text. She is also indebted to her husband, Michael, who let her practice sun avoidance while she worked on this project.

The editors would like to thank Sandra Beberman and her team at Informa Healthcare for their effort and support in bringing this book to fruition.

Henry W. Lim
Zoe Diana Draelos

Contents

SECTION I: HISTORY

SECTION II: UV FILTERS

ix

SECTION III: OTHER PHOTOPROTECTIVE AGENTS

SECTION IV: PHYSICAL PHOTOPROTECTION

SECTION V: EDUCATION

Contributors

Farah K. Ahmed   Personal Care Products Council, Washington, D.C., U.S.A.

Heike Bischoff-Ferrari   Centre on Aging and Mobility, University of Zurich, Zurich, Switzerland

Linda Block   UA Cooperative Extension, The University of Arizona, Tucson, Arizona, U.S.A.

Curtis A. Cole   Johnson & Johnson Consumer and Personal Products Inc., Skillman, New Jersey, U.S.A.

Minas Coroneo   Department of Ophthalmology, University of New South Wales at Prince of Wales Hospital, Sydney, New South Wales, Australia

Brian L. Diffey   Dermatological Sciences, Institute of Cellular Medicine, University of Newcastle, Newcastle upon Tyne, U.K.

Zoe Diana Draelos   Dermatology Consulting Services, High Point, North Carolina, U.S.A.

James Ferguson   Photobiology Unit, Department of Dermatology, University of Dundee, Dundee, Scotland

Anny Fourtanier   L'Oréal Research, Clichy, France

Peter Gies   Australian Radiation Protection and Nuclear Safety Agency, Yallambie, Victoria, Australia

Yolanda Gilaberte-Calzada   Dermatology Service, Hospital San Jorge, Huesca, Spain

Salvador González   Dermatology Service, Memorial Sloan Kettering Cancer Center, New York, New York, U.S.A.; Ramon y Cajal Hospital, Alcalá University, Madrid, Spain

Gary M. Halliday   Discipline of Dermatology, Dermatology Research Laboratories, University of Sydney, Sydney, New South Wales, Australia

Allan C. Halpern   Memorial Sloan-Kettering Cancer Center, Dermatology Division, New York, New York, U.S.A.

Kathryn L. Hatch   Department of Agricultural and Biosystems Engineering, The University of Arizona, Tucson, Arizona, U.S.A.

John L. M. Hawk   St. John's Institute of Dermatology, St. Thomas' Hospital, London, U.K.

Bernd Herzog   Ciba Inc., Grenzach-Wyhlen, Germany

Julian P. Hewitt   Croda Suncare & Biopolymers, Ditton, Cheshire, U.K.

Herbert Hönigsmann   Department of Dermatology, Medical University of Vienna, Vienna, Austria

Henry W. Lim   Department of Dermatology, Henry Ford Hospital, Detroit, Michigan, U.S.A.

Christine Mendrok   DSM Nutritional Products Ltd., Basel, Switzerland

Gillian M. Murphy   National Photodermatology Unit, Beaumont and Mater Misericordiae Hospitals, Dublin, Ireland

J. Frank Nash   Central Product Safety, The Procter & Gamble Company, Sharon Woods Technical Center, Cincinnati, Ohio, U.S.A.

Uli Osterwalder   Ciba Inc., Basel, Switzerland

Rik Roelandts   Photodermatology Unit, University Hospital, Leuven, Belgium

André Rougier   La Roche-Posay Pharmaceutical Laboratories, Asnières, France

Sophie Seité   La Roche-Posay Pharmaceutical Laboratories, Asnières, France

Kenneth A. Smiles   AGI Dermatics, Freeport, New York, U.S.A.

Chanisada Tuchinda   Department of Dtermatology, Faculty of Medicine Siriraj Hospital, Bangkok, Thailand

Juergen Vollhardt   DSM Nutritional Products Ltd., Basel, Switzerland

Steven Q. Wang   Memorial Sloan-Kettering Cancer Center, Dermatology Division, New York, New York, U.S.A.

Daniel B. Yarosh   AGI Dermatics, Freeport, New York, U.S.A.

1
History of Photoprotection

Rik Roelandts
Photodermatology Unit, University Hospital, Leuven, Belgium

SYNOPSIS

- Historically, sunlight has been considered to be the source of life.
- In 1928, the first commercially available sunscreen was introduced, containing benzyl salicylate and benzyl cinnamate.
- During World War II, soldiers used red veterinary petrolatum as sunscreen.
- The first UVA filter, a benzophenone, was introduced in 1962.
- In 1978, the FDA published guidelines on sunscreens and adapted SPF as an assessment method of sunscreens.
- Long UVA filter, dibenzoylmethane derivatives, became available in 1979.
- Micronized inorganic filters became available in 1989 (titanium dioxide) and in 1992 (zinc oxide)

IN THE BEGINNING THERE WAS LIGHT

The sun has always been of vital importance for life on earth. It gives light, warmth, and energy. All vegetation on which life on earth depends is dependent on the sun for carbon and water. Life would be impossible without the sun.

Fossil records show that all early life originated in the sea and that life on land became possible only when the ozone layer covered the earth (1). In the beginning the earth had little oxygen and no ozone layer. Therefore, life on the earth's surface was not possible because of the UVC rays. The visible light needed for photosynthesis and oxygen could penetrate water up to a certain depth where UV rays could not penetrate. Early life was thus possible only by living underwater. Photosynthesis led to a rise in oxygen. With mineral crusts from iron, silica, or clay functioning as primitive sunscreens, early life may first have been able to exist in more shallow water and then even out of water. Therefore, from the start, life has always been connected with photoprotection.

Life became possible because nature provided an additional sophisticated system of protection. The short and most damaging solar radiations are prevented from reaching the

1

earth's surface by two protective shields, or hollow spheres of gas enclosing the earth. The outer one is the ionosphere, reflecting the X rays back into space. The inner one is the ozone layer, absorbing the shorter UV rays. In addition, a great part of the infrared radiation is absorbed by the water vapor in the atmosphere.

FROM ADMIRATION TO ADORATION: THE DAWN OF CIVILIZATION

Since the early part of human history, sunrise and sunset were among the first phenomena to have been noted and admired. Sunrise announced light and became associated with the good, brightness, and warmth. Sunset was the end of light and the beginning of darkness and became associated with the evil. Later on, sunrise became associated with life, and sunset with death.

However, it was not only a question of admiration. Sun exposure and photoprotection were probably an important element in evolution. Even if there were no differences in skin type as we know them nowadays, those with pale skin would have encountered a lot of challenges in sunny climates, while the darker skin types would have had a higher probability for vitamin D deficiency if they lived in less sunny parts of the world. This could have led to the paler skin types living farther away from the equator and the darker ones closer to the equator. Photoprotection by skin color in such circumstances was more a matter of survival.

In the beginning humankind mainly lived of hunting, which was not much affected by seasonal variations. About 10,000 years ago (8000 BC), agriculture became more established; therefore, humans lived a more settled life, becoming more dependent on the weather and on the sun and its seasons for their harvest (2). The earliest farming villages started in the hilly country surrounding the Tigris and Euphrates valleys in Mesopotamia, in what is now Iraq. The ground there was so fertile that the seasons and the influence of the sun were less important; life seemed to come from the earth rather than from the sun. On the contrary, in peak summer, the sun burned all vegetation and made human life difficult. It seems logical that the worship of the sun in such circumstances was less important. This changed when villagers became citizens, not only beside the Tigris and Euphrates but also beside the Nile and Indus. From that time on, worshipping the sun became part of most civilizations, and this is reflected in a large number of solar symbols. In many cases, the sun was conceived of as a disc transported by humans or animals, or as a god. Probably the earliest known solar symbol can be found in Ghassul in the Jordan valley in Israel and is about 6000 years old (3). It was discovered not far from the oldest known settlement in the world at Jericho. As cities grew in importance, the responsibility for communicating with the sun gods also became more important and, as such, even required a professional priesthood and the building of temples in honor of the sun gods (3).

The first important large-scale civilization started around 3000 BC (5000 years ago) in Mesopotamia with the arrival of the Sumerians, who came from Iran. This was the beginning of an unknown cultural evolution, with the discovery of the wheel, the script, the plow, and the technique of bronze making (2). The technique of making bronze already dates back to about 3800 BC (5800 years ago) and was the beginning of the Bronze Age. It came just in time to provide symbols for the sun gods and their temples. Gold was one of the first metals to be worked on by man. Because of its color and its brightness, it was recognized as the metal of the sun (3). The adoration of the sun declined with the growing power of kingship in Mesopotamia. Around 1200 BC (3200 years ago), the center of civilization moved more to the north, to the Assyrians, whereby the sun god gained in importance again. When the Assyrian Empire was overthrown late in the seventh century BC by the Babylonians, the sun god remained dominant. The defeat of the Persians under Cyrus by the Babylonians in 539 BC represented the fall of the ancient world of Bronze Age civilization and the ancient gods.

In Egypt most people were dependent on a green fertile stretch of ground near the Nile. When about 3000 BC (5000 years ago) the whole land became united under the Pharaohs, the sun god was worshipped but under different titles and meanings. This was partly due to the different theology schools at Memphis, Heliopolis, and Thebes. Symbols of the sun can be found in the pyramids, in the obelisks, in the sun temples, and in the numerous paintings throughout the country. The sun crossed the Nile by boat from sunrise to sunset. Egypt became the first really great and rich kingdom in history. When about 3375 years ago Achnaton succeeded to the throne after the death of his father, Amenophis III, the sun god became the one and only god and the Pharaoh became the reincarnation of the sun. His was a religion of love and had much in common with early Christianity. However, Achnaton and his religion were soon pushed aside. When the power and prosperity of Egypt declined, people turned more and more to the cult of Osiris. He could offer the best hope for resurrection. Nevertheless, the sun god still remained important, as is proven by the building of the temple of Abu Simbel by Ramses II (3).

Both civilizations in Mesopotamia and in Egypt started about 5000 years ago. At that time, weaving was discovered, which enabled photoprotection through clothing. However, photoprotection at that time had a completely different meaning. It was mainly a question of avoiding heat by looking for some shade or by staying inside when the sun was at its brightest.

About 2000 to 3000 years after the beginning of both civilizations in Mesopotamia and in Egypt, some civilizations in Central and South America also had a religion related to the sun. It took some time before these civilizations reached their top. The Maya civilization, in what is now Honduras, Guatemala, and Yucatan, reached its top between the third and ninth centuries AD. The Mayans established one of the most accurate calendars ever known. Their gods were mainly the sun, the moon, and the planet Venus. Probably around 1200 AD, the Incas built the city Cuzco in what is now Peru. By the fifteenth century, they had a real empire with sun temples all over the place. The ruler or Sapa Inca was considered a child of the sun. The royal offspring were the true Incas or Children of the Sun. They had the right to use the lunar silver and the solar gold. They worshipped the sun not only because their harvests high above sea level in the Andes were dependent on the sun but also because the sun was the father of their divine ruler. In the valley of Mexico, a civilization developed in the early centuries AD, associated with the Toltecs. Around the tenth or eleventh century AD, the valley was invaded by various nomadic tribes. Around the thirteenth century, a dynasty among them started the Aztec civilization. In the fifteenth century, the Tenochas Aztecs became the most powerful of the Aztec tribes. In their vision, the sun god came as a skeleton from the underworld and had to be nourished with human lives to revive. If they did not, the sun would die and the seasons would stand still. The Aztecs sacrificed their prisoners to the sun god by cutting out their hearts. They even developed a form of holy war to have enough victims to sacrifice. When the great temple of Tenochtitlan was enlarged, 20,000 prisoners were thus sacrificed (3). Interestingly, the Incas and the Tenochas Aztecs dominated at the same time in history but were unknown to one another.

Sun legends appeared in almost every culture. The sun god of the ancient Greeks was Helios driving a golden chariot through heaven. Chariots are found in many ancient civilizations, such as those of Rome, India, China, Turkestan, Persia, and Denmark. The Pueblo Indians in New Mexico in the United States made ceremonial fires to provide the sun with heat. According to some historians, the cross symbolizes the sun and its rays.

The circle at the center of the Celtic cross also symbolizes the sun. The Japanese sun goddess, Amaterasu, is even considered to be the ancestor of the imperial family (1). The Japanese flag symbolizes a sun disc. Louis XIV in France called himself the Sun King.

FROM ADORATION TO EXPLORATION: THE AGE OF DISCOVERY

It was not logical and difficult to imagine that people would protect themselves from something they adored. In addition, it was common belief that sunburn was a result of the sun's heat, and this could be avoided by seeking shade. However, as the rational capacity of humankind increased, their blind worshipping weakened. This is where science started. Instead of worshipping the sun, people started to discover and later on study and analyze the solar irradiation. It was not always an easy process.

In 1543 the Polish astronomer Copernicus published his treatise *De Revolutionibus Orbium Coelestium.* Until then it was still common belief that the earth was the center of our universe and that the sun revolved around the earth. Copernicus had the idea that not the earth but the sun was the center of our planetary system. This was not a logical proposition in a time of religious troubles, which explains why he dared to publish his treatise only when he was nearly seventy (4). He died the same year.

About 1600, two children who happened to be at the shop of spectaclemaker Lippershey in Middelburg in the Netherlands were playing with his lenses. When they put two lenses together and looked through both at the same time, the weathervane on the church tower was magnified. Lippershey looked for himself and started making telescopes. Very soon the telescope was becoming known and many countries were interested, mainly for military reasons. In Italy, Galileo, a professor of mathematics at the University of Padua who was also an instrument maker, started to make telescopes and improved them until at the end of 1609 he had produced a telescope of 30 powers. In 1610, he turned his telescope toward the heaven; this, at that time, was nearly blasphemy. That same year he published his *Sidereus Nuncius,* describing his newly discovered satellites circulating around Jupiter, and concluding that there is not just one planet (the moon) revolving about another (the earth) but also four planets circling around Jupiter, while the whole system travels over a mighty orbit around the sun (5). Galileo could thus prove that Copernicus was right and that the earth was not the center of our planetary system. He died in 1642, the year Newton was born.

The instruments used by Galileo and others were all refracting telescopes, employing lenses to magnify the image and bring the light rays to a focus. These instruments were long and had chromatic aberration. Newton in Cambridge, England, made an instrument with concave mirrors instead of lenses. This instrument was much shorter and could produce a greater magnification without chromatic aberration. One of his first experiments was in 1666, when he made a hole in his window shutters to let in a convenient quantity of light and placed a prism at the entrance. He noted the different colors of the rainbow. Through a small hole, he directed a ray of single color toward a second prism. This light was not further dispersed, but remained a single color. He concluded that light itself is a heterogeneous mixture of differently rays. On using a biconcave lens to bring the rays of the complete spectrum to a common focus, the colors disappeared altogether to produce white light (5,6) (Table 1).

After the discovery of the visible spectrum of the sun, it took nearly another century and a half before the invisible parts of the solar spectrum were discovered. Herschel discovered the infrared spectrum in 1800. He was in fact a German army musician who went to England to become an astronomer. He observed some heat production when he

Table 1 History of Discovery of Electromagnetic Radiation

Year	Investigator(s)	Discovery
1666	Newton	Spectrum of visible light
1800	Herschel	Infrared
1801	Ritter	UV rays
1922	Hausser and Vahle	Action spectra of erythema and pigmentation
1932	Coblentz	Division of UV into UVA, UVB, and UVC

focused his telescope above the visible red light. He did some experiments with a thermometer to evaluate which colors of the visible solar spectrum had the highest temperature. He noted that the thermometer registered a higher temperature above the red visible light and thus discovered the infrared spectrum (7,8).

The discovery of the UV rays by the German Ritter in 1801 was partly based on previous experiments by Scheele in Sweden that were already published in 1777 (9). Scheele showed that paper strips dipped in a silver chloride solution became black after exposure to the sun and that this was more pronounced with blue light than with red light. Ritter noted that the paper strips became even darker when exposed to invisible wavelengths shorter than that of the visible blue light and thus discovered the UV spectrum, which he called "infraviolet" (10,11).

Although the discovery of UV rays was a vital step in the evolution for future photoprotection, it took many years before the importance of the UV rays really became clear. This was mainly due to the common belief that sunburn was a result of heat damage. It changed in 1820, when Home in England exposed one of his own hands to the sun and covered the other with a black cloth. He noted a sunburn on the exposed hand, although a thermometer registered a higher temperature on the other hand (12). In 1889, Widmark in Sweden published the experimental proof that UV radiation caused erythema (13). After Home's experiment and Widmark's publication, it was some time before it became generally known that UV rays induced sunburn. Even in 1891, Kaposi still believed that the sun's heat induced sunburn and pigmentation (7). As late as 1900, Finsen in Denmark repeated Home's experiment without knowing about his work. However, gradually the damaging effects of UV radiation became better known.

During World War I, Hausser and Vahle in Germany made the first detailed action spectrum studies for erythema and pigmentation for human skin. They showed that erythema and pigmentation depend on the wavelengths of the UV radiation and that the effect is mainly due to the wavelengths shorter than 320 nm. In 1922, they published the action spectra for the induction of erythema and pigmentation in human skin, using a monochromator and an artificial mercury lamp (14,15). During the Second International Congress on Light, which took place in Copenhagen, Denmark, in 1932, Coblentz proposed to divide the UV spectrum into three spectral regions: UVA (315–400 nm), UVB (280–315 nm), and UVC (<280 nm) (7).

FROM EXPLORATION TO PROTECTION:
THE AGE OF PREVENTION

Some kind of photoprotection has always existed among humans. This has been done in different ways by wearing appropriate clothing, veils, hats, and turbans, by using umbrellas, by avoiding bright sunlight, by looking for some shade and by using different powders. Historically many substances have probably been tried out as photoprotectors. In ancient Egypt, olive oil was used as a sunscreen, and women used lead paints and chalks to whiten their faces. This was also the case in Greece and Rome. By the middle of the tenth century, arsenic became the preferred skin whitener (16). In sixteenth-century England, Queen Elizabeth I was in the habit of applying arsenic and mercury derivatives on her face to obtain a white complexion. This was most probably done for cosmetic reasons, but maybe also as sun protection.

Much more recently, Parisian women would go horseback riding with their faces covered with veils to prevent tanning, as Renoir has so gracefully shown us in his paintings. Skin color had social importance. Through centuries, pale skin has indicated that one had the luxury of staying indoors, while darker skin has indicated a life of outdoor labor. With the industrial revolution, the complexion of the working classes changed from a dark to a much more pale skin tone. The reason was that many people gave up farming to work inside in factories and coalmines. At the turn of the nineteenth and the twentieth centuries, the upper classes went on holiday to the seaside and to the South, partly for health reasons. A tanned skin thus gradually became associated with health and wealth and, more recently, with the winter sports there is an additional sportive element as well.

As far as we know, the first scientific report on photoprotection dates from the end of the nineteenth century. Most of this early work was done in Germany. In 1887 Veiel reported the use of tannin as a photoprotector, but its use was limited because of its staining potential (17) (Table 2). In 1891 Hammer published a monograph discussing photoprotection and experimenting with different topical agents to prevent sunburn (18); he was the first to recommend the use of chemical sunscreens to prevent sunburn (19). At the beginning of the twentieth century, petrolatum and vegetable oils combined with zinc oxide, magnesium salts, and bismuth were all used for sun protection. It was a common practice to apply zinc oxide on the nose. In 1911, Unna first used Hammer's acidified quinine sulfate, but later used esculin as a sunscreen material (20). This was a chestnut extract, which had been used in folk medicine (19).

Table 2 History of Photoprotection

Year	Advances
1887	Veiel started using tannin as photoprotector
1891	Hammer studied various topical photoprotective agents
Early 1900s	Zinc oxide, magnesium salts, bismuth were used as photoprotective agents
1928	First commercial sunscreen with benzyl salicylate and benzyl cinnamate became available (United States)
1943	PABA patented
1944	Green developed red veterinary petrolatum, used by soldiers during World War II as sunscreen
1948	PABA esters became available
1962	First UVA filter, a benzophenone, was introduced
1974	Greiter popularized "SPF," which was first proposed by Schulze in 1956
1977	First waterproof sunscreen became available
1978	FDA published guidelines on sunscreens, and adapted SPF method to assess sunscreens
1979	Long UVA filter, dibenzoylmethane derivatives, became available
1989– 1992	Micronized inorganic filters became available (titanium dioxide in 1989, zinc oxide in 1992)

Abbreviations: PABA, para-aminobenzoic acid; SPF, sun protection factor; FDA, Food and Drug Administration.

Photoprotection did change with the advent of fashion. In the 1920s, the French designer Gabrielle Coco Chanel developed a tan on a cruise from Paris to Cannes aboard the yacht of the Duke of Westminster (21). At the same time, women started to enjoy outdoor life with picnics and lawn tennis. A tan became a new trend in fashion, stimulated also by the caramel complexion of Josephine Baker, a singer who became increasingly popular in Paris at that time (21). However, obtaining a tan also included the risk of sunburn. When Hausser and Vahle in 1922 reported that sunburn in human skin is caused by a specific part of the UV spectrum between 280 and 315 nm (22), it became theoretically possible to protect the skin by filtering out these specific wavelengths. The idea was very tempting. This resulted in a growing interest in a variety of different sunscreening agents.

Before the first sunscreens became commercially available, people already used preparations usually made by a local pharmacist and mostly based on olive oil or almond oil. The first commercial chemical sunscreen appeared on the market in 1928 in the United States (23). It was an emulsion containing benzyl salicylate and benzyl cinnamate (24,25). During the next years, sunscreens were not widely available and hence not used on a large scale. In Germany, the first commercial sunscreen became available in 1933 (26). It was an ointment containing benzylimidazole sulfonic acid marketed as Delial by IG Farben. It is surprising to realize that during the winter of 1934–1935, at least 75% of the people on the beaches of Florida in the United States were reported to use an oil, cream, or other preparations, but this was probably more for emollient than for protective purposes (27). In France, the first commercial sunscreen became available in 1936 (28). This was an oil preparation containing benzyl salicylate and was marketed as Ambre Solaire by Schueller, the future founder of L'Oréal. The preparation became a great success because it was launched the same year as paid holidays were granted in France. In Austria, the founder of the Piz Buin Company Greiter developed an effective sunscreen in 1938, the Gletscher crème. In 1943, para-aminobenzoic acid (PABA) was first patented but was only marketed as a sunscreen much later (29,30).

The first widely used sunscreen was Red Vet Pet or red veterinary petrolatum, which was produced in 1944 by Greene in the United States, an airman and later pharmacist and founder of Coppertone. During World War II, there was a great need for good sun protection for soldiers engaged in tropical warfare. Red veterinary petrolatum turned out to be one of the most practical and effective such agents and was used as standard equipment (31). It was a physical blocker with a limited effectiveness, and it was a disagreeable red sticky substance. It had to be put on thickly to be effective. Many soldiers developed sunburn in areas where they did not apply it thick enough.

After the war, lifestyle changed in many countries. Women's magazines gradually promoted sun tanning. Pinup girls like Betty Grable and Rita Hayworth were pictured in bathing suits showing their tanned skin (16). A number of filters were synthesized, tested, and marketed. In many cases these filters were used in less effective oil preparations, apparently with the sole purpose of promoting tanning. In 1947, the absorption spectra for several metal oxides were published, including zinc oxide and titanium dioxide (32). By 1948, more effective para-aminobenzoate esters became available (33). In 1955, the majority of sunscreens on the U.S. market contained PABA derivatives or salicylic acid derivatives (34). In 1962, a benzophenone, 3-benzyl-4-hydroxy-6-methoxy-benzenesulfonic acid, was introduced as a sunscreen material (19).

During the 1970s, holidays to sunny areas steadily became more popular greatly because of the cheaper charter flights. This resulted in an increasing demand for sunscreens with better and broader protection, which became possible by incorporating UVB filters into milks and creams instead of oils. In 1977, the first waterproof sunscreen became available (21). In 1978, the Food and Drug Administration (FDA) in the United States published a Federal Register with the guidelines for formulating and evaluating sunscreens (35). These guidelines were further revised in 1993 (36) and in 1999 (37).

In 1979, good UVA filters became available. From that time on, it became possible to commercialize sun products with a broad protection against UVB and UVA at the same time. This became necessary because sunscreens were also used more and more to prevent skin ageing and skin cancer and to protect photosensitive skin, which was much more than just preventing sunburn. The first long UVA filters were the dibenzoylmethane derivatives. In 1980, only 1% of the sunscreens in Europe contained dibenzoylmethane derivatives (38). In 1985, the American Academy of Dermatology introduced the first education program about the risks of overexposure to the sun (16). By 1990, 35% of the sunscreens in Europe did contain dibenzoylmethane derivatives (39). A further advance was the introduction of micronized inorganic powders such as titanium dioxide in 1989 and zinc oxide in 1992 (40). In the meantime, a variety of different UVB and UVA filters have become available.

With the increasing use of sunscreens, there was also an increasing need to find a good method to evaluate their protection. In the early years, no clinical methods were used and the usual way was to determine the absorption spectrum of the sunscreen. This changed in 1934, when Ellinger in Germany proposed to use a biological method by determining the minimal erythema dose in protected and unprotected skin using both forearms (41). He concluded that the method of choice was the way in which the minimal erythema dose could be decreased. He used a mercury lamp as the light source that was not the right irradiation source. In 1956 Schulze in Germany proposed to test commercially available sunscreens by giving them a protection factor (42). The protection factor was obtained by dividing the exposure time needed to induce erythema with sunscreen by the exposure time needed without sunscreen. This was done by applying a series of increasing UV doses (40% increases) on both protected and unprotected skin. The light source was a series of Osram-Ultra-Vitalux lamps, which was much more similar to the solar spectrum than the light source used by Ellinger. The method was further improved in 1974 by Greiter in Austria (43), who popularized the concept of the sun protection factor (SPF) (19). In 1978, this method was adopted by the FDA in the United States (35) and became internationally accepted. At that time, sunscreens were mainly used not only to avoid sunburn but also to prolong the exposure time in order to tan. Therefore sunscreens got a lot of criticism. The main concern was that they could give a false feeling of security.

The evaluation of the UVA protection of a sunscreen is much more difficult than the evaluation of the UVB protection because erythema cannot be used as the endpoint. The UVA protection factor will vary according to the parameter that has been used in the evaluation (44,45). While UVB protection is mostly against erythema, UVA protection can be against a variety of different endpoints. Ideally UVA protection should be evaluated with the endpoint for which the sunscreen will be used. This explains why standardization of the UVA evaluation method is so difficult.

FROM PROTECTION TO SATISFACTION: THE FUTURE

Although nowadays we have much more possibilities to protect our skin against short-term and long-term solar damage than ever before, there is still significant room for improvement. The human mind does not always follow the most logical way, but rather the easiest and most popular one. Common sense is not necessarily the driving force in human behavior. This is especially true concerning photoprotection. For the dermatologist, the gratification of successful photoprotection lies in the prevention of skin lesions induced by sun exposure. For the general population, however, photoprotection could still be viewed as an unwanted nuisance, a compromise necessary to enjoy outdoor life and holidays. Even more important than having the tools is public education on photoprotection, which includes the use sunscreens. All means of making photoprotection easier will therefore be appreciated by caregivers and the general public. This will be our main challenge for the future.

REFERENCES

1. Giese AC. Living with Our Sun's Ultraviolet Rays. New York: Plenum Press, 1976.
2. Gutbrod K. Cantecleer Geschiedenis van de oudste kulturen. Nederland: Cantecleer, de Bilt, 1976.
3. Hawkes J. Man and the Sun. New York: Random House, 1962.
4. Bronowski J. The Ascent of Man. Science Horizons, 1973.
5. Boorstin DJ. The Discoveries. New York: Harry N. Abrams, 1991.
6. Newton I. New theory about light and colours. Philos Trans R Soc Lond 1672; 7(80):3075–3087.
7. Lentner A. Geschichte der Lichttherapie. Aachen, Germany: Foto-Druck Mainz, 1992.
8. Herschel W. Investigation of the powers of the prismatic colours to heat and illuminate objects. Philos Trans R Soc Lond 1800; 90:255–283.
9. Scheele CW. Chemische Abhandlung von der Luft und dem Feuer. Swederus, Crusius, Upsala, Leipzig, Sweden, Germany, 1777.
10. Ritter JW. Physisch-chemische Abhandlungen in chronologischer Folge. B II. Leipzig, 1806:81–107.
11. Ritter JW. Entdeckungen zur Elektrochemie, Bioelektrochemie und Photochemie. Ostwalds Klassiker der exakten Wissenschaften. Band 271. Leipzig, Germany: Akademische Verlagsgesellschaft Geest & Portig K.-G, 1986.
12. Home E. On the black rete mucosum of the Negro, being a defense against the scorching effect of the sun's rays. Philos Trans R Soc London 1820; 111:1.
13. Widmark EJ. Über den Einfluss des Lichtes auf die Haut. Hygiea, Festband 3. Stockholm: Samson and Wallin, 1889:1–22.
14. Hausser KW, Vahle W. Sonnenbrand und Sonnenbräunung. Wiss Veröff Siemens-Konzern 1927; 6:101.
15. Urbach F, Forbes PD, Davies RE, et al. Cutaneous photobiology: past, present and future. J Invest Dermatol 1976; 67:209–224.
16. Sikes RG. The history of suntanning. J Aesth Sci 1998; 1(2):6–7.
17. Henschke U. Untersuchungen an Lichtschutzmitteln. Strahlentherapie 1940; 67:639–668.
18. Hammer F. Uber den Einfluss des Lichtes auf die Haut. Stuttgart, Germany: F. Enke, 1891.
19. Urbach F. The historical aspects of sunscreens. J Photochem Photobiol B 2001; 64:99–104.
20. Unna PG. Über einen neuen farblosen Schutz gegen unerwünschte Wirkungen des Sonnenlichtes auf die Haut. Med Klin 1911; 7:454–456.
21. Thomas L, Lim HW. Sunscreens. J Drugs Dermatol 2003; 2:174–177.
22. Hausser KW, Vahle W. Die Abhängigkeit des Lichterythems und der Pigmentbildung von der Schwingungszahl (Wellenlänge) der erregenden Strahlung. Strahlentherapie 1922; 13:47–71.
23. Shaath NA. Evolution of modern sunscreen chemicals. In: Lowe NJ, Shaath NA, eds. Sunscreens, Development, Evaluation, and Regulatory Aspects. New York: Marcel Dekker, 1990:3–35.
24. Jass HE. Cosmetic suntan products. Cutis 1979; 23:554–561.
25. Owens DW, Knox JM, Freeman RG. A clinical evaluation of sunscreens. Clin Med 1967; 74:45–46.

26. Finkel P. Lichtschutzmittel. In: Umbach W, ed. Kosmetik. Stuttgart – New York: Georg Thieme Verlag, 1995:147–163.
27. Stambovsky L. Comments on solar shields. Drug Cosmet Ind 1935; 36:551–554.
28. Rebut D. The sunscreen industry in Europe: past, present and future. In: Lowe NJ, Shaath NA, eds. Sunscreens, Development, Evaluation, and Regulatory Aspects. New York: Marcel Dekker, 1990:161–171.
29. Safer and more successful suntanning. Consumers Guide. New York: Wallaby Pocketbooks, 1979:31–33.
30. Mackie BS, Mackie LE. The PABA story. Australas J Dermatol 1999; 40:41–53.
31. MacEachern WN, Jillson OF. A practical sunscreen 'Red Vet Pet'. Arch Dermatol 1946; 89:147–150.
32. Grady LD. Zinc oxide in face powders. J Soc Cosmet Chem 1947; 1:1.
33. Kumler WD, Daniels TC. Sunscreen compounds. J Am Pharm Assoc Sci Ed 1948; 37:474–476.
34. Wikipedia. Sunscreen. Available at: http:/en.wikipedia.org/wiki/Sunscreen.
35. Department of Health, Education and Welfare, Food and Drug Administration. Sunscreen drug products for over-the-counter human use. Fed Regist 1978; 43:38206–38269.
36. Department of Health, Education and Welfare, Food and Drug Administration. Sunscreen drug products for over-the-counter human use: Tentative final monograph: proposed rule. Fed Regist 1993; 58:28194–28302.
37. Department of Health, Education and Welfare, Food and Drug Administration. Sunscreen drug products for over-the-counter human use: Final Monograph: final rule. Fed Regist 1999; (64)98: 27666–27693.
38. Roelandts R, Vanhee J, Bonamie A, et al. A survey of ultraviolet absorbers in commercially available sun products. Int J Dermatol 1983; 22:247–255.
39. Schauder S. Änderungen lichtfilterhaltiger Produkte der Bundesrepublik Deutschland zwischen 1988 und 1989/90. Z Hautkr 1990; 65:1152–1160.
40. Roelandts R. Advances in sunscreen technology: choosing the sunscreen to suit. Curr Opin Dermatol 1995; 2:173–177.
41. Ellinger F. Zur Frage der Wertbestimmung von Lichtschutzmitteln. Arch Exp Path u Pharmakologie 1934; 175:481–488.
42. Schulze R. Einige Versuche und Bemerkungen zum Problem der handelsüblichen Lichtschutzmittel. Parf u Kosmet 1956; 37:310–315.
43. Greiter F. Sonnenschutzfaktor – Entstehung, Methodik. Parf u Kosmet 1974; 55:70–75.
44. Roelandts R, Sohrabvand N, Garmyn M. Evaluating the UVA protection of sunscreens. J Am Acad Dermatol 1989; 21:56–62.
45. Lim HW, Naylor M, Hönigsmann H, et al. American Academy of Dermatology Consensus Conference on UVA Protection of Sunscreens: Summary and Recommendations. J Am Acad Dermatol 2001; 44:505–508.

2
Chemistry and Properties of Organic and Inorganic UV Filters

Uli Osterwalder
Ciba Inc., Basel, Switzerland

Bernd Herzog
Ciba Inc., Grenzach-Wyhlen, Germany

SYNOPSIS

- Similar to shade and covering-up, the ideal sunscreen should protect uniformly throughout UVB, UVA-II, and UVA-I radiation.
- UV filters are the heart of every sunscreen, but good UV protection also requires UVA assessment, SPF, and UVA-standards and, most importantly, compliance of the sunscreen user.
- The major protection mechanism of organic and inorganic UV filters is absorption of UV radiation and subsequent conversion to less harmful energy.
- UVA-I protection has improved over the years, mainly thanks to stabilized forms of the UVA-I filter, avobenzone.
- Outside the United States, further improvement toward the ideal sunscreen was made possible by new UVA-I and broad-spectrum UV filters and new UVA regulations.
- State-of-the-art UVB and broad-spectrum UV filters are awaiting FDA approval in 2008/2009.

SUMMARY

Seeking shade and covering-up are the top two means of sun protection. The ideal sunscreen should protect similarly, i.e., uniformly protect against UVB and UVA radiation. The four requirements for good UV protection are (*i*) technology, (*ii*) assessment of performance, (*iii*) standard, and (*iv*) compliance. The highest UVA category (4 stars) of the Food and Drug Administration (FDA)-proposed rule (Federal

Register, 27 Aug 2007) is already very close to the ideal sunscreen. Absorption is the major mechanism of protection by UV filters. Scattering of particulate UV filters contributes a maximum of 5% to 10% to the protection; a higher percentage would lead to the undesired "whitening effect." The UV filters available in the United States absorb mainly in the UVB/UVA-II range. Avobenzone is the only efficient UVA-I filter in the United States. At the time of this writing, four additional UVB and two broad-spectrum UV filters are awaiting FDA approval. The design of UV filters is described with the example of development of the broad-spectrum UV filter bemotrizinol. Variation of substituents to the aromatic ring system of the molecule leads to photostabilization and different UV absorption spectra. The molecular weight of all new UV filters that are not yet available in the United States is generally higher than 500 Dalton.

In sunscreen products, a combination of different UV filters is commonly used. The performance of a particular UV-filter combination can be calculated from the UV absorption of the individual UV filters, its incorporation level, and an assumption regarding the irregular sunscreen film on the skin. Clinically relevant information is how much and what kind of UV radiation is transmitted through the sunscreen into the skin. Thus, besides the absorption property of the UV filters, the galenic properties of a sunscreen can play a major role, e.g., the sun protection factor (SPF) of a water-in-oil (w/o) emulsion is higher than that of an oil-in-water (o/w) emulsion for the same amounts of UV filters. The important question of the relationship between SPF and the amount of sunscreen applied also needs to be considered. The majority of the sunscreens exhibit a quasi-linear SPF/amount relationship because most do not contain good filters that cover the full spectrum of UVA.

In commercial sunscreens, only a fraction of all theoretically available UV filters are actually used. The major reason is efficacy, i.e., UV absorption capacity, water resistance, or compatibility in a particular sunscreen formulation. Sunscreen manufacturers have four basic requirements regarding the use of sunscreen actives: (*i*) efficacy, (*ii*) safety, (*iii*) registration, and (*iv*) patent freedom. These requirements restrict the use of certain UV filters or combinations of UV filters. Furthermore, branded UV filters such as Parsol®, Mexoryl®, or Tinosorb® and UV filter complexes such as Avotriplex®, Helioplex®, or Sunsure® are explained. It is also shown what extra benefit the use of the latest generation of broad-spectrum technology could add to U.S. sunscreens, e.g., the possibility of achieving the highest four stars UVA category of the proposed FDA rule.

INTRODUCTION

Prevention of sunburn, photoaging, and eventually skin cancer is practiced in most cultures by avoiding the sun and covering up. In these forms of protection, solar radiation is reduced uniformly without preference for either UVB or UVA. Consequently, the spectrum of solar radiation to which the human skin has adapted to is essentially maintained.

Yet, with the introduction of topical UV sunscreens and more so with the SPF relating mainly to UVB, photoprotection became biased toward UVB. This imbalance fostered the argument that extensive use of sunscreens may promote rather than prevent skin cancer (1). As early as 1991, Diffey advocated for uniform UV protection; this at a time when the importance of UVA in photoaging and skin cancer was not yet of general consideration (2). The important role of UVA in photoaging and photocarcinogenesis is now better understood. Nonetheless, only few sunscreens provide practically uniform UV protection (3). The ideal sunscreen should provide uniform UVB/UVA protection, because this assures that the natural spectrum of sunlight is attenuated without altering its

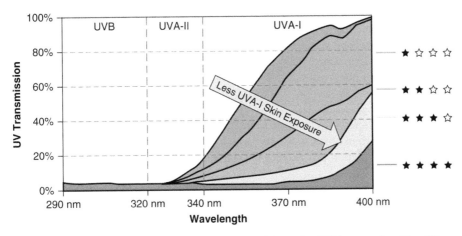

Figure 1 UV transmission of SPF 30 sunscreens with varying UVA protection. The difference is in UVA-I transmission; sunscreens with four stars would protect against UVA-I 10 times better than one-star sunscreens. *Abbreviation*: SPF, sun protection factor.

quality. New broad-spectrum sunscreens will eventually lead us back toward uniform UV protection that sun avoidance and covering-up provided all along.

The four requirements for good uniform protection are as follows:

1. Sunscreen technology, in particular availability of UVA and broad-spectrum UV filters
2. Assessment of performance, in particular SPF and UVA methods
3. Standards set by industry or authorities, in particular regarding UVA protection
4. Compliance of the sunscreen user

This chapter will focus on the first requirement, the heart of the sunscreen technology, the UV filters, and how these UV filters translate into the performance of a sunscreen by illustrating its clinical benefit. The second and third requirements, the actual performance assessment and the standards are discussed in other chapters of this book (chaps. 5 and 4, respectively). Figure 1 shows how different combinations of UV filters lead to varying degrees of UVA protection, up to four stars (4), i.e., UVA-I/UV ratio greater than and equal to 0.95, as rated by the proposed FDA rule; as shown in the Figure 1, a four-star product transmits 10 times less UVA-I radiation than a one-star sunscreen with a UVA-I/UV ratio less than 0.40. A three-stars rating corresponds to the European recommendation (5). Whereas sunscreens with less than three stars provide little UVA protection, those with four stars come close to the ideal uniform UVB/UVA protection. All these examples are SPF 30 sunscreens assessed according to the international SPF method, calculated on a "sunscreen simulator" (6).

The fourth requirement for good, uniform sun protection, namely, compliance of the sunscreen user, depends to a large extent on whether he or she likes the sunscreen, i.e., how it feels on the skin during application, and how easily it can be applied. This in turn depends on the skills of the sunscreen formulator and the available UV filters. With the availability of highly efficient UV filters, which can be used in a smaller amount, it will be easier to make an elegant, cosmetically pleasing sunscreen.

There are other reasons beyond achieving better UVA protection to advocate uniform sun protection. Because UVA-II contributes to UV-induced erythema, for a given SPF, sunscreen with an efficient UVA filter would require less amount of UVB filter to achieve the SPF value; therefore, that sunscreen would have a higher UVB transmission and, in turn, a lower probability of interfering with vitamin D_3 production. It is known that many UVB-biased sunscreens are three times more efficient in suppressing vitamin D_3 production than suppressing erythema (7). Furthermore, because the emission spectrum of solar-simulated radiation source required by regulatory agencies to assess the SPF is weighted toward UVB, for a given SPF, this leads to an underestimation of the protection against UVA, hence the protection against the full spectrum of sunlight.

In the following sections, it will be shown how the UV filters contribute to the performance of a sunscreen. In addition to the absorption spectrum, we will elaborate on the transmission spectrum of the sunscreen, which is more meaningful for skin protection, as after all, the UV radiation that reaches the skin matters more than the one absorbed by the UV filters.

MECHANISMS OF UV ATTENUATION

In sunscreens, three mechanisms of UV attenuation may be distinguished: absorption, scattering, and reflection (backward scattering). Therefore, principally, there are two ways electromagnetic radiation may interact with matter: absorption and scattering. In the case of scattering, the radiation has no resonance frequencies with energy transitions of the molecule, but the electric dipole of the molecule or of the particle oscillates with the frequency of the radiation. The oscillating dipoles will then emit radiation of the original frequency in diverse directions, leading to attenuation of the radiation in the incident direction. With absorption, there is a resonance between the exciting radiation and the energy transition of the molecule, resulting in the transfer of energy to the molecule. When both mechanisms are relevant, for instance, for TiO_2 particles, as they are used in sunscreens, the total effect can be described as the extinction being the sum of absorption and scattering:

$$\text{Extinction} = \text{Absorption} + \text{Scattering} \qquad (1)$$

The strength of the extinction per mol is characterized by the molar decadic extinction coefficient ε(L/mol·cm). A measure related to the amount of the filter in terms of weight is the specific extinction $E_{1,1}$ referring to a 1% solution (or dispersion) of the absorber at 1 cm optical path length. The relationship between both measures is given in the following relationship [M = molar mass (g/mol)]:

$$E_{1,1} = \varepsilon[\text{L}/(\text{mol} \times \text{cm})] \cdot \frac{10(\text{g/L})}{M(\text{g/mol})} \cdot 1(\text{cm}) \qquad (2)$$

By the absorption of a UV photon, an organic absorber molecule goes from the electronic ground state (S_0) to the first excited electronic state (S_1). This absorbed energy can be eliminated via several pathways (Fig. 2) (8). From the S_1 state, it may be lost directly via fluorescence (a radiative transition) or by undergoing photoreactions. There are also radiationless transitions by which the absorbed energy is redistributed inside the molecule: intersystem crossing (ISC) leads to the first triplet state T_1 and internal conversion (IC) to the state S_0^*, which is the electronic ground state but with the excitation energy now migrated into vibrational modes of the molecule. From the first triplet state T_1, the energy may be dissipated by emission of a photon (phosphorescence), by energy transfer to other molecules (sensitization), or via photoreactions. The fate of the energy after IC to the vibrationally excited ground state S_0^* can be emission of infrared (IR) photons (i.e., heat), or collisional deactivation of the vibrational modes via collisions with surrounding molecules. Since the rate constant for emission of IR quanta is very

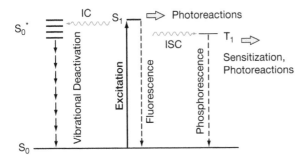

Figure 2 Jablonski diagram showing excitation of organic molecules by photons and deactivation pathways. *Abbreviations*: IC, internal conversion; ISC, intersystem crossing; S_0, ground state; S_0^*, electronic ground state, but with the excitation energy migrated into vibrational modes; S_1, first excited state; T_1, first triplet state.

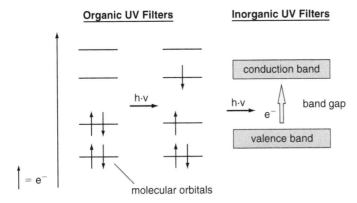

Figure 3 Mechanisms of absorption with organic and inorganic UV filters.

small, collisional deactivation will be the main process after IC, rendering the molecule in its electronic ground state S_0. Hence, in terms of photostability, absorbers showing a high rate of IC are most desirable (9).

In photoreactions, structural changes occur, which may be reversible, as with isomerizations (cis/trans or keto/enol), or irreversible. Irreversible changes leading to decomposition would result in an UV absorber with a photoinstability problem.

The inorganic oxides TiO_2 and ZnO function mainly by absorption of UV radiation (10), although this main effect is superimposed by some scattering (11). Being small particulate crystals, these materials are semiconductors with high bandgap energy between the valence and conduction band. The bandgap of the bulk crystals is in the range of an energy corresponding to wavelengths between 380 and 420 nm, but this may alter with the size of the primary particles (the smaller the primary particles, the higher the bandgap energy). UV radiation is absorbed by elevating an electron from the valence to the conduction band (Fig. 3). The primary particle sizes of TiO_2 for sunscreen applications are between 10 and 30 nm. However, in dispersion, the particles form aggregates with sizes of about typically 100 nm. With ZnO, primary particle sizes from 10 to 200 nm are available, but mainly the grades with larger particles are used. The ratio of light attenuation due to scattering and absorption depends strongly on the particle size: the larger the particle size, the higher is the scattering-to-absorption ratio. With the nano-grades used in sunscreen applications, the absorption is by far dominating.

CHEMISTRY OF UV FILTERS

Overview of UVB, UVA-II, UVA-I, and Broad-Spectrum UV Filters

UV filters that are currently used in sunscreens for the protection of human skin are shown in Tables 1 to 4 (12); in Figures 4 to 7, the UV spectra of the UV filters listed in Tables 1 to 4 are depicted as specific extinction $E_{1,1}$ versus wavelength.

Not every filter substance may be used anywhere in the world, but their use may be limited to specific regions. The most important regions for the registration of UV filters are Australia, Europe, Japan, and the United States. The status of registration in these regions is also given in the Tables. In Tables 1 and 2, the currently used UVB and UVA-II filters are listed; Table 1 shows filters that are oils, i.e., in a liquid state under normal conditions, and Table 2 shows filters that are solids at normal conditions. UVB/UVA-II filters are the only ones that can be present in an oily liquid state. The reason for this is that chromophores absorbing light in the UVB/UVA-II range are generally small, so that intermolecular forces tend to be lower. However, there are also UVB/UVA-II absorbers in the solid state, which have either larger chromophores or contain ionic groups. All known UVA-I or UV broad-spectrum absorbers are solids under normal conditions.

Two filters, bisdisulizole disodium and meradimate, have their absorption maximum at the border between the UVA II and UVA-I range; they are listed and depicted together with the UVA-I absorbers. UV filters available in the United States are marked in bold. There are 10 UVB/UVA-II filters commonly used in the United States. The main reason why UVA protection in the United States is lagging behind the rest of the world is that only one UVA-I filter (avobenzone) and one broad-spectrum UV filter (zinc oxide) are generally allowed to be used in formulations. Another UVA-I filter (ecamsule) is available only in specially approved sunscreen formulations of L'Oréal companies. In Europe and most other parts of the world, two other UVA-I filters and three broad-spectrum UV filters are available. Four UVB/UVA-II filters (amiloxate, ethylhexyl triazone, diethylhexyl butamido triazone, and enzacamene) and two broad-spectrum UV filters (bisoctrizole and bemotrizinol) are currently awaiting FDA approval via the TEA process (material Time and material Extent Application). Under the TEA procedure, the FDA can approve cosmetic ingredients or formulations with five-year foreign marketing experience outside the United States in countries that mirror the U.S. population, after reviewing their efficacy and safety. However, since the TEA procedure became final in 2002, not one ingredient has been approved as yet by the FDA.

MOLECULAR DESIGN OF A BROAD-SPECTRUM UV FILTER

In the year 2000, the first UV filter based on hydroxyphenyltriazine (HPT) technology was added to the approved list of European cosmetic UV filters [International Nomenclature of Cosmetic Ingredient (INCI): bis-ethylhexyloxyphenol methoxyphenyl triazine (BEMT); USAN: bemotrizinol; trade name, Tinosorb S, Ciba Inc.]. BEMT is a new oil-soluble filter with strong broad-spectrum protection in the UVA and UVB regions. BEMT represents a new generation of cosmetic UV filters; its structure and UV spectrum after an elaborate development process are depicted in Figure 8 (case D) (13).

The strong absorption tri-phenyl-triazines show in the UVB range (Fig. 8, case A) has $\pi\pi^*$-character. A $n\pi^*$-transition may also contribute to this band (14). As a first orthohydroxy group is introduced (Fig. 8, case B), a UVA band emerges, which is because of an intramolecular charge transfer ($\pi\pi^*$-CT). With two ortho-hydroxy groups at different phenyl moieties, this UVA absorption increases (Fig. 8, case D), and with three,

Table 1 Current UVB and UVA-II Filters—Liquid at Room Temperature

Colipa No.	INCI—name (and abbreviation)	USAN	Structure	λ_{max}	Registration status, maximal incorporation level (%)			
					U.S.A.	Japan	Europe	Australia
S 8	Ethylhexyl dimethyl PABA (ED-PABA)	Padimate-O		311 nm	8	10	8	8
S 12	Homosalate (HMS)	Homosalate		306 nm	15	10	10	15
S 20	Ethylhexyl salicylate (EHS)	Octisalate		305 nm	5	10	5	5
S 27	Isoamyl methoxycinnamate (IMC)	Amiloxate		308 nm	TEA	10	10	10
S 28	Ethylhexyl methoxycinnamate (EHMC)	Octinoxate		311 nm	7.5	20	10	10
S 32	Octocrylene (OCR)	Octocrylene		303 nm	10	10	10	10
S 74	Polysilicone-15 (BMP)	"Polysilicone-15"		312 nm	-	10	10	10

Abbreviations: Colipa, European Cosmetics, Toiletry and Perfumery Trade Association; INCI, International Nomenclature of Cosmetic Ingredient; USAN, United States Adopted Name; TEA, Time and Extent Application (U.S. Food and Drug Administration application).

Table 2 Current UVB and UVA-II Filters—Solids

Colipa No.	INCI—name (and abbreviation)	USAN	Structure	λ_{max}	U.S.A.	Japan	Europe	Australia
						Registration status, incorporation level (%)		
S 38	Benzophenone-3 (B-3)	Oxybenzone		324 nm	6	5	10	10
S 40	Benzophenone-4 (B-4)	Sulisobenzone		324 nm	10	10	5	10
S 45	Phenyl benzimidazole sulfonic acid (PBSA)	Ensulizole		302 nm	4	3	8	4
S 60	4-Methyl benzylidene camphor (MBC)	Enzacamene		300 nm	TEA	-	4	4
S 69	Ethylhexyl triazone (EHT)	"Octyltriazone"		314 nm	TEA	3	5	5
S 75	Titanium dioxide (TiO₂)	Titanium dioxide	TiO_2	≥290 nm	25	No limit	25	25
S 78	Diethylhexyl butamido triazone (DBT)	"Dibutamidot riazone"		311 nm	-	-	10	-

Abbreviations: Colipa, European Cosmetics, Toiletry, and Perfumery Trade Association; INCI, International Nomenclature of Cosmetic Ingredient; USAN, United States Adopted Name; TEA, Time and Extent Application (U.S. Food and Drug Administration application).

Table 3 Current UVA-I Filters (All Solids)

Colipa No.	INCI—name (and abbreviation)	USAN	Structure	λ_{max}	Registration status, maximal incorporation level (%)			
					USA	Japan	Europe	Australia
–	Menthyl anthranilate (MA) *Meridamate*	*Merodimate*		336 nm	5	–	–	5
S 66	Butyl methoxy dibenzoyl methane (BMDBM) *Avobenzone*	*Avobenzone*		357 nm	3	10	5	5
S 71	Terephtalidene dicamphor sulfonic acid (TDSA)	*Ecamsule*		345 nm	NDA	10	10	10
S 80	Disodium phenyl dibenzimidazole tetrasulfonate (DPDT)	*Bisdisulizole disodium*		335 nm	–	–	10	10
S 83	Diethylamino hydroxybenzoyl hexyl benzoate (DHHB)	*"Aminobenzo-phenone"*		354 nm	–	–	10	–

Abbreviations: Colipa, European Cosmetics, Toiletry, and Perfumery Trade Association; INCI, International Nomenclature of Cosmetic Ingredients; USAN, United States Adopted Name; NDA, New Drug Application (U.S. Food and Drug Administration application).

Table 4 Current UV Broad-Spectrum Filters (All Solids)

Colipa No.	INCI—name (and abbreviation)	USAN	Structure	λ_{max}	Registration status, maximum incorporation level (%)				
					U.S.A.	Japan	Europe	Australia	
S 73	Drometrizole trisiloxane (DTS)	-		303 and 341 nm	-	10	15	15	
S 76	Zinc oxide (ZnO)	Zinc oxide	ZnO	≥ 360 nm	25	No limit	Under review	20	
S 79	Methylene bis-benzotrazolyl tetramethyl-butylphenol (MBBT) Bisoctrizole	Bisoctrizole		305 and 360 nm	TEA	10	10	10	
S 81	Bis-ethylhexyloxy methoxyphenyl triazine (BEMT), Bemotrizinol	Bemotrizinol		310 & 343 nm	TEA	3	10	10	

Abbreviations: Colipa, European Cosmetics, Toiletry, and Perfumery Trade Association; INCI, International Nomeclature of Cosmetic Ingredients; USAN, United States Adopted Name; TEA, Time and Extent Application (U.S. Food and Drug Administration application).

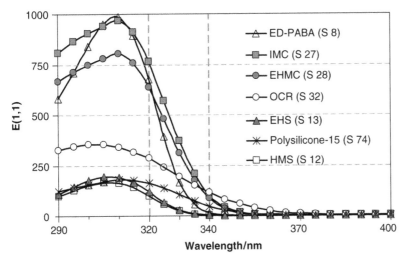

Figure 4 UV spectra of liquid UVB/UVAII filters (see Table 1).

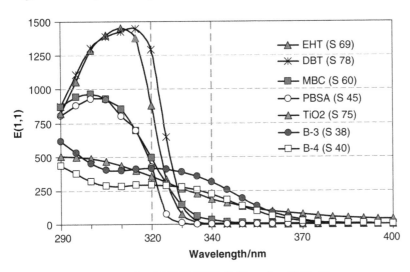

Figure 5 UV spectra of solid UVB/UVA-II filters (see Table 2).

even more (Fig. 8, case C). The optimized broad-spectrum structure was obtained with case D (Fig. 8) referring to bemotrizinol (BEMT), which shows absorption maxima at 310 and 343 nm with ε_{max} = 42800 and 47500 $M^{-1}cm^{-1}$, respectively, measured in ethanol.

Because of the two hydroxyl groups in ortho-position, BEMT contains two intramolecular hydrogen bridges that enable an excited-state intramolecular proton transfer (phototautomerism) after photoexcitation. This is followed by IC and rapid energy dissipation, resulting in inherent photostability. Thus, the presence of ortho-hydroxy groups not only influences the shape of the absorption spectrum, but also the photostability. The photostabilizing effect of an ortho-hydroxy group is also discussed by Shaath (15).

Trend Toward Higher Molecular Weight UV Filters—the 500-Dalton Rule

Over the past decades, the general development of new sunscreen actives was moving toward higher molecular weight filters. The "500-Dalton rule," known from the

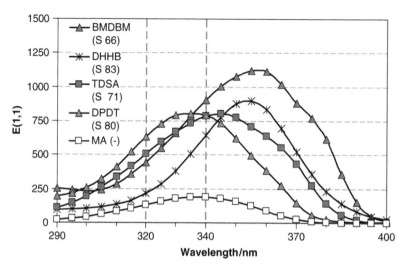

Figure 6 UV spectra of UVA-I filters (see Table 3). DPDT and MA are also taken into this category, although the maximum absorption in these cases is slightly below 340 nm. *Abbreviations*: DPDT, disodium phenyl dibenzimidazole tetrasulfonate; MA, menthyl anthranilate.

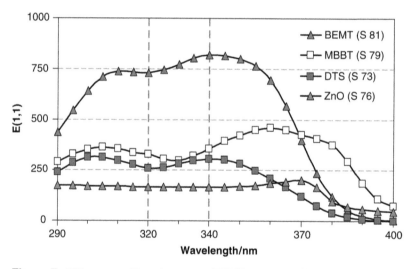

Figure 7 UV spectra of broad-spectrum UV filters (see Table 4). BEMT and DTS measured in ethanol. MBBT, TiO$_2$, and ZnO measured in aqueous dispersion. *Abbreviations*: BEMT, bis-ethylhexyloxy methoxyphenyl triazine; DTS, drometrizole trisiloxane; MBBT, methylene bis-benzotrazolyl tetramethyl-butylphenol.

development of transdermal drugs, can be seen as a common denominator. The 500-Dalton rule for the skin penetration of chemical compounds and drugs states that when topical dermatological therapy or percutaneous systemic therapy is the objective, the development of new innovative compounds should be restricted to molecular weights below 500 Dalton (16). Conversely, one may postulate a 500-Dalton rule for the development of sunscreen actives, which says that the development of new innovative compounds should be restricted to molecular weights above 500 Dalton, where UV filters remaining on, rather than penetrating through, the skin is the objective. As shown in Figure 9, product development over the past 50 years has clearly been heading in the

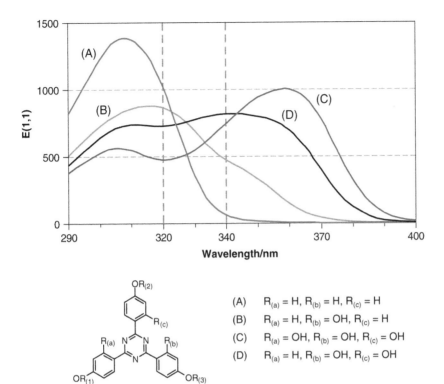

Figure 8 UV spectral performance of phenyl triazine derivatives as function of substitution; $R_{(1)}$ and $R_{(3)}$ = ethyl hexyl and $R_{(2)}$ = methyl.

direction of higher molecular weights above 500 Dalton. However, it should be noted that the 500-Dalton rule alone is neither a necessary nor a sufficient condition for the safety of a new sunscreen active.

PERFORMANCE OF UV FILTERS IN A SUNSCREEN

Performance of UV Filters

UV filters are the actives in sunscreens, which are needed to protect against solar radiation. In most cases, sunscreens contain a blend of UV filters. The overall absorbance spectrum of a sunscreen is determined by the superposition of the UV spectra of the individual filters according to their amounts in the formulation. This is illustrated in Figure 10 with the example of the European Cosmetics, Toiletry, and Perfumery Trade Association (Colipa) P3 standard formulation, which contains 0.5% avobenzone (BMDBM), 3% octinoxate (EHMC), and 2.78% ensulizole (PBSA) (17,18).

However, what is decisive for the protection of the skin is the attenuation of the UV radiation by the film of absorbing material. This attenuation can be characterized by the residual UV radiation, which is still transmitted through the film in relation to the incident radiation, called the UV transmission. The transmission of the film is mainly influenced by the absorbance spectrum of the sunscreen, and to a lesser extent, scattering of incident radiation. However, human skin is not a flat or homogeneous substrate; therefore, the resulting film will be uneven and irregular (Fig. 11). An irregular film structure has a

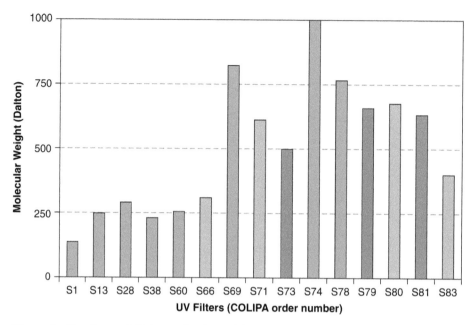

Figure 9 Trend toward higher molecular weight UV Filters (Colipa number). The 500-Dalton rule—a common denominator in the development of UV absorbers (UVB = red, UVA = green, broad-spectrum = blue).

#	UVB/UVA-II filters	#	UVA-I/broad-spectrum UV filters
S1	PABA	S66	Avobenzone
S13	Octisalate	S69	Octyl triazone
S28	Octinoxate	S71	Terephthalylidene dicamphor sulfonic acid
S38	Oxybenzone	S73	Drometrizole trisiloxane
S60	Enzacamene	S79	Bisoctrizole
S74	Polysilicone-15	S80	Bisdisulizole disodium
S78	Dibutamido triazone	S81	Bemotrizinol
		S83	Aminobezophenone

Abbreviation: Colipa, European Cosmetics, Toiletry, and Perfumery Trade Association.

strong impact on the UV transmission. Models for the calculation of the SPF must take this fact into account (18–20).

When the UV transmission spectrum through a sunscreen film with a realistic irregular profile is known, e.g., from calculations, the SPF may be obtained as the factor by which the erythemal effectiveness spectrum is reduced. The erythemal effectiveness spectrum is obtained by multiplication of the sun intensity spectrum (21) by the action spectrum for erythema (22), which is demonstrated in Figure 12.

Because the erythemal effectiveness spectrum is the intensity of solar radiation weighted by the erythemal action spectrum, it is a reflection of the risk spectrum for erythema. In the presence of a protecting film on the skin, the erythemal effectiveness is reduced accordingly. This is shown in Figure 13 for the case of the Colipa P3 standard formulation. Calculating the areas under the two curves in the range between 290 and 400 nm and subsequently the ratio of the area without and the area with protection, the SPF is obtained. For the P3 standard, this results in an SPF = 13.

(A)

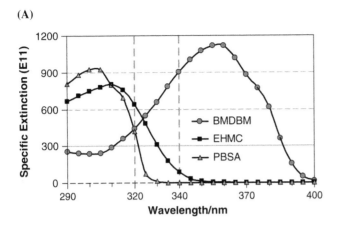

(B)

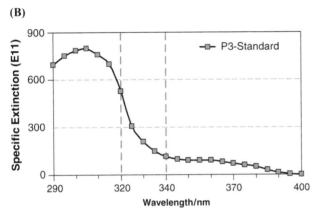

Figure 10 Specific extinction of the individual UV filters used in the Colipa P3 standard (*left*) and of their blend according to the concentrations in the P3 formulation (*right*). *Abbreviation*: Colipa, European Cosmetics, Toiletry, and Perfumery Trade Association.

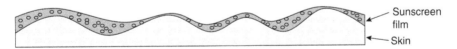

Figure 11 Irregular profile of the sunscreen film on the skin.

Galenics of Sunscreens

Although the main UV protection effect of a sunscreen is the result of properties and concentration of the UV filters, the galenic form can also have great influence; for example, o/w emulsions show generally higher SPFs than w/o emulsions with comparable filter content, because a more uniform sunscreen film is built on the skin.

A sunscreen in most cases comprises the following components:

- sunscreen actives
- a lipid phase (oil phase) containing, e.g., paraffin, fatty acids, fatty alcohols, fatty acid esters, silicon oils, waxes, UV filters, and active ingredients
- an aqueous phase containing, e.g., skin moisturizers, thickeners, polymers, salts, UV filters, and water-soluble actives

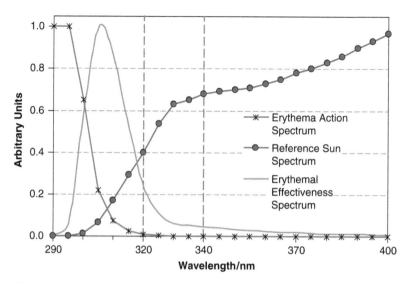

Figure 12 Erythema action spectrum (22), reference sun spectrum (21), and erythemal effectiveness spectrum (values normalized for better visualization).

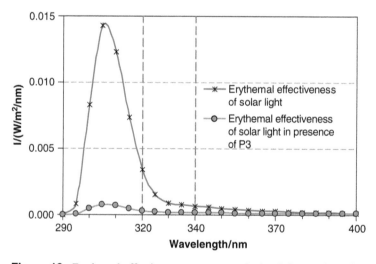

Figure 13 Erythemal effectiveness spectrum calculated from solar reference spectrum (22) and erythemal action spectrum in absence and presence of the Colipa P3 sunscreen standard.

- emulsifiers for o/w systems, e.g., stearic acid, stearic acid esters, ethoxylates, and phosphate emulsifiers; emulsifiers for w/o systems, e.g., polyglycerol, fatty acid esters, and silicone emulsifiers
- polymers that impart water-resistant properties
- stabilizers: preservatives, complexing agents, antioxidants
- perfume

Sunscreens now are available in various forms: creams, gels, lotions, mousse, sprays, sticks, and wipes. The distribution of UV filter in the oil and water phase of an emulsion can play an important role for the uniform distribution of the UV filters on the skin and thus affects the SPF and the UVA protection factor (UVA-PF).

Performance of a Sunscreen

Historically, the sole purpose of sunscreens was to prevent sunburn. The SPF is the ratio between the minimal dose that produces perceptible erythema on the skin [i.e., minimal erythema dose (MED)] in the presence or absence of 2 mg/cm^2 of sunscreen, using solar-simulated radiation as a light source (23). The actual protection provided by a sunscreen is a dynamic process. The exposure time is the most important influencing factor for any effect of UV radiation. This is best illustrated in Figure 14, inspired by the Australian Standard document (24). For individuals with skin phototype I to II, one MED is reached within about 10 minutes without sunscreen (i.e., SPF 1). With SPF 15 and SPF 30 sunscreens, the time to reach one MED is prolonged accordingly to 150 and 300 minutes. However, in a proper photoprotection strategy, sunscreen is not used to reach one MED. To the contrary, sunscreen should be used to stay well below one MED. The example in Figure 14 shows that a two-hour exposure of a person with skin phototype I leads to 80%, 40%, or 20% of an MED if a sunscreen of SPF 15, 30, or 60 (in Europe, labeled 50+) is applied, respectively. The same reasoning as shown in Figure 14 for the SPF holds for the UVA-PF as well. However, sunscreens with the same SPF frequently have different UVA-PF; therefore, a high SPF sunscreen may not automatically provide good UVA protection (25). Therefore, over the person's lifetime, the difference in the cumulative amount UV transmitted by using sunscreens with different SPF is potentially quite significant.

It should be noted that the example shown in Figure 14 is based on the assumption that the UV filters are photostable and the sunscreens are applied at a concentration of 2 mg/cm^2 (the worldwide standard used in SPF testing). Many of the currently used UV filters degrade during UV exposure (26). In actual use, consumers apply on average 0.5 to 1.0 mg/cm^2 of sunscreens (27). Some exposed sites are frequently missed, and with

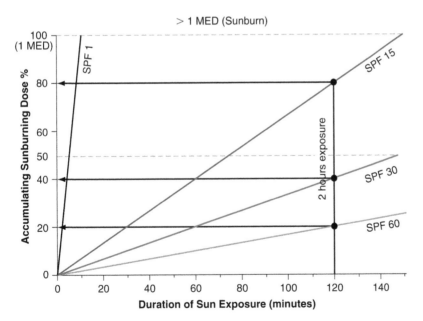

Figure 14 Performance of sunscreens of SPF 15, 30, and 60 in dose versus time diagram; dynamics of the UV dose reaching the skin through sunscreens over time. The example shows the minimal erythema dose received by skin phototype I or II. *Abbreviations*: MED, minimal erythema dose; SPF, sun protection factor.

regular or outdoor activities, sunscreens are rubbed off or washed off with water and sweat exposure.

In vivo studies showed a quasi-linear relationship between the amount applied and SPF (28). In silico calculations explain why this is the case and how the amount of UVA protection actually influences how the SPF depends on the amount applied (Fig. 15). UVB-biased sunscreens [i.e., with low UVA/UVB ratio (29)] lead to a concave SPF/amount curve, whereas uniform UVB/UVA sunscreens exhibit convex SPF/amount curves. This effect is more pronounced at a nominal SPF (e.g., SPF 10 at 2 mg/cm^2) than at SPF 30, the reason being that any sunscreen above about SPF 10 must have some minimal degree of UVA protection, otherwise the freely transmitted UVA radiation would lead to erythema. Hence, the most common sunscreens, which provide some intermediate degree of UVA protection, exhibit a quasi-linear relationship between SPF and amount applied.

An exponential (convex) relationship between SPF and amount applied is only possible if the protection profile is uniform, i.e., if protection against UVB and UVA radiation is the same (also referred to as spectral homeostasis or gray filter). Textiles provide practically uniform protection; therefore, two layers of a UV protection factor (UPF) 5 fabric indeed yield a UPF 25. This can easily be confirmed by a transmission measurement.

The relationship between UVA-PF and application amount is similar to that of SPF and application amount, i.e., it is convex for more uniform sunscreens, concave for UVB-biased sunscreens, and quasi-linear in between. Unlike the SPF that is by definition the same at 2 mg/cm^2, the absolute UVA-PF value varies of course tremendously between a UVB-biased and a uniform sunscreen (Fig. 16A, B).

Figures 17A and B show the ratio UVA-PF/SPF as a function of the application amount. In Europe, sunscreens must have a minimum ratio of 1/3 according to the European Commission (EC) recommendation (5). The figures show that if a sunscreen fulfills this criterion (at the standard 2 mg/cm^2), lower application amount will always lead to a relatively better UVA protection than sunburn protection. This is a very important conclusion. It means that while we need to be concerned about the decline of SPF with lower application amount, the UVA-PF will always decline less.

USE OF UV FILTERS IN COMMERCIAL SUNSCREENS

Basic Requirements for the Use of UV Filters

Sunscreens usually contain between two to seven UV filters, depending on their intended SPF and degree of UVA protection. Even in the United States, there are more then seven UV filters available on the sunscreen monograph (30). So, why is it that only a fraction of the available UV filters is actually used? The major reason is efficacy, i.e., UV absorption capacity, but also water resistance or compatibility in a particular sunscreen formulation. As mentioned earlier in this chapter, in addition to efficacy, sunscreen manufacturers have to consider three other basic requirements: safety, registration, and patent freedom. If any of these four requirements is not fulfilled, a UV filter will not be used.

Efficacy

An efficient sunscreen active shows good absorption, at the very least, in parts in the relevant UV range between 290 and 400 nm. Efficacy also means that the UV absorber must be easily incorporated in any kind of formulation. If not, it may become difficult to achieve formulations that are also cosmetically acceptable. This, in turn, would negatively influence

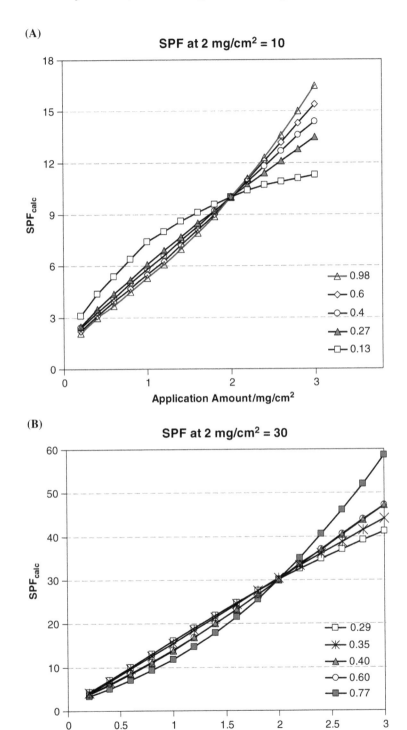

Figure 15 (**A**) SPF versus application amount for SPF 10 sunscreens and various UVA/UVB ratios, calculated with the Ciba Sunscreen Simulator. (**B**) SPF versus application amount for SPF 30 sunscreens and various UVA/UVB ratios, calculated with the Ciba Sunscreen Simulator.

(A)

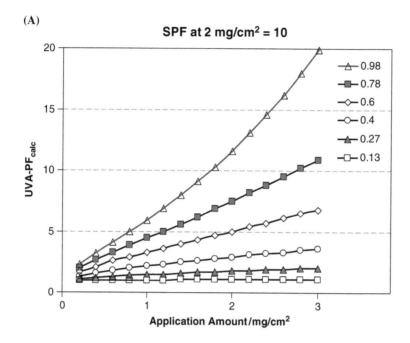

(B)

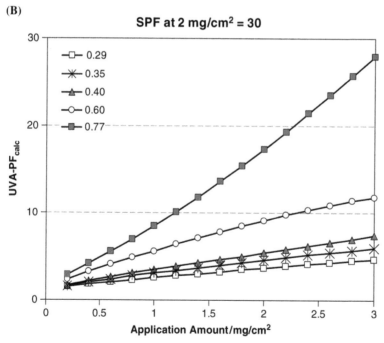

Figure 16 (**A**) UVA-PF versus application amount for SPF 10 sunscreens and various UVA/UVB ratios, calculated with the Ciba Sunscreen Simulator. (**B**) UVA-PF versus application amount for SPF 30 sunscreens and various UVA/UVB ratios, calculated with the Ciba Sunscreen Simulator.

the compliance of the sunscreen user. Efficacy may also mean good solubility of a UV absorber in different emollients relevant to cosmetics. Other major characteristic-influencing efficacy is the photostability of the UV absorber, which can be determined by irradiating a sunscreen sample in the laboratory (31). Unstable sunscreen actives lose efficacy and may

(A)

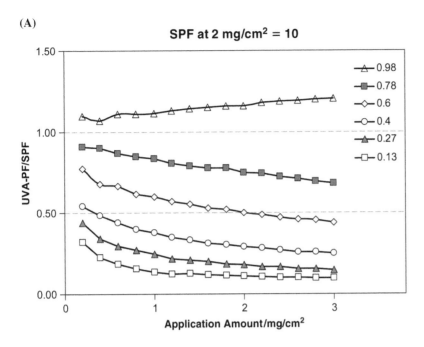

(B)

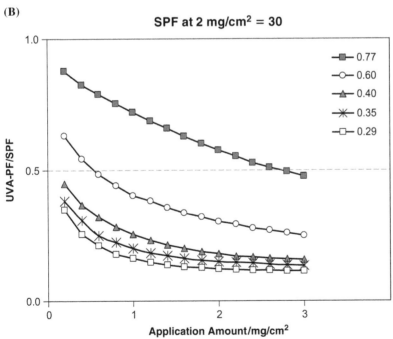

Figure 17 (**A**) Ratios of UVA-PF/SPF versus application amount for SPF 10 sunscreens and various UVA/UVB ratios, obtained from results of Figures 15 and 16. (**B**) Ratios of UVA-PF/SPF versus application amount for SPF 30 sunscreens and various UVA/UVB ratios, obtained from results of Figures 15 and 16.

Table 5 Typical International Safety Dossier of a New Sunscreen (32)

- Acute oral and dermal toxicity
- Dermal, ocular irritation, skin sensitization
- Photoirritation, photosensitization
- Subchronic oral and topical toxicity
- Chronic toxicity
- Fertility, early embryonic development
- Embryofetal toxicity and peri-/postnatal toxicity
- In vitro and in vivo percutaneous absorption
- Topical and oral pharmacokinetic and metabolism
- In vitro and in vivo genetic toxicity
- Carcinogenicity
- Photocarcinogenicity
- Safety and efficacy in man

even lead to safety concerns upon irradiation. Furthermore, the UV absorber substance must be compatible with all other ingredients in a formulation; there should be no discoloration of skin and hair, no staining of textiles, and no odor. For water-resistant claim, the UV absorber should be insoluble in water. Last but not least, the UV filter should be economical in its use. These parameters are all part of the efficacy requirement.

Safety

Sunscreen actives should have no adverse effect on humans and environment. Although direct comparison with a new pharmaceutical drug is not appropriate, the development of a new sunscreen active for global use is nearly as demanding. The toxicological studies required for a global registration are listed in Table 5.

Registration

In order to exploit the full economic potential of a UV filter, UV absorber manufacturers are aiming for global registration. In Europe, South America, Asia, and South Africa, where sunscreens are considered as cosmetics, approval is possible within one to two years of filing. In Australia, New Zealand, Japan, and the United States, it takes longer. In 2002, the United States introduced a new procedure, TEA (33), to accelerate the process. So far, six UVB filters that are widely used outside the United States have received the status of "eligibility to enter the Sunscreen Monograph" (34). By end of 2008, none of them have yet been added to the sunscreen monograph.

Patent Freedom

Patenting of sunscreen actives and their applications deserve special attention in this chapter. Patent freedom means the free use of sunscreen actives by any sunscreen manufacturer, i.e., without any uncertainty about whether any third-party patent rights are infringed by the use of a particular ingredient.

Until about 15 years ago, UV absorber manufacturers protected their inventions by simple substance patents that included the basic applications, e.g., "invention of a novel UV absorber for the incorporation in personal care formulations for the protection of skin and hair." The innovative cosmetics manufacturers would then file their own patents on

Table 6 Examples of Specially Emphasized UV Filters

Brand/drug name (manufacturer)	Product (ingredient) information
Mexoryl® SX Ecamsule (L'Oréal)	L'Oréal patented ecamsule first, in 1982. It was approved by the European Union (EU) in 1991. Sunscreens based on ecamsule have been available in Europe, Canada, and other parts of the world since 1993 and were given approval by the FDA in the United states in July 2006 (36) This approval only extends to ecamsule-containing sunscreens registered under a new drug application, not ecamsule itself (37).
Mexoryl XL Drometrizol (L'Oréal)	Mexoryl XL is a photostable broad-spectrum UVB/UVA filter. It is not yet approved by the FDA, although Mexoryl XL-containing products are widely available in many parts of the world. Products marketed as excellent broad-spectrum sunscreens (38).
Optisol™ Titanium Dioxide (Croda)	The Optisol technology involves the doping of titanium dioxide with a low level of manganese; the manganese ions are located both within the structural lattice of the TiO_2 and at the surface of the particles. This results in absorption of UVA radiation without the concurrent formation of free radicals. Furthermore, while providing balanced UVA and UVB protection, Optisol also provides additional benefits in absorbing free radicals that may be generated by other components of the sunscreen formulation; it also enhances formulation stability (39).
Parsol® 1789 Avobenzone (DSM)	Avobenzone was patented in 1973 and was approved in the EU in 1978. It was approved by the FDA in 1988. Its use is approved worldwide (40). Avobenzone has been shown to degrade significantly upon exposure to UV, resulting in less protection over time. This degradation can be reduced by using a photostabilizer, such as octocrylene. Other photostabilizers include Tinosorb® S, Tinosorb M, butyloctyl salicylate, Mexoryl SX, Corapan® TQ, and others (41).
Tinosorb M Bisoctrizole (Ciba)	Tinosorb M is the first representative of a new class of UV absorber, i.e., organic microfine particles that absorb, reflect, and scatter. The commercial form Tinosorb M is produced as a 50% aqueous dispersion of colorless organic microfine particles (42).
Tinosorb S Bemotrizinol (Ciba)	Tinosorb S was specifically designed to meet the needs of the cosmetic industry. Besides the excellent performance as a photostable broad-spectrum UV filter, it is compatible with organic and inorganic filters, meets the high safety requirements, and is oil soluble for high water resistance (43).
Z-Cote® Zinc oxide (BASF)	Z-Cote is a broad-spectrum UVB-UVA filter. Its physical characteristics are such that products that are elegant and transparent can be formulated (44).
ZinClear™ Zinc oxide (Adv. Nano Techn.)	Patented process stabilizes particle surface, minimizing agglomeration, and resulting in cosmetically transparent SPF 30+ sunscreens containing only zinc oxide as the UV absorber (45).

specific applications and technologies that they had invented and were using to differentiate themselves from their competitors. This system allowed both the supplier and the manufacturer of sunscreens to create new business by protecting their respective inventions. In the mid-1990s, important cosmetics manufacturers started to patent not

Table 7 Examples of Specially Emphasized UV Filter Complexes

Brand name, Manufacturer	Patent information
Avotriplex®, Banana Boat®	Boat sun care products with AvoTriplex technology last longer in the sun. This means you can stay out longer and enjoy your day worry-free. Products marketed to provide photostable UVA/UVB protection (46). US Patent 7,014,842 (abstract) There is provided a composition comprising one or more photoactive compounds and one or more optimization agents. The composition requires a small amount of optimization agent to efficiently optimize the polarity, critical wavelength, SPF, PFA, Star Rating, photostability, or any combinations thereof. Subsequently, an efficient sunscreen composition is achieved.
Helioplex®, Neutrogena® (J&J)	Helioplex is a proprietary name for a formulation of broad-spectrum UVA/UVB skin protection containing avobenzone and oxybenzone (47). US Patent 6,444,195 (abstract) The present invention relates to a method of photostabilizing a composition comprising (a) one or more dibenzoylmethane derivative UV-A absorbing agent(s); (b) one or more benzophenone derivative(s); and (c) a diester or polyester of a naphthalene dicarboxylic acid and a method of protecting mammalian skin or hair from UV radiation comprising topically applying to the skin or hair such a composition.
Sunsure®, Hawaiian Tropic®	SunSure technology uses less chemical sunscreens to achieve a higher SPF with longer-lasting protection (48). US Patent 7,309,481 (Abstract) The present invention relates to photostable compositions that provide protection from ultraviolet radiation ("UVR"). The invention particularly relates to the sunscreens avobenzone, octocrylene and oxybenzone, forming a triplet combination. Compositions of the present invention are free of diesters or polyesters of naphthalene dicarboxylic acid and also are substantially free of substantial amounts of other sunscreens and substantial amounts of optimizing agents. Sunscreens of the invention may be essentially free of, or free of, lower monohydric alcohol and/or acrylates/C.sub.12-22 alkylmethacrylate copolymer in an effective non-pilling amount used to gel a C.sub.1-C.sub.4 alcohol. The triplet combination surprisingly provides and substantially maintains the initial SPF value of the sunscreen composition throughout the period of UVR exposure. Compositions of the invention are photostable such that each of sunscreen active in the triplet combination does not appreciably photodegrade. The present invention accurately communicates the amount of UVR photoprotection actually provided in natural sunlight.

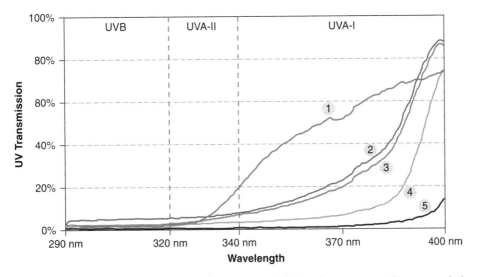

Figure 18 Commercial sunscreens on the way towards the ideal sunscreen profile—transmissions of typical US sunscreens with 0%, 1%, 2%, and 3% avobenzone (49) and European BOOTS 5-star sunscreen containing broad-spectrum UV filters bisoctrizole and bemotrizinol.

Sunscreen			UV filter composition	
#	SPF	UVA[a]	UVB/UVA-II	UVA-I/broad-spectrum
1	50	Low	Homosalate 15%, octinoxate 7.5%, octisalate 5%, titanium dioxde 2.4%	-
2	50	Medium	Octocrylene 8%, oxybenzone 3.5%	Avobenzone 1%
3	45	Medium	Homosalate 15%, octioxate 7.5%, octisalate 5%, oxybenzone 6%	Avobenzone 2%
4	45	High	Homosalate 13%, octisalate 5%, octocrylene 7%, oxybenzone 4%	Avobenzone 3%
5	60[b]	Highest	Octocrylene, titanium dioxide	Bisoctrizole, bisdisulizole disodium, bemotrizinol

[a]The evaluation of the UVA category is tentative since the proposed FDA method for the determination of the UVA-I/UV ratio is not yet finalized.
[b]SPF according to International Harmonized Method (others according to FDA method); in Europe SPF > 60 are labeled 50+ (EC recommendation).

only their specific technologies but also generic combinations of different ingredients without the intention for use. This "blocking strategy" was aimed to keep competitors from using new technology that emerged in the market (35). This strategy is not only limiting the potential of competing sunscreen manufacturers, it is also detrimental to the supplier who suddenly sees the potential market of his new sunscreen active shrinking because of patent restrictions. As a consequence, suppliers had to react and rethink the patenting strategy and the whole innovation process, especially in the realization phase and the market introduction. A strategy to avoid blocking situations is to publish all sorts of combinations of ingredients and claims that may never become relevant before the identity of the new ingredient becomes publicly known. Institutions to publish quickly now exist on the Internet, e.g., www.ip.com. The site enables innovative companies to quickly and easily protect their inventions by the rapid publication and creation of prior art in the form of technical disclosures.

Sunscreen Manufacturer-Specific Technology

Sunscreen manufacturers are branding several UV filters and various technologies to physicians, patients, and consumers; some of the examples are listed in Tables 6 and 7, respectively. UV filters or complexes that provide stable or stabilized UVA protection are the major examples.

Improvement of UVA Protection in Commercial Sunscreens

Over the last 20 years, since the approval of avobenzone by the FDA, products with good UVA protection have steadily been increasing worldwide. In the United States, because of lack of a UVA regulation, many different UVA claims are made on products. The new proposed FDA UVA star-rating system will allow a correlation of UVA-I protection with the amount of photostablized avobenzone that is used in a sunscreen. Figure 18 shows U.S. sunscreens with 0%, 1%, 2%, and 3% avobenzone (49). In addition, a European sunscreen is shown that contains new broad-spectrum UV filters bisoctrizole and bemotrizinol. Such compositions come very close to the ideal of uniform UVB/UVA protection and should be able to achieve the four-star rating of the proposed FDA UVA star-rating category.

REFERENCES

1. Haywood R, Wardman P, Sanders R, et al. Sunscreens inadequately protect against ultraviolet-a induced free radicals in skin: implications for skin aging and melanoma?. J Invest Dermatol 2003; 121:862–868.
2. Diffey BL. The need for sunscreens with broad spectrum protection. In: Urbach F, ed. Biological responses to ultraviolet a radiation. A symposium on UV-A radiation. San Antonio, TX, June 1991. Overland Park, KS: Valdenmar Publication Co., 1992:321–328.
3. Moyal D, Fourtanier AM. Broad-spectrum sunscreens provide better protection from solar ultraviolet-simulated radiation and natural sunlight-induced immunosuppression in human beings. J Am Acad Dermatol 2008; 58(5):S149–S154.
4. Sunscreen Drug Products for Over-the-Counter Human Use; Proposed Amendment of Final Monograph. Fed Regist 2007; 72(165):49069–49122 (Proposed Rules).
5. European Commission Recommendation on the efficacy of sunscreen products and the claims made relating thereto. OJ L265, 20067647/EC, 39–43.
6. Sun Care—UV Protection. Available at: https://www.ciba.com/sunscreen-simulator. Accessed May 20, 2008.
7. Sayre RM, Dowdy JC. Darkness at noon: sunscreens and vitamin D3. Photochem Photobiol 2007; 83(2):459–463.
8. Barltrop JA, Doyle JD. 1975 Excited States in Organic Chemistry. London: John Wiley & Sons, 1975.
9. Ottersted JE. Photostability and molecular structure. J Phys Chem 1973; 58:5716–5725.
10. Kollias N. The absorption properties of "physical" sunscreens. Arch Dermatol 1999; 135:209.
11. Schlossmann D, Shao Y. Inorganic ultraviolet filters. In: Shaath NA, ed. Sunscreens—Regulations and Commercial Development, Cosmetic Science and Technology Series 28, 3rd ed. New York: Taylor & Francis Group, 2005:239–279.
12. Steinberg DC. Regulations of sunscreens worldwide. In: Shaath NA, ed. Sunscreens—Regulations and Commercial Development, Cosmetic Science and Technology Series 28, 3rd ed. New York: Taylor & Francis Group, 2005:173–198.
13. Herzog B, Hueglin D, Osterwalder U. New sunscreen actives. In: Shaath NA ed. Sunscreens—Regulations and Commercial Development, Cosmetic Science and Technology Series 28, 3rd ed. New York: Taylor & Francis Group, 2005:291–320.

14. Stueber GJ, Kieninger M, Schettler H, et al. Ultraviolet stabilizers of the 2-(2′-hydroxyphenyl)-1,3,5-triazine class: Structural and spectroscopic characterization. J Phys Chem 1995: 99:10097–10109.

15. Shaath NA. Evolution of modern sunscreen chemicals. In: Lowe NJ, Shaath NA, Pathak MA, eds. Sunscreens: Development, Evaluation, and Regulatory Aspects, 2nd ed. New York: Marcel Dekker, 1997:17.

16. Bos JD, Meinardi MM. The 500 Dalton rule for the skin penetration of chemical compounds and drugs. Exp Dermatol 2000; 9(3):165–169.

17. COLIPA sun protection factor test method. Ref. 94/289. The European Cosmetic Toiletry and Perfumery Association—COLIPA; Oct. 1994; Rue du Congrès, Brussels.

18. Herzog B. Prediction of sun protection factors by calculation of transmissions with a calibrated step film model. J Cosmet Sci 2002; 53:11–26.

19. Ferrero L, Pissavini M, Marguerie S, et al. Efficiency of a continuous height distribution model of sunscreen film geometry to predict a realistic sun protection factor. J Cosmet Sci 2003; 54:463–481.

20. Herzog B. Models for the calculation of sun protection factors and parameters characterizing the UVA protection ability of cosmetic sunscreens. In: Tadros TF, ed. Colloids in Cosmetics and Personal Care. New York: Wiley–VCH, 2008:275–308.

21. Diffey BL, Robson J. A new substrate to measure sunscreen protection factors throughout the ultraviolet spectrum. J Soc Cosmet Chem 1989; 40:127–133.

22. McKinlay AF, Diffey BL. A reference action spectrum for ultraviolet-induced erythema in human skin. CIE J 1987; 6:17–22.

23. United States Food and Drug Administration, HHS. Sunscreen drug products for over-the-counter human use; final monograph. Final rule. Fed Regist 1999; 64(98):27666–27693.

24. Australian/New Zealand Standard™, Sunscreen products—evaluation and classification. Originated in Australia as AS 2604:1983; Previous ed. AS/NZS 2604:1997; 5th ed. 1998.

25. Fourtanier A, Moyal D, Maccario J, et al. Measurement of sunscreen immune protection factors in humans: a consensus paper. J Invest Dermatol 2005; 125:403–409.

26. Maier H, Schauberger G, Brunnhofer K, et al. Change of ultraviolet absorbance of sunscreens by exposure to solar-simulated radiation. J Invest Dermatol 2001; 117:256–262.

27. Kullavanijaya P, Lim HW. Photoprotection. J Am Acad Dermatol 2005; 52:937–958.

28. Bimczok R, Gers-Barlag H, Mundt C, et al. Influence of applied quantity of sunscreen products on the sun protection factor—a multicenter study organized by the DGK taskforce sun protection. Skin Pharmacol Physiol 2007; 20:57–64.

29. Boots UK limited. Measurement of UVA: UVB Ratios According to the Boots Star Rating System. Nottingham, UK, 2008.

30. Shaath NA. The chemistry of ultraviolet filters, chapter 13. In: Shaath N, ed. Sunscreens: Regulations and Commercial Development, 3rd ed. Cosmetic Science and Technology Series, Vol 28. Boca Raton, FL: Taylor & Francis Group, 222.

31. Sayre RM, Dowdy JC. Photostability testing of avobenzone. Cosmetics and Toiletries 1999; 114(5):85–91.

32. Nohynek G, Schaefer H. Benefit and risk of organic ultraviolet filters. Regul Toxicol Pharmacol 2001; 33:1–15.

33. Food and Drug Administration. Additional criteria and procedures for classifying over-the-counter drugs as generally recognized as safe and effective and not misbranded. 21 CFR Part 330. [Docket No. 96N–0277], RIN 0910–AA01, Federal Register/Vol. 67, No. 15/Wednesday, January 23, 2002/Rules and Regulations, 3060–3076.

34. Food and Drug Administration. Over-the-counter drug products; safety and efficacy review; additional sunscreen ingredients. [Docket No. 2003N–0233], Federal Register/Vol. 68, No. 133/Friday, July 11, 2003/Notices, 41386–41387.

35. Rudolph M, Specific UV filter combinations and their impact on sunscreen efficacy. Presented at: International Sun protection conference, Commonwealth Institute; March 9–10, 1999; London.

36. Search for "ecamsule." Available at: http://www.accessdata.fda.gov/scripts/cder/drugsatfda/. Accessed May 29, 2008.
37. Ecamsule. Available at: http://en.wikipedia.org/wiki/Ecamsule. Accessed May 20, 2008.
38. Sunscreen. Available at: http://en.wikipedia.org/wiki/Sunscreen. Accessed May 20, 2008.
39. About OPTISOL™ UV Absorber. Available at: http://www.oxonica.com/materials/materials_optisol.php. Accessed May 20, 2008.
40. Avobenzone. Available at: http://en.wikipedia.org/wiki/Avobenzone. Accessed May 20, 2008.
41. Skin breaks-drugs-avobenzone overview. Available at: http://www.kosmix.com/Health/skin_breaks-Drugs-Avobenzone-s. Accessed May 20, 2008.
42. Bisoctrizole. Available at: http://en.wikipedia.org/wiki/Bisoctrizole. Accessed May 20, 2008.
43. Bemotrizinol. Available at: http://en.wikipedia.org/wiki/Bemotrizinol. Accessed May 20, 2008.
44. BASF. Available at: http://www.basf.com/corporate/news2005/050905_Z-Cote_Max.htm. Accessed May 20, 2008.
45. ZinClear™. Available at: http://www.antaria.com/index.php?page=zinclear. Accessed May 20, 2008.
46. AvoTriplex™. Available at: http://www.playtexproducts.com/avo/. Accessed May 20, 2008.
47. Helioplex. Available at: http://en.wikipedia.org/wiki/Helioplex. Accessed May 20, 2008.
48. SunSure® Technology. Available at: http://www.hawaiiantropic.com/SunFacts/SunSure-Technology.aspx. Accessed May 20, 2008.
49. Wang SQ, Stanfield JW, Osterwalder U. In vitro assessments of UVA protection by popular sunscreens available in the United States. J Am Acad Dermatol 2008 Oct 1; [Epub ahead of print].

3
Formulation and Stability of Sunscreen Products

Curtis A. Cole
Johnson & Johnson Consumer and Personal Products Inc., Skillman, New Jersey, U.S.A.

Juergen Vollhardt and Christine Mendrok
DSM Nutritional Products Ltd., Basel, Switzerland

SYNOPSIS

- This chapter provides a brief history of how sunscreen products came into being and discusses the many challenges facing the modern day sunscreen formulator and developer. Creating a successful sunscreen product requires a complex blend of photoprotection science, consumer insights, aesthetic art, global regulatory knowledge, and photochemistry understanding. The chapter describes a deeper look inside the formulation laboratory to see the creation process for today's modern sunscreens.

INTRODUCTION AND HISTORY OF SUNSCREENS

From the earliest use of mud and clays to protect skin from the sun's burning rays, today's sunscreen products have come a long way in efficacy, convenience, and elegance. In the late 1930s, Dr. Franz Greiter, a Swiss chemist and amateur mountain climber, was annoyed by being frequently sunburned at high altitudes and started compounding sunscreening lotions in his laboratory to protect himself from sunburn. This led ultimately to the founding of the Greiter company, which marketed products under the Piz Buin® brand. Veterans from the Pacific Theater may remember the "red veterinary petrolatum" provided in life rafts and survival kits as a sunscreen, a heavy greasy ointment containing an undefined UV-absorbing contaminant, which was quite substantive against water exposure, for obvious reasons. Unfortunately, the UV protection was more limited compared with its wash resistance. This compound and improved sunscreen formulations are credited to

Dr. Benjamin Greene, a Florida physician, who needed a sunscreen to protect his balding pate. His discoveries resulted in the brand known today as Coppertone® (1).

The "modern day" sunscreens began their appearance in the 1960s with simple alcoholic solutions of para-aminobenzoic acid and benzophenones, and giving only modest protection. The rating system for classifying their protective capabilities was also evolving, with credit given again to Dr. Franz Greiter, for the concept of the sun protection factor (SPF) testing system in 1962 (1). The SPF testing methodology has been refined by numerous industry and regulatory agencies and has been adopted around the globe as the means to communicate the efficacy of sunscreen products to consumers.

Early "modern" sunscreen products were almost exclusively ultraviolet B (UVB)-blocking sunscreens with minimal SPF (below 10), without waterproofing agents to provide resistance to water or sweat exposure. It was not until the early 1980s that use of waterproofing systems based on polymeric resins became available for use in oil-in-water emulsions that provided SPF protection after 80 minutes of water exposure. Numerous polymeric film formers and polymeric emulsifiers are now available for and used extensively for waterproofing sunscreen preparations. Examples of polymeric emulsifiers include PEG-30 dipolyhydroxystearate, acrylates/C10-30 alkyl acrylate cross polymer, TEA-diethanolaminoethyl polyisobutenylsuccinate, and lauryl PEG/PPG-18/18 methicone.

During this infancy period of "modern sunscreen products," the understanding of the extent of damage caused by ultraviolet exposure to the skin grew substantially as photobiologists studied the effects of first ultraviolet B (UVB: 290–320 nm radiation), and then ultraviolet A radiation (UVA: 320–400 nm radiation) on exposed skin. The two sciences of sunscreen formulation and photobiology grew simultaneously in depth and breadth of knowledge, with the newly acquired understanding of the effects of ultraviolet radiation on skin feeding the dermatologist's push for higher- and broader-spectrum protection in sunscreen products. An SPF horsepower "race" ensued in the mid-1980s with SPFs starting at a maximum of 15, then to 23, 30, 45, 55, during the early 2000s, and most recently in the United States to a maximum of 85 in 2008.

Also in the mid 1980s, the role of UVA in affecting the skin's immune function, skin cancer, and structural proteins was starting to emerge. At about the same time, a powerful, new, UVA absorber, avobenzone [butyl methoxydibenzoylmethane (BMDM)], was introduced to the European market and later adopted into the U.S. monograph in 1996, providing the first truly broad-spectrum UVA absorber for sunscreen products. Along with the development of products with substantial UVA protection, came the need to quantitate the extent (both breadth and magnitude) of that UVA protection, resulting in numerous UVA testing methods that are only now (2008) beginning to coalesce to a few standard test methods. A second horsepower race, this time for UVA protection, ensued in the mid-2000s with companies claiming UVA protection factors (UVA-PFs) in the 20 to 30s. Through all of this, history shows clearly that knowledge and understanding of the dangers of UV exposure have led to greater and greater protection of product offerings in the marketplace, and the consumers are the main winners, acquiring the ability to play and enjoy themselves in the sun with less fear of painful sunburn and longer-lasting skin damage.

FORMULATING FOR CONSUMER COMPLIANCE

Product Aesthetics

While the sunscreen industry manufacturers have been consistently developing products with better and better protection potential, the fact remains that unless the consumers actually apply the product to their skin, in appropriate quantities over the entire surface, they will not get the benefits of true sun protection. The reason most often quoted by consumers for not using sunscreen products relates to the tactile and aesthetic properties of the sunscreen products—"they're too greasy and icky." In fact, most of the sunscreens, both recreational and daily wear moisturizers with SPF, use oil-soluble UV filters, as they are the most easily "waterproofed" as well as the easiest to formulate. The most commonly used UVB filters are all oil soluble, octyl methoxycinnamate (octinoxate), octocrylene, and the salicylates (homosalate and octisalate). Similarly, the most commonly used UVA filters oxybenzone and avobenzone are also oil soluble. The inorganic or particulate sun filters, titanium dioxide and zinc oxide, can be either oil dispersed or water dispersed, depending on the surface coating applied by the supplier. The result is that the oil portion of the formulation becomes an increasingly higher proportion of the SPF of the product, taxing the ability of the formulator to develop a "nongreasy" formulation. Compounding the problem for recreational sunscreen products, a waterproofing polymer is necessary to help "stick" the oils to the surface of the skin to resist wash-off or sweating-off of the product in use. Examples of waterproofing polymers include acrylates/polytrimethylsiloxymethacrylate copolymer, Bis-PEG-18 methyl ether dimethylsilane, cetyl dimethicone, trimethylsiloxysilicate, butylated PVP, VP/hexadecene copolymer, VP/eicosene copolymer, triacontanyl PVP, and acrylates/octylacrylamide copolymer—ingredients that actually form physical film over the surface of the skin to help hold the sunscreen-absorbing oils onto the skin's surface, but also add to the "ick" factor experienced by many consumers. Improperly formulated, these film formers can form little "pils," like those experienced on sweaters that can ball up on the surface of the skin when rubbed. Clearly this does not lead to the desired consumer experience and enthusiasm to slather on sunscreens on every outdoor occasion.

Approaches to diminish the greasy and icky feel of sunscreen products have led formulators to incorporate a host of ingredients, including silicones, silicas, and other slip agents to diminish the heavy and tacky feeling left by oily sunscreen filters and waterproofing polymers. Polymeric surfactants, such as acrylate cross polymers now available, can play a dual role to emulsify as well as to provide wash resistance for recreational products, with excellent rapid emulsion-breaking characteristics for ease of spreading on skin and skin feel after drying.

Daily-wear moisturizers with SPF (non-recreational) typically use the same oil-based sun filters used in recreational products, but typically do not incorporate the polymeric film formers used for waterproofing purposes. In addition, since wash resistance is not a critical performance criterion, water-soluble filters can be more readily incorporated into these types of products. Providing UV protection into both the water and oil portions of the emulsion can help fill in the "holes" left by evaporation of water in an "oil filter only" sunscreen product. The lower oil phase content of a hybrid water-soluble filter and oil-soluble filter system can provide for a less "greasy" product with user-preferred aesthetic properties. The most widely used water-soluble filter is ensulizole, a high absorbtivity UVB filter. Water-soluble filters, sulizobenzone and dioxybenzone, provide modest levels of absorbtivity in the UVB as well as the shortwave UVA2 region (324–340 nm radiation).

The sunscreen industry has done an excellent job of developing and providing sun protection in the widest possible variety of product forms to help make their use more enjoyable and convenient. One of the most effective means to provide meaningful and consistent sunscreen protection use has been the incorporation of sun filters with SPF into daily moisturizer products, typically applied in the morning before sun exposure can occur. This category of product usage began in the late 1980s with a brand called "Purpose®," starting initially with only SPF 12 protection. This category has grown enormously over the past 20 years such that virtually every line of facial moisturizer offers an SPF version of the product. SPFs offered in this category are now typically above SPF 15, and as high as SPF 45. These products contain essentially the same UV filters used in recreational sunscreen products, but do not contain the waterproofing polymers and are formulated for a light texture, compatible with use of makeup.

Sunscreen filters have also made their way into lip products, under-eye treatments, and specialized stick application products for protecting noses and ears, for example. The oil-soluble UV filters are readily incorporated into wax-based sticks and provide convenient controlled application to specific areas. To prevent other topical sunscreens from running or "creeping" into one's eye, one can use a stick product to create a protective barrier ring around the eye socket that the topical sunscreens will not cross. Some manufacturers have offered a combination cream with stick package to offer both forms in a single package.

Convenience of application has further driven innovation in packaging, with offerings of small convenience-size packages, and more notably a spray application format. The spray sunscreen products use pressurized "cans" containing either emulsion formulations or alcohol or emollient-based clear sunscreens that apply either as a stream of product that requires hand spreading or as a fine mist that covers the skin and does not require hand spreading. This "no-hands" application form has been a real hit with the consumer, particularly for application to children. Spray rates are critical for this form of product; if the mist is too fine, application density is too low, and protection is compromised. Application with the spray should leave the skin "glossy" with the product to insure adequate coverage at a sufficient application density. Again, the intent is to provide the consumer with the most convenience and best aesthetics to encourage regular and convenient product usage.

FORMULATING FOR BALANCED PROTECTION

UVB and UVA Protection—Broad Spectrum

Photobiology learnings over the past 30 years have shown that broad-spectrum UVB and UVA protection is critical to adequate sunscreen protection. In addition to well-documented effects of UVB radiation on skin, UVA radiation, once thought innocuous, has been shown to be important in suppression of the skin's natural immune function (2–5), an important factor in modulating skin cancer initiation and promotion. UVA radiation has also been implicated in the aging processes of skin, leading to matrix degradation felt to result in the leathery qualities of photo-damaged skin and ultimately the wrinkles and sagging properties associated with extensive sun overexposure (6–11). UVA radiation penetrates further into the skin, into the dermal matrix, and can react with oxygen to create free radicals that cause inflammation, collagen cross-linking, and damage to fibroblasts. Until 1996, the benzophenone filters were the primary filters used in the United States to provide any level of UVA protection, having limited filtering capability in the long-wave UVAI region of the solar spectrum (340–400 nm). UVA-PFs as measured by persistent pigmentation testing (12–15) [or persistent pigment darkening (PPD) test methods—similar to SPF ratings, but only evaluating UVA protection] were only in the range of 3 to 4. Addition of titanium dioxide or zinc oxide gave some modest additional UVA protection, but can cause unacceptable whitening of the skin and undesirable skin feel and high concentrations. Recent improvements in formulation have helped to improve the aesthetic properties of these inorganic or mineral filters, but in general, the UVA protection that they provide is only modest compared with avobenzone or other filters such as the ingredients (i.e., Tinosorb S®—USAN—bemotrizanol and Tinosorb M® USAN—bisoctrizole or Uvinul A+—diethylamino hydroxybenzoyl hexyl benzoate). In 1996, avobenzone was included in the U.S. monograph up to 3%, but was only allowed to be used in combination with a limited number of other sun filters. With avobenzone available for use, formulators have the ability to do more meaningful development of truly broad-spectrum sunscreen products, which will be further enhanced with approvals of pending new ingredients currently undergoing the time and extent application (TEA) evaluations by the Food and Drug Administration (FDA).

One of the fundamental questions facing formulators with regard to balancing UVB and UVA protection is "what is the right balance, and how do I measure it?" Depending on the regulatory requirements or the specific marketing claim desired, one would have a different answer and formulation approach. It has been well established that a balance of UVA protection with the UVB is desirable. For "broad-spectrum" protection, it is commonly accepted that a critical wavelength (16) of around 370 is appropriate to substantiate this claim. This measure evaluates the area under the spectrophotometric absorbance curve (AUC) and requires that 90% of the AUC is below the "critical wavelength" after some level of pre-irradiation of the sample with solar-simulated radiation. To meet this criterion typically requires addition of at least 0.5% avobenzone to the formulation, or significant levels of zinc oxide or titanium dioxide.

The European Commission has required that products sold in the European Union (EU) claiming UVA protection must provide a UVA-PF [as measured by the PPD test protocol or the new Colipa (European Cosmetic Association) in vitro test method] (12,13) to SPF rating of at least 1:3, such that there is a constant proportionality of UVA protection relative to the SPF of the product. In addition, only distinct SPF numbers can be claimed, particularly for the high-protection region: for example, "30" or "30+" and "50" or "50+." For example, this would require a protection factor in UVA (PFA) result of at least 5 for a product with SPF 15, or at least 10 for an SPF 45 (to be claimed as SPF 30+) product. Attaining such high levels of UVA protection requires high levels of UVA blockage across the UVA spectrum, typically obtained by using high levels of avobenzone (in Europe allowed at 5% level) and in combination with other UVA filters such as combinations of avobenzone and ecamsule or combinations of avobenzone and bemotrizanol, bisoctrizole, zinc oxide, or titanium dioxide.

In the United Kingdom, products sold through the Boots chain of stores are required to be labeled for UVA protection according to the Boots "star" rating system (17). This rating system measures the ratio of the spectrophotometric measured average AUC for UVA absorbance divided by the average UVB absorbance and awards stars for packaging claims accordingly. A higher ratio closest to 1 is awarded five stars (flatter absorbance curve), while a product with proportionately low UVA/UVB absorbance ratio has few, if any, stars. With this system, the formulator has two choices to achieve higher star ratings—boost UVA protection significantly to try to achieve "flatness" or to diminish UVB protection to achieve flatness while still trying to maintain adequate overall protection for the desired SPF rating of the product. This illustrates one of the flaws of this success criteria measurement, as it infers that UVB radiation is equally as damaging as UVA radiation, and UVA protection must be equivalent to UVB protection. Photo-biological research has clearly found that UVB radiation is much more damaging with longer-term consequences [particularly skin cancer (18)] compared with equivalent amounts of UVA radiation.

Similarly, the recent FDA Proposed Amendment to the Sunscreen Monograph (19) indicated the intent to label sunscreen products according to their UVA protectiveness (as measured by PFA), and the extent of UVA1 absorbance relative to the total UV absorbance of the product measured in vitro. To achieve high star ratings, the product must approach a "flat" absorbance spectrum. Unfortunately, the capabilities and permitted use concentrations of the currently approved UV filters do not allow achievement of the highest UVA rating (UVA1/UV absorbance ≥ 0.95), and products will be labeled with lower ratings than is indicated by their UVA-PF performance. This is particularly true for products with SPF ratings much above 15. To achieve high UVA ratings and to maintain the flatness of the curve, the formulator must start to diminish the UVB protection, which makes it impossible, at least currently, to offer high SPF (30 and higher) with highest star rating.

The primary UVA filters for achieving a "balanced" broad-spectrum protection are typically combinations of avobenzone with oxybenzone or alternatively combinations of oxybenzone with titanium dioxide and zinc oxide (since the combination of avobenzone with either titanium dioxide or zinc oxide combination is not approved by the FDA). For Europe and most of the rest of the world, the choices are much broader, including combinations of avobenzone, bemotrizanol, bisoctrizole, ecamsule, drometrizole trisiloxane, diethylamino hydroxybenzoyl hexyl benzoate, as well as zinc oxide or titanium dioxide. Making a balanced protection product requires sequential formulation and in vitro testing, coupled with in vivo SPF evaluation, to determine the optimal concentrations of UVB filters and choice and concentrations of the UVA filters. This adds to the complexity, cost, and time required for development of new sunscreen products. In addition, UVA labeling rules in various regions (proposed in the United States), Japan, and Europe (SPF/PFA ratio) require additional in vivo testing to confirm achievement of the required UVA protection to substantiate the labeling claims. With all these requirements to consider, the formulator must carefully build formulations step by step knowing that minor changes to the carrier ingredients, or even processing changes, can effect the overall balance or magnitude of protection provided by the formula.

FORMULATING FOR PHOTOSTABILITY

As indicated earlier, in the past few years the sun care market has experienced a race toward higher and higher SPF products. Currently the majority of the sunscreen business consists of products with SPF of at least 30, with a significant volume with SPF numbers above 50 and 50+. Given the detrimental effects of solar UVB and the trend for consumers to participate in more and more outdoor activities, the need for higher performance in protection is really necessary for meaningful protection of human skin and health. But with high levels of UVB protection, significant proportional amounts of UVA protection are also needed. There are several possibilities to provide adequate UVA protection and to reach the 1:3 ratio of UVA-PF/SPF value as demanded in Europe. Avobenzone provides the highest and broadest absorption, and it is possible to make combinations of it with other filters for maximal UVA protection. To use avobenzone's full potential, the formulator needs to take into account that this global UVA filter is not photostable on its own or in combination with some specific filters (26,27), and it deteriorates during sunlight exposure outdoors.

While this may be a desirable property environmentally, it is not desirable to have it behave this way on skin where it is meant to protect against UVA radiation. Avobenzone breaks down to other molecules that do not absorb UVA, so that a formulation built on the superior absorption power of avobenzone, but not adequately photostabilized, will quickly lose a great deal of its protective UVA effect. To counteract avobenzone's photo-instability and find suitable stabilizers, it is important to ask the questions "why does this happen?"

In general, when a UV filter molecule absorbs radiation, its electrons accept the energy and jump from a ground state to an "excited state," like using a fast elevator in a skyscraper. When it has arrived on the "100th floor," it has several options to get down and repeat the process over and over again. Typically, it loses its energy in the form of heat or sometimes as visible radiation (fluorescence). However, particularly in case of avobenzone, the molecule can perform an intersystem crossing from the singlet state into a triplet state. To stay with this skyscraper model is like jumping from the 100th floor to another somewhat lower building nearby—only to find out that this building has no good elevator down. A molecule in a triplet state waits a considerably longer time to be quenched or to be dropped down to the ground (state). This waiting time opens the door for chemical reactions using the high-preserved energy of the triplet excited state within the molecule to break its own chemical bonds, and as a result, the avobenzone breaks into pieces. In addition, for some molecules "the 100th floor" is a good meeting place to form new "alliances" with other molecules. This is the way that avobenzone reacts with octinoxate yielding new compounds, which unfortunately do not absorb UV light anymore. In this case, the excited state of one molecule (avobenzone) actually destroys two UV filters (avobenzone and octinoxate) in each reaction, which leads to a loss in both UVB *and* UVA performance (Fig. 1A). This combination of octinoxate with avobenzone has been the basis for many sunscreen products, as they are the most powerful UVB and UVA absorbers, respectively, and are registered globally, but unfortunately is the least photostable combination of UV filters. The formulator has to be aware of unfavorable filter combinations that react with each other in the presence of UV exposure to avoid them. The formulator has to be aware of this unfavorable filter combination and avoid it. UV filter suppliers offer guidance to formulators as to which combinations of filters will provide good photostability.

A less detrimental pathway for octinoxate to discharge its excited energy is through a process called E/Z-isomerization. Octinoxate, when freshly used in a formulation, exists

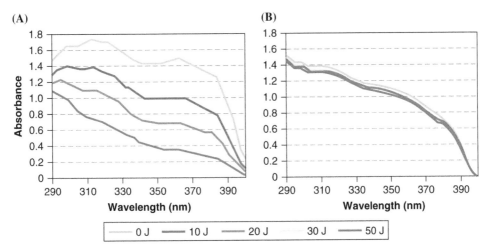

Figure 1 (**A**) Absorbance spectrum of a non-photostable formulation containing 7.5% octinoxate plus 3% avobenzone. The sample was prepared in a thin film (0.75 mg/cm^2) and exposed to a solar simulator UV radiation for 0, 10, 20, 30, and 50 J/cm^2. The loss of absorbance and protection is evident. (**B**) Absorbance spectrum of a photostable formulation containing 3% avobenzone and the photostabilizing components DEHN plus oxybenzone with other UVB filters to provide full spectrum protection. The sample was prepared and irradiated as described for Figure 1(**A**), with little loss of absorbance across the entire spectrum. *Abbreviations*: UV, ultraviolet; DEHN, diethylhexyl 2, 6 naphthalate; UVB, ultraviolet B.

in a specific molecular shape. Radiation with UVB light and the excitation energy allows the molecule to undergo shape changes. It goes from the E to the Z form and back. After only 10 to 15 minutes, there is a constant equilibrium of both compounds, but the new Z-form has somewhat lower absorption power. Therefore, while the UVB performance shrinks compared with the starting value, this process does not destroy the molecule and, because it leads after a short radiation time back to a constant absorbance, the in vivo SPF is not negatively influenced by this effect.

The intrinsic photoinstability of avobenzone calls for a solution, keeping in mind that it is the only worldwide-approved UVA filter with unmatched level of performance. Having a technical solution to its photoinstability would significantly improve the level and longevity of the protection provided in sunscreen products. Staying again in our skyscraper model, the molecule needs either to be picked up from the 100th floor (singlet state) or when it already has jumped down a bit from the triplet state before it breaks down. Typically, the "pick up" or "release" from the triplet state is more effective as this energy state has a longer life span.

Singlet state quenching is another possible elevator ride down to ground for an excited avobenzone molecule. The singlet state-quenching process always works better if the quenching molecule has an excited state that is close to that of the excited molecule, or in other words, the quenching neighbor molecule needs to have its own energy level in the area around the 100th floor. The same is actually true also for the triplet state, only the energy level is somewhat lower. Then the excited avobenzone molecule can be brought safely to the ground, and the quenching molecule is now elevated into the excited state. This then requires that the quencher be able to lose its newly acquired energy very fast and in a nondestructive process so that it can repeat the process again and again.

A variety of suitable quenchers have been discovered meanwhile to quench the triplet state of avobenzone as well as some singlet state quenchers (Table 1). Most of these are also UV filters [octocrylene (OC), methylbenzilidine camphor (MBC), bis-ethylhexyloxphenol methoxyphenyltriazine (BEMT), polysilicone-15] and can be used to

Table 1 Percent of Remaining Nondegraded Avobenzone After Exposure of a Thin Film (2 mg/cm^2) of Formulation to 25 MEDs of UV Radiation (50 J/cm) from a Solar Simulator, as Measured by HPLC Analysis. Photostabilizing Additives Added to This Formulation with Avobenzone show Varying Levels of Ability to Photostabilize the Avobenzone

4% avobenzone plus:	Percent of avobenzone remaining after 25 MEDs of UV exposure
No stabilizer	23%
Octocrylene 3.6%	90%
4-Methylbenzilidine camphor 5% (ex. United States)	87%
Bemotrizanol (5%) (ex. United States)	81%
Oxybenzone 5%	80%
Diethylhexyl syringylidenemalonat 0.8%	73%
Polysilicone 15 4% (ex. United States)	53%
Tris(tetramethylhydroxypiperidinol)citrate 2%	53%
Butyloctyl salicylate 5%	50%
Polyester 8 3%	50%
Diethylhexyl-2,6-naphthalate 5%	47%

Abbreviations: UV, ultraviolet; MEDs, minimal erythema doses.

Table 2 Samples Prepared as Described in Table 1 with Binary Combinations of Photostabilizing Ingredients can Yield High Levels of Photostabilization of Avobenzone

	Filter concentrations				
Avobenzone	4%	4%	4%	4%	4%
Octocrylene	3.6%	3.6%	3.6%	3.6%	3.6%
Bemotrizanol (ex. United States only)		4%			
4-Methylbenzylidene camphor (ex. United States only)			2%	4%	
Polysilicone 15 (ex. United States only)					4%
Content avobenzone after 25 MEDs	**90%**	**100%**	**95%**	**100%**	**95%**

Abbreviation: MEDs, minimal erythema doses.

create high-performing sunscreen formulations. One of the most popular additives is octocrylene. Because effective photostabilizing combinations are of great economic interest, allowing the formulation of light-stable and high-performance broad-spectrum protection, numerous patents have been filed and granted to claim combinations in this area. The formulator of a sunscreen needs to carefully check the materials they intended to use together in the formula to avoid violation of intellectual property rights.

More recently other materials also have been offered for stabilization purposes. Table 1 gives values from a screening assay using binary mixtures of 4% avobenzone (butyl methoxydibenzoylmethane, BMDBM) and recommended use of levels of stabilizers in an oil base after radiation of 25 minimal erythema doses (MEDs) of ultraviolet radiation and analysis by high-pressure liquid chromatography (HPLC) and spectrophotometric quantification (20). Besides the group of triplet quenchers, oxybenzone also turns out to be very effective at higher concentrations acting as a singlet-quenching agent.

In addition to binary combinations of agents, the formulator can choose to use ternary or even more complex mixtures as outlined in Table 2 to achieve an almost 100% stabilization of avobenzone.

In emulsion systems like O/W (oil in water) lotions, the stabilization effect is somewhat reduced as the gel network of the emulsion seems to limit the free interaction of the chromophores to a certain extent. However, with suitable combinations of photostabilizers added to the formulation, a level of stabilization of avobenzone can be reached where a reduction of the adsorption upon UV irradiation is virtually zero with no negative impact on the UVA-PF or star rating.

Particularly, a recently developed blend of avobenzone with oxybenzone and an emollient, diethylhexyl 2, 6 naphthalate (DEHN), are worth mentioning as they ensure excellent photostability under long radiation times. Figure 2 shows the photostabilizing effects of each of these ingredients alone, and then in combination at different concentrations of the oxybenzone. The DEHN provides triplet energy quenching, which with the singlet quenching of oxybenzone, provides photostabilization of the avobenzone at levels above 80%. Commercial products with this blend also benefit from the additional triplet energy quenching of octocrylene to yield photostability up to and above 90% as measured by UVA-PF values before and after irradiation with 50 J/cm^2 of UV irradiation (Fig. 1B).

From a product design perspective, the development of a new UV-stable high-performance formulation starts with three to five conceptual designs regarding UV filter combinations. For this "paper" design process information such as an XY table is very helpful, but it never replaces experimental proof of the concepts. There are numerous other

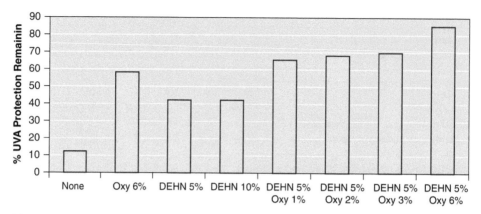

Figure 2 Percent of remaining UVA-PF value for a water-in-oil formulation containing 3% avobenzone plus the various additive photostabilizing components of DEHN or oxybenzone, or combinations of the two at various concentrations (21). *Abbreviations*: UVA-PF, ultraviolet A protection factor; DEHN, diethylhexyl 2, 6 naphthalate.

factors that can influence the overall photostability of the formulation in both directions. The result is that the formulator is required to create and test seemingly endless combinations of filters, stabilizers, emollients, and even preservative systems, changing one variable at a time to ultimately achieve the desired cosmetic aesthetic attributes, physical stability parameters, biological efficacy, microbial robustness, and photostability properties.

FORMULATING WITH PIGMENTS

Another category of UV filter materials is inorganic pigments. Not many years ago, there were only inorganic pigments available like titanium dioxide and zinc oxide, but recently an organic pigment (BEMT) has also been introduced in Europe and in other regions. Inorganic pigments, especially titanium dioxide, were particularly viewed as safe as they do not penetrate into the skin. This has been shown in skin penetration studies (22,23). From an optical physics point of view, they scatter and reflect light, but more importantly, they actually absorb UV light (24). With scattering the optical pathway of a light ray through a UV filter film on skin, the pathway does not remain straight, and the path length for scattered light becomes much longer, increasing the effective absorbance of the filters. Therefore combinations of pigments and organic-soluble filters are very useful, because the absorption is directly dependent on path length, and with the inclusion of the inorganic pigments, the path length is now longer with more interactions of the UV photons with the filters. This scattering phenomenon is strongly wavelength dependent. In general, the size of the particle should be half of the radiation to be scattered. In case of titanium dioxide, the ideal particle size would be in the 150 nm region. If the particle size is much larger (e.g., in wall paints), it will also scatter visible light and lead to a white coloration on the skin. Titanium dioxide comes in a variety of "primary" particle sizes; however, during the manufacturing process, these primary crystals quickly associate to larger agglomerates and will even not disintegrate under the high sheer mixing during emulsification process. If these agglomerates are not properly dispersed, they will accumulate, and the formulation will start to become visible on skin, particularly depending on the concentrations used in the formulations. For the formulator, the challenge is to maintain the size of these agglomerates throughout the manufacturing process such that the pigment stays finely dispersed and stabilized within the formulation. Wetting agents, specific coatings, or high-sheer-mixing machinery are helpful to accomplish the task, and manufacturing processes must be carefully followed to provide consistent results from batch to batch.

Pure titanium dioxide crystals have photoreactivity properties that are not desirable in sunscreen formulations. The photoreactive nature of titanium dioxide can produce oxidative stress, particularly if crystal imperfections, doped or spiking materials, are present. Therefore, titanium dioxide needs to be fully and tightly coated to fully prevent photoreactivity processes. There are some simple experiments for the formulator to check if a material is sufficiently coated. When a formulation is spread in a thin film on a glass plate and exposed to sunlight, a poorly coated titanium material will react to form a grayish-blue color. One can also check for oxidative stress using the vitamin C derivative, ascorbyl palmitate. When added to a formulation containing a poorly coated titanium oxide material, the formulation will turn brown when exposed to UV radiation. With simple test like these, the formulator could easily check the titanium dioxide products that are suitable for sun care formulations. Numerous coatings are used by titanium dioxide manufacturers to address this photoreactivity (25), such as silicon dioxide, stearic acid, and alumina stearate, for example.

Zinc oxide offers another option for extending UVA protection in sunscreen products and is often combined with titanium dioxide to provide a longer critical wavelength rating. The absorbance spectrum for zinc oxide is relatively flat across the UVB and the UVA, with a distinct drop in absorbance around 372 nm. Zinc oxide is often thought of as an opaque barrier material for coating lips and noses; however, even in high concentrations with high visibility, the protection provided can be very modest, in the range of SPF 5, with UVA-PF values of only 4 to 5. The visibility becomes a positive attribute as it allows one to see when it has been rubbed off and requires reapplication, unlike traditional organic filter-based sunscreens whose invisibility leaves one guessing whether or not they have been rubbed or washed off the skin.

It is erroneously thought that titanium dioxide and zinc oxide are protective because they act as physical barriers or scatterers of the UV radiation from sunlight. In fact, the primary mechanism of protection by these inorganic filters is actually the same as the organic-soluble sun filters, direct absorption of the photons, excitation to a higher-energy state, with release of the energy through heat energy, fluorescence, or internal conversion (24).

The formulator is severely challenged to balance the aesthetic properties desired by the consumer against the protection provided, as the inorganic sunscreen filters pose great difficulty in achieving ease of spreading, evenness of the application on skin, the dragginess of the filters, and the often white or "blue" hue given to the skin. Moderate SPF values of 15 and below can achieve quite nice aesthetic properties, with higher SPFs having less desirable aesthetic properties. In fact, the primary use of titanium dioxide and zinc oxide has been as additives at relatively low concentrations to the organic filters to boost the SPF and UVA protection characteristics of these products. The "whitening" disadvantage needs only to be considered in the U.S. and E.U. markets. It is of less importance in the Asian sun care market as the beauty target for women is to have an almost white skin tone. Even some clearly visible zinc oxide qualities can be used for Asian sun care formulations.

FORMULATION CHALLENGES

In summary, the formulator approaching the laboratory bench faces tremendous challenges in creating a competitive and consumer-preferred new product. They must know the desired consumer aesthetic attributes and relate them to a huge library of chemical ingredients to choose the right combination and proportions of oils and emollients to create just the right feel of the product on the skin. Inherent to knowing these ingredients, they must be versed in the patent landscape associated with each of these ingredients to prevent creating formulations that would infringe on others' intellectual property. This challenge becomes more daunting in this highly competitive field of cosmetic chemistry.

They must also understand the nature of the action of the sunscreen filters on the skin, how other formulation components—the emollients, the emulsifiers, and the thickeners—can influence the film integrity of the filters on the skin, and the polymer waterproofing agents. They must know the filter wavelength absorption properties to create the desired balance of UVB and UVA protection and what combinations of filters and proportions will deliver the desired SPF and UVA-PF values. They must know and test the physical stability of the products they have created to assure uniformity of product consistency in adverse conditions such as would be encountered in car trunks through summer and winter seasons. And last, but certainly not least, the formulator is now typically producing formulations that will be sold internationally, where the rules for UVB to UVA balance are likely different, where the filters permitted and the allowed concentrations and combinations, as well as testing methods and requirements for waterproof claims will be different.

When we look back over the past 30 years of "modern sunscreens," the progress in the protection provided has been incredible. More importantly, the formulator has been able to balance all these critical protection needs with the art of creating products that are beautiful and pleasant to wear, helping to insure that the consumer is willing to use this critical form of protection that will help preserve the skin's health and beauty for a lifetime.

REFERENCES

1. Wikipedia, Sunscreen History. Available at: http:/en.wikipedia.org/wiki/Sunscreen.
2. Moyal D, Fortanier A. Broad-spectrum sunscreens provide better protection from solar ultraviolet simulated radiation and natural sunlight-induced immunosuppression in human beings. J Am Acad Dermatol 2008; 58(suppl 2):S149–S154.
3. Ulrich S, Nghlem D, Khaskina P. Suppression of an established immune response to UVA—a critical role for mast cells. Photochem Photobiol 2007; 83(5):1095–1100.
4. Halliday G, Byrne S, Kuchel J. et al. The suppression of immunity by ultraviolet radiation: UVA, nitric oxide and DNA damage. Photochem Photobiol Sci 2004; 3(8):736–740.
5. Moyal D, Fortanier A. Efficacy of broad-spectrum sunscreens against the suppression of elicitation of delayed-type hypersensitivity responses in humans depends on the level of ultraviolet A protection. Exp Dermatol 2003; 12(2):153–159.
6. Yaar M, Gilchrest B. Photoageing: mechanism, prevention and therapy. Br J Dermatol 2007; 157(5):874–887.
7. Seite S, Zucchi H, Septier D, et al. Elastin changes during chronological and photoaging: the important role of lysozyme. J Eur Acad Dermatol Venereol 2006; 20(8):980–987.
8. Vielhaber G, Grether-Bech S, Koch O, et al. Sunscreens with an absorption maximum of > or =360 nm provide optimal protection against UVA1-induced expression of matrix metalloproteinase-1, interleukin-1, and interleukin-6 in human dermal fibroblasts. Photochem Photobiol Sci 2006; 5(3):275–282.
9. Photostability of sunscreen products influences the efficiency of protection with regards to UV-induced genotoxic or photoaging-related endpoints. Br J Dermatol 2004; 151(6):1234–1244.
10. De Gruijl FS. Carcinogenesis: UVA vs UVB radiation. Skin Pharmacol Appl Skin Physiol 2002; 15(5):316–320.

11. Krutmann J. The role of UVA rays in skin aging. Eurl J Dermatol 2001; 11(2):170–171.
12. Japan Cosmetic Industry Association Technical Bulletin. Measurement standards for UVA protection efficacy. Issued November 21, 1995.
13. Agence Franaise de sécurité sanitaire des produits de santé (AFSSAPs) Determination of the UVA protection factor based on the principles recommended by the JCIA. January 13, 2006.
14. Moyal D, Chardon A, Kollias N. Determination of UVA protection factors using the persistent pigment darkening (PPD) as the end point. (Part 1). Calibration of the method. Photodermatol Photoimmunol Photomed 2000; 16(6):245–249.
15. Moyal D, Chardon A, Kollias N. UVA protection efficacy of sunscreens can be determined by the persistent pigment darkening (PPD) method. (Part 2). Photodermatol Photoimmunol Photomed 2000; 16(6):250–255.
16. Diffey BL, Tanner PR, Matts PJ, et al. In vitro assessment of the broad-spectrum ultraviolet protection of sunscreen products. J Am Acad Dermatol 2000; 43:1024–1035.
17. Diffey BL. A method for broad-spectrum classification of sunscreens. Int J Cosm Sci 1994; 16:47–52
18. Cole C, Forbes PD, Davies RE. An action spectrum for UV photocarcinogenesis. Photochem Photobiol 1986; 43:275–284.
19. Federal Register. Sunscreen Drug Products for Over-the-Counter Human Use; Proposed Amendment to the Final Monograph; Proposed Rule. CFR 21, 72(165): Parts 347–352,49071–49122, 2007.
20. Gonzenbach H, Hill TJ, Truscott TG. The triplet energy levels of UVA and UVB sunscreens. J Photochem Photobiol 1992; 16(3–4):377–379.
21. Cole C, Natter F. Sunscreen compositions containing a dibenzoylmethane derivative. US Patent 6444195B1. September 3, 2002
22. Lademann J, Weigmann H, Rickmeyer C, et al. Penetration of titanium dioxide microparticles in a sunscreen formulation into the horny layer and the follicular orifice. Skin Pharmacol Appl Skin Physiol 1999; 12(5):247–256.
23. Nohynek GJ, Lademann J, Ribaud C, et al. Grey goo on the skin? Nanotechnology, cosmetic and sunscreen safety. Crit Rev Toxicol 2007; 37(3):251–277.
24. Kollias N. The absorption properties of "physical" sunscreens. Arch Derm 1999; 135(2):209–210.
25. Lademann J, Weigmann H, Schaefer H, et al. Investigation of the stability of coated titanium microparticles used in sunscreens. Skin Pharmacol Appl Skin Physiol 2000; 13(5):258–264.
26. Gaspar LR. Maia Campos PM Evaluation of the photostability of different UV filter combinations in a sunscreen. Int J Pharm 2006; 307(2):23–28.
27. Sayre RM, Dowdy JC, Gerwig AJ, et al. Unexpected photolysis of the sunscreen octinoxate in the presence of the sunscreen avobenzone. Photochem Photobiol 2005; 81(2):452–456.

4

Assessment of Photoprotective Properties of Sunscreens

Brian L. Diffey
Dermatological Sciences, Institute of Cellular Medicine, University of Newcastle, Newcastle upon Tyne, U.K.

James Ferguson
Photobiology Unit, Department of Dermatology, University of Dundee, Dundee, Scotland

SYNOPSIS

- SPF is the ratio of the least amount of UV energy required to produce a minimal erythema on sunscreen-protected skin to the amount of energy required to produce the same erythema on unprotected skin.
- There are many in vitro and in vivo methods for assessing the UVA protection of sunscreens. Worldwide harmonization has not been achieved; however, in vivo PPD method has been widely used in many parts of the world.
- The ability of sunscreen products to protect against immunosuppression is the basis for IPF determination. However, a simple method of IPF determination has yet to be developed.
- Consumers apply sunscreens at much lesser amount than that used in testing ($2 \ mg/cm^2$). This stresses the importance of the development of sunscreens with excellent cosmetic "feel" and public education on photoprotection.

INTRODUCTION

Topical sunscreens act by absorbing or scattering ultraviolet (UV) radiation and are widely available for general public use as a consumer product. Because of the deleterious effect of visible light in some photodermatoses (1), sunscreens that offer a degree of protection at wavelengths beyond 400 nm have been described (2,3) in this book but will not be considered in this chapter.

As described in chapter 1, the first use of sunscreens was reported in 1928 (4) and, since then, they have become increasingly popular, particularly during outdoor recreation in which as little clothing as possible is worn, such as at the seaside (5,6). When their application is commensurate with exposure, sunscreens undoubtedly protect against sunburn. A 4.5-year study, with an 8-year follow-up, of over 1600 individuals in Queensland, Australia, demonstrated that the use of sun protection factor or sunburn protection factor (SPF) 16 broad-spectrum sunscreen decreased the incidence of squamous cell carcinoma by 38% and basal cell carcinoma by 25%, although the latter was not statistically significant (7).

The core ingredient of a sunscreen is, of course, the UV absorber(s), but other factors such as the vehicle for the UV filters and optimization of the sunscreen in terms of attributes such as water resistance and photostability will also affect the efficacy and performance of the product (4).

The protection provided by a sunscreen is universally expressed by its SPF. This metric is valid only as a measure of the ability of a sunscreen to protect against sunburn; for other biological endpoints, different protection factors, such as the immune protection factor (IPF) (8), will be more appropriate.

The SPF is popularly interpreted as how much longer skin covered with sunscreen takes to burn compared with unprotected skin, but a more rigorous definition is that it is the ratio of the least amount of UV energy required to produce a minimal erythema on sunscreen-protected skin to the amount of energy required to produce the same erythema on unprotected skin.

HISTORY OF SPF METHOD

Historically, the first known studies establishing the basis for the SPF or index of protection began more than half a century ago (9,10). These and other studies led to the first standard method for SPF determination and labeling, which was issued by the Food and Drug Administration (FDA) in the United States in 1978 (11), followed in 1984 by the DIN67501 norm in Germany (12), which was applied mainly in Europe.

These two standards differed principally in respect of the type of UV source used (xenon arc lamp or mercury arc lamp) and the rate of product application on skin (2.0 or 1.5 mg/cm^2), which led to some discrepancies in measured protection factors. Following agreed rationalization, all standards issued subsequently stipulated the use of an optically filtered xenon lamp as the UV source and an application density of 2.0 mg/cm^2.

Standards similar to the FDA were issued by the Standards Association of Australia in 1986 (13), which included both SPF and water resistance testing, and by the Japan Cosmetic Industry Association (JCIA) in 1991 (14). Since their introduction, both the Australian and Japanese standards have undergone revision. The New Zealand Standards joined the Australian Standards for their joint new version (AS/NZS 2604:1993) in 1993 (15) and their revised version in 1998 (16).

The European Cosmetic, Toiletry and Perfumery Association (Colipa), in its 1994 SPF test method (17), introduced new techniques to characterize and specify the emission spectrum of the UV source and to assign skin types based on skin color. At the same time, two high SPF standard products were proposed to take into account the increase in SPF values that were appearing commercially.

Colipa, together with the standards' authorities in Japan and South Africa, began discussion on the harmonization of the SPF measurement method in 2000 and reached a joint agreement of the International SPF Test Method in October 2002 and updated in 2006 by the European, Japanese, American, and South African industries (18).

Most recently, on August 27, 2007, the FDA published its long-awaited Final Proposed Rules for sunscreens (19). One of the proposed changes of note is that the SPF will now be an acronym for "sunburn protection factor" (formerly sun protection factor), and it is proposed to be capped at 50+ as opposed to the current not-implemented proposal of 30+. In addition, for the first time, FDA also proposed assessment and labeling of UVA protection of sunscreens, using a combination of in vitro (UVA1/UV absorbance ratio) and in vivo [(persistent pigment darkening (PPD)] methods.

MEASUREMENT OF THE SPF

The SPF determined in vivo is now a universal indicator of the efficacy of sunscreen products against sunburn, and as reviewed above, detailed protocols are available.

The measurement of the SPF requires the exposure of both sunscreen-protected and sunscreen-unprotected skin in a cohort of volunteers to a series of different UV doses, with the respective exposure doses of UV resulting in just a perceptible reddening of skin observed 16 to 24 hours after exposure and is taken as the endpoint in each instance. The ratio of these two UV doses is numerically equal to the SPF.

FACTORS AFFECTING MEASUREMENT OF THE SPF

A number of factors affect the determination of SPF, and some of these are discussed below. The numerical values that appear in the following subsections (e.g., number of test subjects) are taken from the International SPF Test Method (18); in some cases, the FDA method (19) will stipulate different numerical values.

Test Subjects

The test panel should consist of fair-skinned individuals with sun-reactive skin types according to the Fitzpatrick classification (20) of I, II, or III, with the back chosen as the anatomical region for the test area. Between 10 and 20 test subjects should be recruited for each test. As an example of the lack of international consistency, the FDA method (19) stipulates that for products with an expected SPF under 30, the test panel should consist of 20 to 25 subjects with at least 20 subjects producing valid data for analysis. And for products with an expected SPF of 30 or over, 25 to 30 subjects are required for the test panel with at least 25 subjects yielding valid data for analysis.

For results to be acceptable, the International SPF Test Method (18) stipulates that it is necessary for the 95% confidence interval (95% CI) of the mean SPF to be within ±17% of the mean SPF. So, for example, if the mean SPF is 10.0, the 95% CI should fall within the range 8.3 to 11.7.

Source of UV Radiation

The UV radiation source used in the phototesting must be a xenon arc solar simulator. The output from the solar simulator should be stable, spatially uniform across the output beam, and suitably optically filtered to create a spectral quality that is a close match to a defined solar spectrum in the UV wave band and complies with required acceptance limits (18).

SPF of Standard Sunscreen Products

Ideally, a sunscreen formulated in a standard way should be used as a methodological control to verify the test. This requires that one standard sunscreen be assayed on the same day as the products that are being tested. For example, the FDA mandates that 8% homosalate be used as the standard. Results from the test product should only be accepted if the measured SPF for the standard sunscreen falls within prerequisite limits.

Amount of Product Applied

The amount of test and standard product applied to the skin before spreading is universally taken as 2 mg/cm^2. This amount was selected to ensure even application of the product over the test area; it was considered more difficult to achieve even application with lower amount. Care must be taken to prevent evaporative loss of volatile components when the product is being weighed and before application to the skin.

Mode of Delivery

To aid uniform coverage, droplets of the product should be deposited with a syringe or pipette and then spread over the test site with light pressure using a finger cot.

Time Between Sunscreen Application and UV Exposure

Sunscreen is normally allowed to dry for 15 to 30 minutes before commencing exposure of the test site to the sequence of UV doses.

UV Exposures

The test subsites intended for UV exposure should be free from blemishes and have an even skin tone. The minimum acceptable area of each exposure subsite is 0.5 cm^2, although the recommended area is at least 1 cm^2 (18).

Incremental Progression of UV Dose

For the unprotected site, the center of the total UV dose range should be established using the subject's estimated minimal erythema dose (MED). A minimum of five subsites centered on the estimated MED is exposed with incremental UV doses using a recommended geometric progression of either 1.12 or 1.25.

For the product-protected site, the center of the UV dose range is that of the unprotected MED multiplied by the expected SPF of the product. Again, a minimum of five subsites centered on the expected (protected) MED is exposed with incremental UV doses using a geometric progression with the same dose increment, but for products with an expected SPF greater than 25, the dose increment is reduced to 1.12 (18).

Assessment of MED

The MED, expressed in radiometric units of J/cm^2 or mJ/cm^2, is normally assessed visually when the erythemal response is optimal, that is, between 16 and 24 hours after exposure. Both the International SPF Test Method (18) and the most recent FDA method (19) define the MED as the lowest UV dose that produces the first perceptible unambiguous erythema with defined borders.

ALTERNATIVE METHOD FOR SPF DETERMINATION

Determining sunscreen SPFs on products designed to provide high levels of protection is problematic and can be time consuming, especially if multi-port solar simulators are not used. As an alternative to exposing a number of subsites to a series of increasing UV doses, SPF assessment, using a single exposure on sunscreen-protected skin of volunteers to arrive at a reliable estimate of the mean SPF of a test product, has been proposed (21), as it might find applications for endpoints other than sunburn (8).

UVA PROTECTION

There are a number of in vivo, ex vivo, and in vitro methods that have been described to measure UVA, or broad-spectrum, protection of sunscreens; these are summarized in Table 1.

The current position internationally is that in vivo SPF determination remains the criterion standard for the magnitude of protection (18,19). On the other hand, methods for the assessment of the level of UVA protection have been a matter of debate for almost 20 years (31), and even now there are differing recommendations from a European and North American perspective.

European Perspective

In Europe, a consensus appears to be near in that the European Commission favors in vitro to in vivo assays for UVA protection (cheaper, faster, safer), and there is agreement within the European sunscreen industry on an in vitro method, based on the UVA Index (30), to determine UVA protection. Guidelines were published in March 2007 (32), and these are currently with stakeholders for consideration.

The basis of the UVA Index to evaluate the UVA protection of sunscreens is to measure the transmission of UV radiation through a layer of product applied to a

Table 1   **Methods to Assess UVA Protection**

Test method	Reference
In vivo	
Sensitise skin to UVA, e.g., 8-MOP	22
UVA erythema in unsensitized skin	23
PPD	24
Diffuse reflectance spectroscopy	25
Ex vivo	
Excised human epidermis	26
Excised mouse epidermis	27
In vitro	
UVA:UVB absorbance ratio	28
UVA I:UV absorbance ratio	19
Critical wavelength	29
UVA Index	30
Dilute solution/thin film	16

Abbreviations: UV, ultraviolet; PPD, persistent pigment darkening.

roughened glass substrate and then calculate an in vitro UVA PPD protection factor while taking into account the in vivo SPF value of the product. The UVA Index is calculated as the in vivo SPF divided by the in vitro UVA PPD protection factor (32). To ensure adequate broad-spectrum protection, the European Commission (33) recommends a UVA Index of at least 3 and a critical wavelength (29) of 370 nm.

U.S. Perspective

The FDA (19) has expressed concern that use of the in vivo PPD method alone could result in some sunscreen products yielding high UVA protection factors without exhibiting broad absorbance throughout the entire UVA radiation spectrum due to strong influence of the short-wavelength UVA (UVA II: 320–340 nm) in PPD response. In other words, a sunscreen could absorb high levels of UVA II but very little long-wavelength UVA (UVA I: 340–400 nm) and achieve a high UVA rating under the PPD method. To militate against this, the FDA has proposed that an in vitro method be used (to assess the breadth of absorbance across the UV radiation spectrum) in conjunction with the PPD method to assess more fully the broad-spectrum properties of a sunscreen.

The proposed method (19) is a modified version of a method first introduced by Diffey (28) and which forms the basis of the Boots star rating system used since 1992 in the United Kingdom. The modified FDA method calculates the ratio of the mean UVA I absorbance to the mean absorbance over the full solar-UV spectrum (290–400 nm) to provide a measure of the relative UVA I radiation protection provided by a sunscreen. The FDA believes that this test, in combination with the PPD method, provides a better assessment of overall UVA radiation protection.

Finally, in terms of labeling a product, the FDA proposes that the UVA category assigned to a product shall be the lower of either the UVA I/UV ratio category determined in vitro or the UVA-PPD protection factor determined in vivo. Technical details of how these respective categories (either "low," "medium," "high" or "highest") are assigned can be found in reference 19. If the product does not attain at least a 'low' category rating for both the UVA-PPD protection factor and the UVA I/UV ratio, the product is not permitted to display a UVA claim. Otherwise, the final combined category rating (i.e., the lower of either the UVA I/UV ratio or UVA-PPD protection factor categories) is displayed on the product packaging along with the corresponding number of stars (1 star for low through to 4 stars for highest) for the appropriate combined category.

ASSESSMENT OF WATER RESISTANCE OF SUNSCREENS

This is done by immersing test subjects in water for a prescribed period of time, and measuring the SPF before and after water immersion. For "water-resistant" products, the FDA requires two 20-minutes moderate activity in water, separated by a 20-minutes rest period without wiping the test sites; for "very water-resistant" products, the requirement is four 20-minutes water immersion (19). The use of the term "waterproof" is strongly discouraged by the FDA.

SUNSCREEN IPFs

It is increasingly accepted that sunscreens should protect against UV-induced immunosuppression, with an index of protection that can be compared with the SPF. Current methods for evaluating the IPF in humans rely on the ability of a sunscreen to inhibit UV-induced local suppression of the contact hypersensitivity response or the delayed-type hypersensitivity response, using either the induction or the elicitation arms of these responses.

A consensus was arrived at by five groups of immunoprotection researchers who reviewed current techniques and protocols and concluded that there is a need for a new simpler method of IPF determination that will require validation against existing models (8). In the absence of adequate knowledge into the relationship between the modulation of the skin's immunity by solar UV and human skin cancer, the consensus was that it is prudent to propose that sunscreen use should not substantially alter the relationship between UV-induced erythema and immune modulation. This can only be achieved if the SPF and IPF of a sunscreen are comparable, and this relationship should be maintained even when the sunscreen is applied such that it will not achieve the labeled SPF, as is often the case in practice.

THE MISMATCH BETWEEN EXPECTED AND DELIVERED PROTECTION

The SPF of a sunscreen is assessed after phototesting in vivo at an internationally agreed application thickness of 2 mg/cm^2. Yet a number of studies have shown that consumers apply much less than this, typically between 0.5 and 1.0 mg/cm^2 (Fig. 1). Figure 2 illustrates that application thickness has a significant effect on protection with most users probably achieving a mean value of between 20% and 50% of that expected from the product label as a result of common application thickness (41). That the protection achieved is often less than that expected depends on a number of other factors apart from amount applied, such as uniformity of application; cosmetic "feel" of sunscreen; resistance to water immersion and sand abrasion; and when, where, and how often sunscreen is reapplied (42). Furthermore studies of sunscreen use by beachgoers highlight other important behavioral considerations, including failure to apply sunscreen prior to exposure and failure to apply to all exposed skin (43).

This mismatch between expected and delivered photoprotection has led many commentators into the trap of believing that consumers use inadequate amounts of sunscreen for protection. The reality is the reverse. People use the quantity they feel

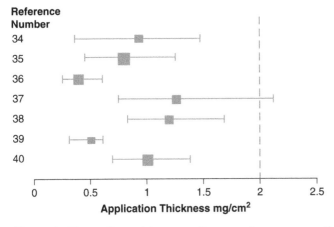

Figure 1 The median and inter-quartile range of sunscreen application from seven user studies. The vertical dashed line indicates the standard application thickness of 2 mg/cm^2 used in laboratory determination of the SPF. *Abbreviation*: SPF, sun protection factor.

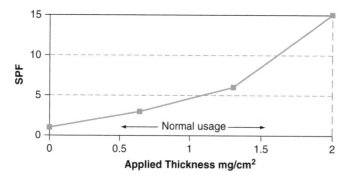

Figure 2 The variation of delivered SPF with application thickness for a sunscreen of nominal SPF 15 (41). *Abbreviation*: SPF, sun protection factor.

comfortable with and in this sense are using the "correct" amount; it is the labeled SPFs that are misleading. As one study found (44), 78% of the volunteers taking part in a beach study did not like the feeling of sunscreens on their skin and only used them so that they did not sunburn.

So from a public health perspective it is clear that the UV exposure of sunscreen-protected skin depends not just on the absorption characteristics of the product but also on a number of other factors to do with application. A mathematical study (45) that examined the relative importance of three of these factors—amount applied, how it is spread, and UV-absorbing properties of sunscreens—found that in a population of sunscreen users most of the variance in UV protection achieved depends on issues of compliance—how much sunscreen is applied and how well it is applied—with the technical performance of the product (how well it absorbs UV) contributing only about 10% of variance. Consequently, the efficacy of a product depends not just on the technical performance of its active UV filters but also on whether the product is pleasing to use (*compliance*).

One consequence of the trend for higher SPFs is that, in general, the water content of the formulation decreases as the concentration of UV filters increases to deliver the higher protection, with the result that in many cases the product is more difficult to spread and users compensate by applying a smaller amount than they might do with lower SPF products. That the formulation of the product has a significant impact on quantity applied, and hence protection delivered, was demonstrated in a user study of two sunscreens with equal labeled SPFs but different formulations (38). As manufacturers strive for greater photoprotection in their products, this needs to be accompanied by close attention to cosmetic (or galenic) attributes so that the improved UV-absorbing properties of the products are translated to the user. So should tests that measure qualitatively and quantitatively various sensory attributes of sunscreen products be introduced (46) so that we move from a purely in vivo SPF assay to a process that is in vivo veritas?

THE LABELING OF SUNSCREENS

In September 2006, the European Commission issued a recommendation (33) to ensure that as of 2007 the sunscreen industry applies standardized, simple, and understandable labeling of sunscreen products. These recommendations included the following ways to improve the labeling:

- To enable consumers to compare products, UVA protection should be indicated in a uniform way based on standardized testing methods.

- Claims giving the impression of total protection, such as "sunblock," should disappear.
- Labels should bear clear and understandable warnings and usage instructions for the consumer on how to use a sunscreen product correctly.

In particular, the Commission supported a proposal made six years previously (47) that labeling using one of four categories (low, medium, high, and very high) provides for a simpler and more meaningful indication of the efficacy of sunscreen products than a variety of different numbers and recommended that this ordinal scale should be labeled at least as prominently as the SPF, which is based on an interval scale.

REFERENCES

1. Mahmoud BH, Hexsel CL, Hamzavi IH, et al. Effects of visible light on the skin. Photochem Photobiol 2008; 84:450–462.
2. Kaye ET, Levin JA, Blank IH, et al. Efficiency of opaque photoprotective agents in the visible light range. Arch Dermatol 1991; 127:351–355.
3. Moseley H, Cameron H, MacLeod T, et al. New sunscreens confer improved protection for photosensitive patients in the blue light region. Br J Dermatol 2001; 145:789–794.
4. Shaath NA. Sunscreen evolution. In: Shaath NA, ed. Sunscreens: Regulations and Commercial Development, 3rd ed. Boca Raton FL: Taylor & Francis Group, 2005:3–17.
5. Koh HK, Bak SM, Geller AC, et al. Sunbathing habits and sunscreen use among white adults: Results of a national survey. Am J Public Health 1997; 87:1214–1217.
6. Robinson JK, Rademaker AW. Sun protection by families at the beach. Arch Pediatr Adolesc Med 1998; 152:466–470.
7. van der Pols JC, Williams GM, Pandeya N, et al. Prolonged prevention of squamous cell carcinoma of the skin by regular sunscreen use. Cancer Epidemiol Biomarkers Prev 2006; 15:2546–2548.
8. Fourtanier A, Moyal D, Maccario J, et al. Measurement of sunscreen immune protection factors in humans: a consensus paper. J Invest Dermatol 2005; 125:403–409.
9. Blum H, Eicher M, Terus W. Evaluation of protective measures against sunburn. Am J Physiol 1945; 146:118–125.
10. Schulze R. Einige Versuche und Bemerkungen zum Problem der handelsüblichen Lichtschutzmittel. Parf u Kosm 1956; 37:310–315.
11. FDA Department of Health and Human Services Food & Drug Administration, USA. Sunscreen drug products for over the counter use: proposed safety, effectiveness and labelling conditions. Fed Regist 1978; 43(166):38206–38269.
12. Deutsches Institut für Normung: Experimentelle dermatologische Bewertung des Erythemschutzes von externen Sonnenschutzmitteln für die menschliche Haut. DIN 67501. 1984.
13. Standard Association of Australia. Sunscreen products, evaluation and classification. AS 2604-1986.
14. Japan Cosmetic Industry Association (JCIA). Standard SPF Test Method (revised version), 1999.
15. Standards Australia, Standards New Zealand. Sunscreen products, evaluation and classification. AS/NZS 2604:1993.
16. Australian/New Zealand Standard. Sunscreen products—evaluation and classification. AS/NZS 2604:1998.
17. COLIPA. Sun Protection Factor Method. Brussels, Belgium: European Cosmetic Toiletry, and Perfumery Association (COLIPA), 1994.
18. COLIPA. International Sun Protection Factor (SPF) Test Method. Brussels, Belgium: European Cosmetic Toiletry, and Perfumery Association (COLIPA), 2006.

19. FDA Department of Health and Human Services Food & Drug Administration, USA. Sunscreen drug products for over the counter use: proposed Amendment of Final Monograph; Proposed Rule. Fed Regist 2007; 72(165):49070–49122.

20. Fitzpatrick TB. Soleil et peau. J Med Esthet 1975; 2:33–34.

21. Diffey BL. Sun protection factor determination *in vivo* using a single exposure on sunscreen-protected skin. Photodermatol Photoimmunol Photomed 2003; 19:309–312.

22. Gange R, Soparkar A, Matzinger B, et al. Efficacy of a sunscreen containing butyl methoxydibenzoylmethane against ultraviolet A radiation in photosensitised subjects. J Am Acad Dermatol 1986; 15:494–499.

23. Cole C, Van Fossen R. Measurement of sunscreen UVA protection: an unsensitized human model. J Am Acad Dermatol 1992; 26:178–184.

24. Moyal D, Chardon A, Kollias N. UVA protection efficacy of sunscreens can be determined by the persistent pigment darkening (PPD) method. Photodermatol Photoimmunol Photomed 2000; 16:250–255.

25. Moyal D, Refrégier JL, Chardon A. *In vivo* measurement of the photostability of sunscreen products using diffuse reflectance spectroscopy. Photodermatol Photoimmunol Photomed 2002; 18:14–22.

26. Marginean G, Fructus AE, Marty JP, et al. A new *ex-vivo* method of evaluating the photoprotective efficacy of sunscreens. Int J Cosmet Sci 1995; 17:233–243.

27. Sayre R, Agin P. A method for determination of UVA protection for normal skin. J Am Acad Dermatol 1990; 23:429–440.

28. Diffey BL. Indices of protection from *in vitro* assay of sunscreens. In: Lowe NJ, Shaath NA, Pathak MA, eds. Sunscreens: Development, Evaluation and Regulatory Aspects. New York: Marcel Dekker, 1996:589–600.

29. Diffey BL. A method for broad spectrum classification of sunscreens. Int J Cosmet Sci 1994; 16:47–52.

30. Wendel V, Klette E, Gers-Barlag H. A new in vitro test method to assess the UVA protection performance of sun care products. SÖFW Journal 2001; 127:12–30.

31. Lim HW, Naylor M, Hoenigsmann H, et al. American Academy of Dermatology Consensus Conference on UVA protection of sunscreens: summary and recommendations. J Am Acad Dermatol 2001; 44:505–508.

32. COLIPA Recommendation N°20. Method for the in vitro determination of UVA protection provided by sunscreen products. March 2007. Available at: http://www.colipa.com/site/index.cfm?SID=15588&OBJ=14409&back=1.

33. European Commission Recommendation on the efficacy of sunscreen products and the claims made relating thereto, OJ L265, 20067647/EC, 39–43.

34. Szepietowski JC, Nowicka D, Reich A, et al. Application of sunscreen preparations among young Polish people. J Cosmet Dermatol 2004; 3:69–72.

35. Neale R, Williams G, Green A. Application patterns among participants randomized to daily sunscreen use in a skin cancer prevention trial. Arch Dermatol 2002; 138:1319–1325.

36. Autier P, Boniol M, Severi G, et al. Quantity of sunscreen used by European students. Br J Dermatol 2001; 144:288–291.

37. Hart GC, Wright AL, Cameron RG. An assessment of the adequacy of sunscreen usage. Radiat Prot Dosim 2000; 91:275–278.

38. Diffey BL, Grice J. The influence of sunscreen type on photoprotection. Br J Dermatol 1997; 137:103–105.

39. Bech-Thomsen N, Wulf HC. Sunbathers' application of sunscreen is probably inadequate to obtain the Sun Protection Factor assigned to the preparation. Photodermatol Photoimmunol Photomed 1993; 9:242–244.

40. Stenberg C, Larkö O. Sunscreen application and its importance for the Sun Protection Factor. Arch Dermatol 1985; 121:1400–1402.

41. Stokes RP, Diffey BL. How well are sunscreen users protected? Photodermatol Photoimmunol Photomed 1997; 13:186–188.

42. Diffey BL. Sunscreens: use and misuse. In: Giacomoni PU, ed. Sun Protection in Man. Amsterdam: Elsevier Science BV, 2001:521–534.

43. Dobbinson S, Hill DJ. Patterns and causes of sun exposing and sun protection behaviour. In: Hill DJ, Elwood JM, English DR, eds. Prevention of Skin Cancer. Cancer Prevention-Cancer Causes, Vol. 3. Dordrecht, NL: Kluwer Academic, 2004:211–240.

44. Lademann J, Schanzer S, Richter H, et al. Sunscreen application at the beach. J Cosmet Dermatol 2004; 3:62–68.

45. Diffey BL. Sunscreens and UVA Protection: a major issue of minor importance. Photochem Photobiol 2001; 74:61–63.

46. Standard Practice for Descriptive Skinfeel Analysis of Creams and Lotions. American National Standards Institute ASTM E1490-03, 2003.

47. Diffey BL. Has the sun protection factor had its day? Br Med J 2000; 320:176–177.

5
Worldwide Regulation of UV Filters: Current Status and Future Trends

Farah K. Ahmed
Personal Care Products Council, Washington, D.C., U.S.A.

SYNOPSIS

> • This chapter provides an overview of regulations surrounding the marketing of sunscreen products, including permitted sunscreen UV filters, in a number of countries around the world.

WORLDWIDE REGULATION OF UV FILTERS: CURRENT STATUS AND FUTURE TRENDS

Ultraviolet (UV) filters are regulated globally as either over-the-counter (OTC) drugs, cosmetics, or quasi drugs. All countries have a listing of permitted UV filters, including maximum concentrations allowed in sunscreens, or they follow a major world regulator or organization such as the Food and Drug Administration (FDA), Colipa (the European cosmetic trade association), or the Japan Cosmetic Industry Association (JCIA).

With respect to SPF (sun protection factor, or sunburn protection factor) and UVA testing and labeling requirements, SPF is fairly well established and somewhat consistent around the world, while UVA is currently prescribed in some, but not all countries, and is under development in others. Regarding UV filtering ingredients, the variety and maximum concentration of permitted UV filters vary from country to country.

UV filter regulations in nine major geographic markets—the United States, Europe, Canada, Australia and New Zealand, China, Japan, South Africa, ASEAN (Association of Southeast Asian Nations) and the MERCOSUR (Member State of the Common Market of South America)—are outlined below.

United States

The Federal Food, Drug, and Cosmetics Act ("FFDCA" or "Act") requires that FDA preapprove all new drugs prior to their entering the market—a very lengthy, involved, and expensive process. However, the Act exempts any drugs that FDA has generally recognized as safe and effective (GRAS/E) from this requirement. In 1972, FDA began the process of recognizing GRAS/E drugs through developing an OTC monograph system. Similar to other types of rulemaking, monograph development involves a number of procedural steps, mainly—Advanced Notice of Proposed Rulemaking → Proposed Rule → Final Monograph—with each step allowing the public an opportunity to submit data and information pertaining to the rulemaking at hand. This process is still underway today for sunscreens and other OTC monograph drugs. The Personal Care Products Council (the Council) (formerly, the Cosmetics, Toiletry, and Fragrance Association) is the trade association representing the U.S. cosmetics industry. Over the years, the Council has submitted a number of substantive and data-driven comments to the agency on a variety of issues and has been heavily engaged in FDA's sunscreen monograph development. An OTC monograph is essentially a recipe for producing certain categories of OTC drugs. Specifically, each OTC monograph identifies a different OTC drug category (e.g., sunscreens, external and internal analgesics, antidandruff shampoos, and antifungal products), and within each category, it specifies permitted active ingredients, labeling requirements, and in some instances, efficacy-testing requirements. In other words, if manufacture is done pursuant to an FDA monograph, filing a New Drug Application (NDA) (for products that do not fit within a specific monograph) is not required. In the United States, FDA primarily regulates the manufacture and sale of sunscreens under the agency's OTC monograph system.[a]

FDA's first rulemaking pertaining to sunscreens occurred in 1978, with the publication of an Advance Notice of Proposed Rulemaking (ANPR) (3). The ANPR assigned a number of active UV filters to one of three categories: Category I (ingredients that are GRAS/E); Category II (ingredients that are not GRAS/E); and Category II (ingredients that require more data before a determination can be made as to whether they are GRAS/E). In 1993, FDA published a Tentative Final Monograph (TFM), which removed a number of active ingredients listed in the 1978 ANPR (4). In 1996, FDA added avobenzone, and in 1998, added zinc oxide as new active ingredients to the TFM. In 1997, FDA allowed for the marketing of sunscreens containing avobenzone (5), and in 1998, added zinc oxide as new active ingredients to the TFM (6). In 1999, FDA finalized the TFM, however, the agency subsequently, in 2001, stayed the effective date of the Final Rule until further notice (7). The 1999 Final (stayed) Sunscreen Rule discusses the ability of a sunscreen to protect against UVB light, but the effective date of the monograph was later stayed until reliable testing methods for protection against UVA light were developed. Table 1 lists UV filters that are permitted in the United States.

On August 27, 2007, FDA published its Proposed Rule to amend the Final (stayed) monograph for OTC sunscreen drug products (8). The Proposed Rule, when finalized, would set standards for formulating, testing, and labeling OTC sunscreen drug products with UVA light and UVB light protection.

A key new aspect of FDA's Proposal Rule is a standard testing method to determine a sunscreen's efficacy for protection against UVA light along with the a one-to four-star labeling system to indicate a sunscreen's level of UVA protection. The UVA level would be derived from two tests the FDA proposes, to assess the effectiveness of sunscreens in providing protection against UVA light. The first test measures a product's ability to

---

[a]with the exception of Mexoryl SX. In July 2006, FDA approved L'Oréal's NDA for Mexoryl SX (ecamsule) in a single cosmetic formulation sold under the name, Anthelios SX.

Table 1   **United States: Permitted UV Filters (Sunscreen Active Ingredients)**[a]

Active ingredient (drug name)	Maximum concentration (%)
Aminobenzoic acid	15
Avobenzone	3
Cinoxate	3
Dioxybenzone	3
Homosalate	15
Meradimate	5
Octocrylene	10
Octinoxate	7.5
Octisalate	5
Oxybenzone	6
Padimate O	8
Ensulizole	4
Sulisobenzone	10
Titanium dioxide	25
Trolamine salicylate	12
Zinc oxide	25

[a]According to the 1999 Final (stayed) Rule.

reduce the amount of UVA radiation that passes through it. The second measures a product's ability to prevent pigment darkening.

Other proposed amendments to the monograph include the following:

1. Revisions to the UVB labeling regulations, including (*i*) the increase of the highest SPF value from SPF30+ to SPF50+; (*ii*) use of the terms "low" and "medium" rather than "minimal" and "moderate" as category descriptors for protection against UVB; and (*iii*) insertion of the term "UVB" before "SPF" and before "sunburn"
2. Renaming of the rating for UVB protection (i.e., SPF) from "sun protection factor" to "sunburn protection factor"
3. Addition of avobenzone with zinc oxide and avobenzone with ensulizole as permitted combinations of active ingredients in OTC sunscreens
4. Placing of the following mandatory warning, in italics, in the "Drug Facts" box on the product label: **UV exposure from the sun increases the risk of skin cancer, premature skin aging, and other skin damage. It is important to decrease the UV exposure by limiting the time in the sun, wearing protective clothing, and using a sunscreen. [bold]**
5. A requirement for a statement to inform consumers about the importance of both UVB and UVA protection
6. Mandatory directions that consumers apply the sunscreen either "liberally" or "generously" and that the sunscreen be reapplied at least every two hours
7. Various modifications to the SPF testing procedures, which are intended to increase protection of persons enrolled in the SPF test and to improve accuracy and reproducibility of the test results

With respect to antiaging indications, in the Proposed Rule, FDA took the position that despite studies supporting the conclusion that exposure to UV rays increases the risk of premature skin aging, the study data fails to show that sunscreen use *alone* helps prevent premature skin aging and skin cancer.

The timing of the publication of a final rule will depend on the number of issues including the number of comments FDA receives as well as the level of detail and amount of data contained in each comment. Comments were due by December 26, 2007 (1). Regarding implementation of a final rule, FDA commented that the agency "understands the seasonal nature of the sunscreen industry and the time required for product testing and relabeling. FDA is also aware that more than 1 year may be needed for implementation. FDA is proposing an 18- to 24-month implementation date and will try to have it coincide with the June/July time period." (2). As of the date of publication of this book, FDA is evaluating comments it received as the public awaits issuance of the agency's Final Sunscreen Monograph.

FDA is also considering requests for the addition of seven new sunscreen active ingredients to the OTC sunscreen monograph. The six requests were made via Time and Extent Applications (TEA). In 2002, FDA established the criteria for requesting the addition of new conditions for marketing ingredients under the OTC drug review process. The basic TEA requirements are that the ingredient should have been marketed for a material time (at least five continuous years in the same country) and in sufficient quantity. In 2003, TEAs were submitted for amiloxate, enzacamene, and octyl triazone (9), in 2005 for bisoctrizole and bemotrizinol (10), and in 2006 for diethylhexyl butamido triazone (11), and in 2008 for terephthalylidene dicamphor sulfonic acid (ecamsule) (12). As of the date of publication of this book, FDA is evaluating all six TEAs, as the public awaits the agency's decision.

European Union

Sunscreen products are cosmetic products according to European Council Directive 76/768/EEC of 27 July 1976 (Cosmetics Directive). The Cosmetics Directive is the overarching legislation that regulates the manufacture and marketing of cosmetic products. It defines a cosmetic as "*any substance or preparation intended to be placed in contact with the various external parts of the human body (epidermis, hair system, nails, lips and external genital organs) or with the teeth and the mucous membranes of the oral cavity with a view exclusively or mainly to cleaning them, perfuming them, changing their appearance and/or correcting body odours and/or protecting them or keeping them in good condition.*"

Colipa collects, evaluates, and presents data on all UV filters used in Europe and accordingly makes recommendations to the European Economic Commission (EEC) for the addition or removal of ingredients. Table 2 lists UV filters that are permitted in Europe.

Canada

In Canada, sunscreens are classified as drugs if they contain at least one ingredient from Table 3. However, if they contain ingredients from Table 4, they are classified as natural health products (NHPs).

Australia and New Zealand

In Australia, sunscreens are primarily regulated as medicines under the Therapeutic Goods Act 1989 (TGA). Most sunscreens currently defined as medicines can be listed; some are exempt from registration or listing and some must be registered in the Australian Register of Therapeutic Goods (ARTG). However, some products containing sunscreen

Table 2   EU: Permitted UV Filters

INCI or other name	Maximum concentration (%)
Benzophenone-3	10
Benzophenone-4	5 (of acid)
Benzophenone-5	5 (of acid)
3-Benzylidene camphor	2
Benzylidene camphor sulfonic acid	6 (expressed as acid)
Bis-ethylhexyloxyphenol methoxyphenyl triazine	10
Butyl methoxydibenzoylmethane	5
Camphor benzalkonium methosulfate	6
Diethylamino hydroxy benzoyl hexyl benzoate	10
Biethylhexyl butamido triazone	10
Disodium phenyl dibenzylmidazole tetrasulfonate	10 (of acid)
Drometrizole trisiloxane	15
Ethylhexyl dimethyl PABA	8
Ethylhexyl methoxycinnamate	10
Ethylhexyl salicylate	5
Ethylhexyl triazone	5
Homosalate	10
Isoamyl p-methoxycinnamate	10
4-Methylbenzylidene camphor	4
Methylene bis-benzotriazolyl tetramethylbutylphenol	10
Octocrylene	10 (expressed as acid)
PABA	5
PEG-25 PABA	10
Phenylbenzimidazole sulfonic acid	8 (expressed as acid)
Polyacrylamido methylbenzylidene camphor	6
Polysilicone-15	10
Terephthalylidene dicamphor sulfonic acid	10 (expressed as acid)
Titanium dioxide	25

Abbreviation: INCI, International Nomenclature of Cosmetic Ingredient.

ingredients are regulated as cosmetics rather than as medicines, because the primary purpose of the product is not sunscreen protection. These cosmetic products are referred to as excluded sunscreens and are not regulated under therapeutic goods legislation.

Exempt sunscreens do not require registration or listing, but are treated as medicines in all other respects. They must comply with all relevant parts of the legislation, such as the Labeling Order (Therapeutic Goods Order No. 69) and the Therapeutic Goods Advertising Code.

Sunscreen products are exempt if (*i*) the claimed SPF is 3 according to testing established by AS/NZS 2604:1984; (*ii*) the label claims comply with AS/NZS 2604:1998; and (*iii*) the product does not contain ingredients of human origin or from cattle, sheep, goats, or mule deer, which are derived from body parts listed in the regulations (e.g., adrenal glands, brain).

In New Zealand, products described as or containing sunscreens are considered cosmetics. Table 5 lists UV filters that are permitted in Australia and New Zealand.

China

In China, sunscreens are classified as "cosmetics for special use," which also include cosmetic products used for hair growth, hair dyeing, hair perming, hair removal, breast

Table 3   Canada: Permitted Drug UV Filters (Drug Medicinal Ingredients)

Medicinal ingredient preferred name	Synonyms and other recognized names	Maximum concentration (%)
Avobenzone	Butyl methoxy dibenzoylmethane	5
Cinoxate	2-Ethoxyethyl p-methoxycinnamate	3
Diethanolamine-methoxycinnamate		10
Dioxybenzone	Benzophenone-8	3
Drometrizole trisiloxane		15
Ensulizole	2-Phenylbenzimidazole-5-sulfonic acid	8
Enzacamene	4-Methylbenzylidene camphor	6
Homosalate	Homomenthyl salicylate	15
Meradimate	Menthyl 2-aminobenzoate,menthyl anthranilate	5
Octinoxate	2-Ethylhexyl methoxycinnamate, octyl methoxycinnamate	8.5
Octisalate	Octyl salicylate2-ethylhexyl salicylate	6
Octocrylene	2-Ethylhexyl-2-cyano-3,3 diphenylacrylate	12
Oxybenzone	Benzophenone-3	6
Padimate-O	Octyl dimethyl PABA	8
Sulisobenzone	Benzophenone-4	6
Sulisobenzone sodium	Benzophenone-5	6
Terephthalylidene dicamphor sulfonic acid[a]	3,3'-(1,4-phenylenedimethylidene) bis[7,7-dimethyl-2-oxobicylclo [2.2.1] hept-1-yl methanesulfonic acid	10
Triethanolamine salicylate	Trolamine salicylate	12

[a]Recognized UVA absorber.

Table 4   Canada: Permitted NHP UV Filters (NHP Medicinal Ingredients)

Proper name(s)	Common name(s)	Maximum concentration (%)
Titanium dioxide	Titanium dioxide	25
Zinc oxide	Zinc oxide	25

beautification, health and beauty (e.g., weight control), deodorization, and removal of freckles. Cosmetics are currently regulated by two agencies: the Ministry of Health (MOH) and the General Administration of Quality Supervision, Inspection, and Quarantine (AQSIQ). On the label of all cosmetic products that declare having sun-protective function, the corresponding SPF, PFA or PA factor, or other sun-protection function indicators must be labeled. All sun-protection function indicators must have a valid testing basis support. SPF, PFA or PA factors must, according to testing procedures of sun protection factor of cosmetic sunscreen issued (or approved) by the Ministry of Health, undergo testing in laboratories recognized by the Ministry of Health or qualified foreign laboratories. Table 6 lists UV filters that are permitted in China.

Table 5   Australia and New Zealand: Permitted UV Filters

AAN	INCI or other name	Maximum concentration (%)
Aminobenzoic acid	PABA	15
Isoamyl methoxycinnamate	Isopentenyl p-methoxycinnamate	10
Butyl methoxydibenzoylmethane	Butyl methoxydibenzoylmethane	5
Cinoxate	Cinoxate	Aus = 6 NZ = 3
Dioxybenzone	Benzophenone-8	3
...	PEG-25 PABA	10
Padimate O	Ethylhexyl dimethyl PABA	8
Oxyl methoxycinnamate	Ethylhexyl methoxycinnamate	10
Oxyl salicylate	Ethylhexyl salicylate	5
Homosalate	Homosalate	15
Menthyl anthranilate	Menthyl anthranilate	5
4-Methylbenzylidene camphor	4-Methylbenzylidene camphor	4
Octocylene	Octocylene	10 NZ = 10 (expressed as acid)
Octyl triazone	Octyl triazone	5
...	Benzylidene camphor sulfonic acid	6 (as acid)
Oxybenzone	Benzophenone-3	10
Phenylbenzimidazole sulfonic acid	Phenylbenzimidazole sulfonic acid	4 NZ = 8
...	Camphor benzalkonium methosulfate	6 (as acid)
Sulisobenzone	Benzophenone-4	10 NZ (of acid)
...	Bezophenone-5	10 NZ (of acid)
Ecamsule	Terephthalylidene dicamphor sulfonic acid	10 NZ (expressed as acid)
Titanium dioxide	Titanium dioxide	25
Triethanolamine salicylate	TEA salicylate	12
Zinc oxide	Zinc oxide	No limit NZ = 25
Bemotrizinol	...	10
Methylene bis-benzotriazolyl tetramethylbutylphenol	Methylene bis-benzotriazolyl tetramethylbutylphenol	10
Drometrizole trisiloxane	Drometrizole trisiloxane	15
Disodium phenyl dibenzimidazole tetrasulfonate	Disodium phenyl dibenzimidazole tetrasulfonate	10 NZ (of acid)
Polysilicone-15	Polysilicone-15	10
	Meradimate methyl anthranilate	5

Abbreviations: INCI, International Nomenclature of Cosmetic Ingredient; AAN, Australian approved name; NZ, New Zealand.

Table 6   **China: Permitted UV Filters**

INCI or other name	Maximum concentration (%)
Benzophenone-3	10
Benzophenone-4	5 (of acid)
Benzophenone-5	5 (of acid)
3-Benzylidene camphor	2
Benzylidene camphor sulfonic acid	6 (of acid)
Bis-ethylhexyloxyphenol ethoxyphenyl Triazine	10
Butyl mthoxydibenzylmethane	5
Camphor benzalkonium methosulfate	6
Diethylamino hydroxy benzoyl hexyl benzoate	10
Diethylhexyl butamido triazone	10
Disodium phenyl dibenzylimidazole tetrasulfonate	10 (of acid)
Drometrizole trisiloxane	15
Ethylhexyl dimethyl PABA	8
Ethylhexyl methoxycinnamate	10
Ethylhexyl salicylate	5
Ethylhexyl triazone	5
Homosalate	10
Isoamyl p-methoxycinnamate	10
4-Methylbenzylidene camphor	4
Methylene bis-benzotriazolyl tetramethylbutylphenol	10
Octocrylene	10 (expressed as acid)
PABA	5
PEG-25 PABA	10
Phenylbenzimidazole sulfonic acid	8 (expressed as acid)
Polyacrylamido methylbenzylidene camphor	6
Polysilicone-15	10
Terephthalylidene dicamphor sulfonic acid	10 (expressed as acid)
Titanium dioxide	25
Zinc oxide	25

Abbreviation: INCI, International Nomenclature of Cosmetic Ingredient.

India

In India, sunscreens are regulated as cosmetic products. India is currently developing its regulations with respect to sunscreen testing and labeling (e.g., maximum SPF). Table 7 lists UV filters that are permitted in India.

Japan

In Japan, sunscreens are regulated as cosmetics. The Japanese regulate all cosmetic products through their Ministry of Health, Labor, and Welfare according to the Pharmaceutical Affairs Law (Law No. 145) adopted in 1960. Japan has adopted a list of prohibited ingredients, a list of restricted ingredients, a positive list of UV filters, and a positive list of preservatives. In Japan, UV filters are permitted in the following three categories: Type 1—all cosmetics; Type 2—rinse-off cosmetics but not mucus membrane application; and Type 3—rinse-off and leave-on cosmetics. Table 8 lists UV filters that are permitted in Japan.

Table 7   India: Permitted UV Filters

INCI or other name	Maximum concentration%
PABA	5
Camphor benzalkonium methosulfate	6
3,3,5-Trimethylcyclohexyl 2-hydroxybenzoate homomenthyl salicylate	10
Benzophenone-3	10
Ensulizole	8 (expressed as acid)
Terephthalylidene dicamphor sulfonic acid	10
Butyl methoxydibenzoylmethane	5
Benzylidene camphor sulfonic acid	6 (expressed as acid)
Octocrylene	10 (expressed as acid)
Polyacrylamidomethyl benzylidene camphor	6
Ethylhexyl methoxycinnamate	10
PEG-25 PABA	10
Isoamyl p-methoxycinnamate	10
Octyl triazone Ethylhexyl triazone	5
Drometrizole trisiloxane	15
Diethylhexyl butamido triazone	10
4-Methylbenzylidene camphor	4
3-Benzylidene camphor	2
Octyl salicylate	5
Padimate O	8
Benzophenone-5	5 (of acid)
Sulizobenzone 2-hydroxy-4-methoxybenzophenone-5-sulfonic acid and its trihydrate	5 (of acid)
Methylene bis-benzotriazolyl tetramethylbutylphenol	10
Disodium phenyl dibenzimidazole tetrasulfonate	10 (of acid)
Bis-ethylhexyloxyphenol methoxyphenyl triazine	10

Abbreviation: INCI, International Nomenclature of Cosmetic Ingredient.

Korea

In Korea, sunscreens are regulated as functional cosmetics. Table 9 lists UV filters that are permitted in Korea.

South Africa

As is done in the EU, South Africa regulates sunscreens as cosmetics. South Africa permits the largest number of UV filters. Table 10 lists UV filters that are permitted in South Africa.

ASEAN

Countries in the ASEAN are Brunei, Cambodia, Indonesia, Laos, Malaysia, Myanmar, Philippines, Singapore, Thailand, and Vietnam. These countries consider sunscreens to be cosmetics. The ASEAN Cosmetic Directive is similar to the EU's Cosmetics Directive and lists permitted UV filters. Table 11 lists UV filters that are permitted in ASEAN.

Table 8   Japan: Permitted UV Filters

INCI or other name	Maximum concentration (%)
Benzophenone-1	10 (not for use on mucus membrane)
Benzophenone-2	10 (not for use on mucus membrane)
	0.05 (allowed for use on mucus membrane)
Benzophenone-3	5 (leave-on and not for use on mucus membrane)
	No limit (rinse-off and not for use on mucus membrane)
Benzophenone-4	10 (not for use on mucus membrane)
	0.1 (allowed for use on mucus membrane)
Benzophenone-5	10 (not for use on mucus membrane)
	1 (allowed for use on mucus membrane)
Benzophenone-6	10 (not for use on mucus membrane)
Benzophenone-9	10 (not for use on mucus membrane)
Beta, 2-glucopyranoxy propyl hydroxy benzophenone	5 (not for use on mucus membrane)
Butyl methoxydibenzoylmethane	10
Cinoxate	5 (leave-on and not for use on mucus membrane)
	No limit (rinse-off and not for use on mucus membrane)
Diisopropyl methylcinnamate	10 (not for use on mucus membrane)
Dimethoxyphenyl-[1-(3,4)]-4, 4-dimethyl 1,3 pentanedione	7 (not for use on mucus membrane)
Drometrizole trisiloxane	15 (not for use on mucus membrane)
Ethylhexyl dimethoxy benzylidene dioxoimidazoline propionate	3 (not for use on mucus membrane)
Ethylhexyl dimethyl PABA	10 (not for use on mucus membrane)
	7 (allowed for use on mucus membrane)
Ethylhexyl methoxycinnamate	20 (not for use on mucus membrane)
	8 (allowed for use on mucus membrane)
Ethylhexyl salicylate	10 (not for use on mucus membrane)
	5 (allowed for use on mucus membrane)
Ethylhexyl triazone	3 (not for use on mucus membrane)
Ferulic acid	10 (not for use on mucus membrane)
Glyceryl ethylhexanoate dimethoxycinnamate	10
Homosalate	10
Isopentyl trimethoxycinnamate trisiloxane	7.5 (not for use on mucus membrane)
	2.5 (allowed for use on mucus membrane)
Isopropyl methoxycinnamate	10 (not for use on mucus membrane)
Methylene bis-benzotriazolyl tetramethylbutylphenol	10 (not for use on mucus membrane)
Octocrylene	10
PABA	4 (as total of acid and its esters)
Pentyl dimethyl PABA	10 (not for use on mucus membrane)
Phenylbenzimidazole sulfonic acid	3 acid only (not for use on mucus membrane)
Polysilicone-15	10
Terephthalylidene dicamphor sulfonic acid	10 (not for use on mucus membrane)
Titanium dioxide	No limit (as scattering agent)
Zinc oxide	No limit (as scattering agent)

Abbreviation: INCI, International Nomenclature of Cosmetic Ingredient.

Table 9   Korea: Permitted UV Filters

INCI or other name	Maximum concentration (%)
PABA	5
3,3,5-trimethylcyclohexyl 2-hydroxybenzoate homomenthyl salicylate	10
Benzophenone-3	5
Ensulizole	4
Terephthalylidene dicamphor sulfonic acid	10 (expressed as acid)
Butyl methoxydibenzoylmethane	5
Octocrylene	10
Ethylhexyl methoxycinnamate	7.5
Isoamyl p-methoxycinnamate	10
Octyl triazone ethylhexyl triazone	5
Drometrizole trisiloxane	15
Diethylhexyl butamido triazone	10
4-Methylbenzylidene camphor	5
Octyl salicylate	5
Padimate O	8
Sulizobenzone 2-hydroxy-4-methoxybenzophenone-5-sulfonic acid and its Trihydrate	5
Benzophenone-4	5
Disodium phenyl dibenzimidazole tetrasulfonate	10 (of acid)
Bis-ethylhexyloxyphenol methoxyphenyl triazine	10
Polysilicone-15	10
Titanium dioxide	25
Cinoxate	5
Benzophenone-8	3
Menthyl anthranilate	5
Zinc oxide	25
Digalloyl trioleate	5
Glyceryl PABA	3
Drometrizole	7

Abbreviation: INCI, International Nomenclature of Cosmetic Ingredient.

MERCOSUR

MERCOSUR include Argentina, Brazil, Paraguay, and Uruguay. MERCOSUR is in the process of harmonizing their respective regulations, including those governing cosmetic products. The EU and MERCOSUR definitions of cosmetic products are very similar, and both consider sunscreens to be cosmetic products. Table 12 lists UV filters that are permitted in MERCOSUR.

REGULATORY SUMMARY

Table 13 provides a brief summary comparing worldwide sunscreen product regulations.

Table 10   **South Africa: Permitted UV Filters**

INCI or other name	Maximum concentration (%)
Benzophenone-1	10
Benzophenone-2	10
Benzophenone-3	10
Benzophenone-4	5 (of acid)
Benzophenone-5	5 (of acid)
Benzophenone-6	10
Benzophenone-8	3
Benzophenone-9	No limit listed
3-Benzylidene camphor	2
Benzylidene camphor sulfonic acid	6
Beta, 2-glucopyranoxy propyl hydroxy benzophenone	5
Bis-ethylhexylopcphenol methoxyphenyl triazine	10
Butyl methoxydibenzoylmethane	5
Camphor benzalkonium methosulfate	6
Cinoxate	5
DEA methoxycinnamate	8
Diethylhexyl butamido triazone	10
Digalloyl trioleate	5
Diisopropyl methylcinnamate	10
Dimethoxyphenyl-[1-(3,4)]-4,4-dimethyl 1,3 pentanedione	7
Ethyl dihydroxypropyl PABA	5
Ethylhexyl dimethyl PABA	8
Ethylhexyl methoxycinnamate	10
Ethylhexyl salicylate	5
Ethylhexyl triazone	5
Ferulic acid	10
Glyceryl ethylhexanoate dimethoxycinnamate	10
Glyceryl PABA	5
Homosalate	10
Isoamyl p-methoxycinnamate	10
Isopropy salicylate	4
Isopropyl methoxycinnamate	10
Menthyl anthranilate	5
Polysilicone-15	10

Abbreviation: INCI, International Nomenclature of Cosmetic Ingredient.

Future Trends: Towards International Harmonization

Consumers want safe products that are available and consistently regulated across the globe, and companies need predictable regulatory regimes to maintain product innovation. To that end, industry and regulators alike are making progress toward international harmonization of standards and regulations. Specifically regarding sunscreens, efforts are currently underway at ISO (International Organization for Standardization) to harmonize worldwide SPF and UVA testing standards. Also, sunscreens were recently added to the International Cooperation on Cosmetics Regulation (ICCR) in a further effort to harmonize regulations products intended to provide protection again the sun. (See below for information on ICCR). In time, we expect more consistency in sunscreen-testing requirements (SPF and UVA), as well as available UV filters.

Table 11   ASEAN: Permitted UV Filters

INCI or other name	Maximum concentration (%)
Benzophenone-3	10
Benzophenone-4	10 Thai[a]
Benzophenone-5	5 (of acid)
Benzophenone-8	3 Thai[a]
3-Benzylidene camphor	2
Benzylidene camphor sulfonic acid	6
Bis-ethylhexyloxyphenol methoxyphenyl triazine	10
Butyl methoxydibenzoylmethane	5
Camphor benzalkonium methosulfate	6
Cinoxate	3
DEA-methoxycinnamate	10
Diethylhexyl butamido triazone	10
Digalloyl trioleate	5 Thai[a]
Disodium phenyl dibenzylmidazole tetrasulfonate	10
Drometrizole trisiloxane	15
Ethyl dihydroxypropyl PABA	5
Ethylhexyl dimethyl PABA	8
Ethylhexyl methoxycinnamate	10
Ethylhexyl salicylate	5
Ethylhexyl triazone	5
Glyceryl PABA	3 Thai[a]
Homosalate	10
Isoamyl p-methoxycinnamate	10
Methyl anthranilate	5 Thai[a]
4-methylbenzylidene camphor	4
Methylene bis-benzotriazolyl tetramethylbutylphenol	10
Octocrylene	10
PABA	5
PEG-25 PABA	10
Pentyl dimethyl PABA	5
Phenylbenzimidazole sulfonic acid	8
Polyacrylamido methylbenzylidene camphor	6
Polysilicone-15	10
Titanium dioxide	25
Terephthalylidene dicamphor sulfonic acid	10
Trolamine salicylate	12
Zinc oxide	20

[a] Indicates permitted only in Thailand.
Abbreviation: INCI, International Nomenclature of Cosmetic Ingredient.

Background on ICCR

The Council has led global industry efforts to establish a formal dialogue between the cosmetics industry and global regulators, similar to what has existed for two decades for medical devices and pharmaceuticals. The Council worked closely with Colipa, JCIA, and the Canadian Cosmetic, Toiletry, and Fragrance Association to develop proposals for an industry–regulators dialogue that would achieve meaningful results towards international

Table 12 **MERCOSUR: Permitted UV Filters**

INCI name	Maximum concentration (%)
Benzylidene camphor sulfonic acid	6 (expressed as acid)
Benzophenone-3	10
Benzophenone-4	10 (of acid)
Benzophenone-5	5 (of acid)
Benzophenone-8	3
3-Benzylidene camphor	2
Bis-ethylhexylopcphenol methoxyphenyl triazine	10
Butyl methoxydibenzoylmethane	5
Camphor benzalkonium methosulfate	6
Cinoxate	3
Diethylamino hydroxy benzoyl hexyl benzoate	10
Diethylhexyl butamido triazone	10
Disodium phenyl dibenzylimidazole tetrasulfonate	10 (of acid)
Drometrizole trisiloxane	15
Ethylhexyl dimethyl PABA	8
Ethylhexyl methoxycinnamate	10
Ethylhexyl salicylate	5
Ethylhexyl triazone	5
Homosalate	15
Isoamyl p-methoxycinnamate	10
Menthyl anthranilate	5
4-Methylbenzlidene camphor	4
Methylene bis-benzotriazolyl tetramethylbutylphenol	10
Octocrylene	10 (expressed as acid)
PABA	15
PEG-25 PABA	10
Phenylbenzimidazole sulfonic acid	8 (expressed as acid)
Polyacrylamido methylbenzylidene camphor	6
Polysilicone-15	10
TEA salicylate	12
Terephthalylidene dicamphor sulfonic acid	10 (expressed as acid)
Titanium dioxide	25
Zinc oxide	25

Abbreviation: INCI, International Nomenclature of Cosmetic Ingredient.

harmonization of regulations. In 2007, ICCR was officially launched. ICCR is a formal dialogue between regulators and industry from the United States, Europe, Canada, and Japan to promote global harmonization of regulations for cosmetics and personal care products. Because regulations in different countries often conflict, increasing costs to manufacturers and straining government resources, the mission of ICCR is to identify ways to better align regulations and remove regulatory obstacles among the regions while maintaining the highest level of global consumer protection.

Table 13 Comparison of International Sunscreen Regulation

	Class	Mandatory efficacy test for UVA	Mandatory efficacy test for SPF	Maximum SPF
USA	Drugs	Unresolved, with newly proposed UVA test method	Yes Monograph	30+, with proposed increase to +50
EU	Cosmetics	Unresolved	Yes Colipa	30+
Canada	Drugs or NHP	Unresolved	Yes Monograph	30+
Australia	Therapeutic or Exempt	Yes	Yes Australia/New Zealand Standard AS/NZS 2604:1998	30+
New Zealand	Cosmetics	Yes	Yes Australia/New Zealand Standard AS/NZS 2604:1998 Not mandatory but encouraged	No limit specified
China	Cosmetics	Yes	Yes MOH TM, equivalent methods (EU, United States, Australia) acceptable; testing lab shall be GLP certified by a recognized regulatory body.	30+ (Hong Kong has no specified limit)

(Continued)

Table 13   **Comparison of International Sunscreen Regulation** (*Continues*)

	Class	Mandatory efficacy test for UVA	Mandatory efficacy test for SPF	Maximum SPF
India	Cosmetics	No	No	Not specified
Japan	Cosmetics or quasi-drug	Yes	Yes	50+
		JCIA measurement standards for UVA protection efficacy (1995) JHPIA	Standard sun protection factor test method (2003 revised version) JHPIA	
Korea	Functional cosmetics	Yes	Yes	50+
		Korean measurement standards for UV protection efficacy (KMSUV) and JCIA are acceptable	Korean measurement standards for UV protection efficacy (KMSUV) and JCIA are acceptable for import	
South Africa	Cosmetics	Unresolved	Yes	30+
ASEAN	Cosmetics	Unresolved	Yes	Not specified
MERCUSOR	Cosmetics	Unresolved	Yes	Unclear

REFERENCES

1. 72 Fed Reg 67264 (November 28, 2007).
2. 72 Fed Reg 49073 (August 27, 2007). FDA extended the original deadline of November 26, 2007 to December 26, 2007.
3. 43 Fed Reg 38206 (August 25, 1978).
4. 58 Fed Reg 28194 (May 12, 1993).
5. 62 Fed Reg 23350 (April 30, 1997).
6. 63 Fed Reg 56584 (November 22, 1998).
7. 66 Fed Reg 67485 (December 31, 2001).
8. 72 Fed Reg 49070 (August 27, 2007).
9. 68 Fed Reg 41386 (July 11, 2003).
10. 70 Fed Reg 72449 (December 5, 2005).
11. 71 Fed Reg 42405 (July 26, 2006).
12. 73 Fed Reg 53029 (September 12, 2008).

6
Sunscreens and Photodermatoses

Zoe Diana Draelos
Dermatology Consulting Services, High Point, North Carolina, U.S.A.

Henry W. Lim
Department of Dermatology, Henry Ford Hospital, Detroit, Michigan, U.S.A.

André Rougier
La Roche-Posay Pharmaceutical Laboratories, Asnières, France

SYNOPSIS

- Photoprotection is an integral part of the management of all photodermatoses, including the use of sunscreens on the exposed areas.
- Because the action spectrum of most photodermatoses includes UVA, the use of broad-spectrum sunscreens is beneficial.
- The ability of sunscreens with photostable UVA filters (ecamsule, silatriazole) in minimizing UV-induced eruption in PLE, LE, and SU has been demonstrated.

Photodermatoses comprise a group of skin diseases exacerbated by solar radiation. Photodermatoses can be classified into four groups: immunologically mediated photodermatoses, drug- and chemical-induced photosensitivity, DNA repair–deficient photodermatoses, and photoaggravated dermatoses (Table 1) (1). For all photodermatoses, an essential component of their management is photoprotection, which consists of seeking shade, the use of photoprotective clothing and wide-brimmed hat, and the application of broad-spectrum sunscreens that protect against UVB and UVA. A number of UVA filters are available in many parts of the world (see chap. 2); however, in the United States, only oxybenzone, sulisobenzone, meradimate, avobenzone, titanium dioxide, zinc oxide, and ecamsule are available. Avobenzone is the only long-wave organic UVA filter available in the United States. The availability of sunscreens with good UVA protection is

Modified from Rougier A, Seite S, Lim HW. Novel developments in photoprotection: Part II. In: Lim HW, Hönigsmann H, Hawk J., eds. Photodermatology. New York: Informa Healthcare, 2007: 297–309.

Table 1	Classification of Photodermatoses

Immunologically mediated photodermatoses
   Polymorphous light eruption
   Hydroa vacciniforme
   Actinic prurigo
   Chronic actinic dermatitis
   Solar urticaria
Drug- and chemical-induced photosensitivity
   Drug- and exogenous chemical-induced photosensitivity
   Cutaneous porphyries
DNA repair-deficient photodermatoses
   Xeroderma pigmentosum
   Bloom syndrome
   Cockayne syndrome
   Rothmund–Thompson syndrome
   Trichothiodystrophy
   UV-sensitive syndrome
Photoaggravated dermatoses
   Lupus erythematosus
   Dermatomyositis
   Pellagra

Source: From Ref. 1.

important in the management of photodermatoses, since the action spectra for most of them do include UVA.

    While it is common practice to use sunscreens as part of the management of patients with photodermatoses, studies to critically evaluate the efficacy of sunscreens in photodermatoses have been done primarily in polymorphous light eruption (PLE), lupus erythematosus (LE), and solar urticaria (SU), using sunscreens containing photostabilized avobenzone, ecamsule (Mexoryl® SX), and silatriazole (Mexoryl XL). These studies will be reviewed in this chapter.

POLYMORPHOUS LIGHT ERUPTION

PLE is one of the most common photodermatoses with an estimated incidence of approximately 3% to 17%. It is diagnosed on the basis of clinical symptoms, location of the lesions, relationship of the occurrence of the lesions to sun exposure, and time course of the lesions (2). It is characterized by a variety of lesions, which may be papular, papulovesicular, eczematous, and plaque-like (3). Moreover, photo-provocation testing has revealed that 75% of PLE patients are sensitive to either UVB plus UVA or UVA alone (4). Ortel and colleagues found that 56% of subjects in their population had an action spectrum in the UVA range, 17% in the UVB range, and 26% in both ranges (5). This emphasizes the importance of broad-spectrum photoprotection as an integral part of the management of PLE (6).

    An article by Gschnait, published in 1983, stated, "topical sunscreens in the majority of cases are sufficient to protect UVB-promoted PLE, but fail in UVA-induced disease"(7). This reflects the inability of the filters available in 1983 to adequately block UVA radiation. Newer UVA filters, most notably avobenzone (butyl methoxydibenzoylmethane), have enhanced UVA photoprotection. Avobenzone is a broad UVA absorber; however, its drawback is photoinstability, which can be avoided by combining it with octocrylene, 4-methylbenzylidene camphor, or oxybenzone and 2,6 diethylhexylnaphthlate (DEHN). The rationale for the photostabilizing property of these combinations is that in the presence of these filters, the excited-state avobenzone can rapidly transfer the energy to the other photostable UV filters, hence minimizing the photodegradation of avobenzone.

Other UVA filters include oxybenzone, meradimate (menthyl anthranilate), and the newly developed ecamsule (terephtalylidene dicamphor sulfonic acid) and silatriazole (drometriazole trisiloxane). Ecamsule, also known as Mexoryl SX, is a strong short UVA photostable absorber, which absorbs UV radiation between 290 and 390 nm with a peak at 345 nm (Fig. 1). Silatrizole, also known as Mexoryl XL, is a broad UV filter against UVA and UVB spectrum (Fig. 2). Mexoryl XL belongs to the photostable group of the hydroxybenzotriazole and is composed of two different chemical groups: hydroxyphenylbenzotriazole, which provides photostable UVA and UVB absorption; and a short siloxan chain, which provides liposolubility of the molecule. Mexoryl XL has two absorption spectra in UVB and UVA range (290–320 nm, λ_{max} 303 nm; and 320–360 nm, λ_{max} 344 nm). By combining the lipophilic Mexoryl XL with hydrophilic Mexoryl SX, a high level of photoprotection can be achieved.

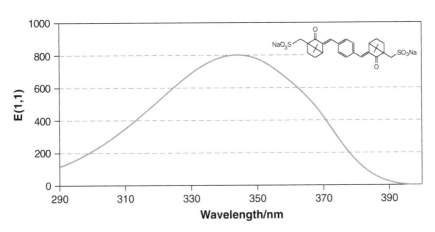

Figure 1   The structure and absorption spectrum of Mexoryl® SX.

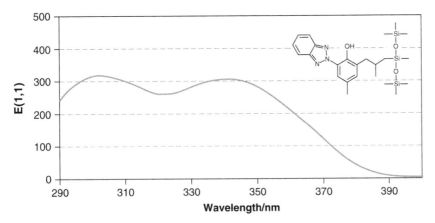

Figure 2   The structure and absorption spectrum of Mexoryl® XL.

The ability of these new sunscreen filters to provide photoprotection in PLE has been studied. Three different sunscreens with high sun protection factors (SPFs), 35, 60, and 75, but different UVA protection factors (UVA-PFs) of 3 to 28, were compared for their ability to prevent the development of skin lesions in PLE patients (8). The sunscreen with SPF 50^+ and UVA-PF 28 (Anthelios XL 50^+ containing octocrylene, Mexoryl SX, Mexoryl XL, avobenzone, and TiO_2) protected the development of PLE in all patients, while sunscreens with high SPFs of 35, 60, and 75 but low UVA-PF values of 3 to 5 protected only 23% to 45 % of the patients. In addition, effective prevention of clinically apparent skin lesions was associated with complete inhibition of UVA-induced expression of ICAM-1 mRNA. Interestingly, all the three products tested had avobenzone as a UVA filter. However, the one with the highest UVA-PF also had Mexoryl SX and Mexoryl XL, indicating that the type of UV filters used is critical for the efficacy of a given sunscreen to provide photoprotection. This observation further supports the concept that PLE represents an abnormal response of human skin toward UVA and UVB, resulting in an increased expression of pro-inflammatory molecules, such as ICAM-1.

LUPUS ERYTHEMATOSUS

LE is an autoimmune disease that is triggered and exacerbated by UVR (9). Sanders et al. found that 93% of LE patients demonstrated an abnormal reaction to UVR and visible light (10). Photosensitivity to wavelengths shorter than 320 nm may involve DNA as the chromophore, while in vitro studies indicate that radiation of 360 to 400 nm activates a photosensitizing compound in the lymphocytes and serum of LE patients (11). As a consequence, photoprotection is one of the measures in the management of these patients (12,13).

Eleven patients with LE were repeatedly exposed to UVA; the ability of sunscreens with high SPFs of 35 to 75 but different UVA-PF of 3 to 28 was studied. Similar to results observed in PLE, sunscreenss with high UVA-PF 28 (Anthelios XL 50^+) prevented the development of lesions in all patients, while those with lower UVA-PF only partially did so (14). High UVA-PF products also prevented the increased expression of ICAM-1 associated with development of lesions (14).

SOLAR URTICARIA

SU is a rare photosensitive disorder with an action spectrum ranging from UVB to UVA and also the visible spectrum. Within 5 to 10 minutes of sun exposure, patients experience itching, erythema, and patchy or confluent whealing. Chronically exposed skin, such as that on the face and arms, is generally less susceptible than normally covered areas. Uetsu found in a study of 40 patients with SU that the disease most commonly appeared during the third decade (15). Thus, photoprotection is an important lifelong need in this population (16).

The protective effect of a high SPF and high UVA-PF product (SPF 60, UVA-PF 12; Anthelios L, containing Eusolex 6300, Mexoryl SX, avobenzone, and TiO_2) was assessed in SU patients ($n = 10$) following 1000 W xenon arc solar simulator exposure (17). The minimal urticarial dose (MUD) on unprotected area was determined for each patient and for each triggering spectral band (UVA1: 360 nm; UVA2: 335 nm; and UVB: 310 nm) by clinical assessment of erythema and swelling in the early minutes following each UV exposure. MUD on protected area was then measured for each triggering spectral band following application (2 mg/cm^2) of either the broad-spectrum sunscreen or

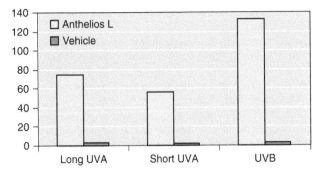

Figure 3 SUPFs in each triggering spectral band. (SUPF = MUD with sunscreen or vehicle/MUD unprotected. *Abbreviations*: SUPF, solar urticaria protection factors; MUD, minimal urticarial dose.

its vehicle, and SU protection factor (SUPF) was determined by dividing the MUD value obtained with the sunscreen or its vehicle by the MUD value obtained without any product. Results showed that the SUPFs of the vehicle were 2.7, 2.0, and 3.3, respectively, in the long UVA, short UVA, and UVB range, whereas these SUPFs were of 75, 56, and 133 on the broad-spectrum sunscreen-treated areas (Fig. 3).

These experiments confirm that the different parts of the UV spectrum can elicit SU. Moreover, it was found that most of the patients react to very low doses of UV, particularly in the UVA domain, confirming the extreme skin sensitivity of this photodermatosis. The results also indicate that the use of broad-spectrum sunscreens with highly efficient UV filters can be considered as an option in the management of patients with SU with action spectra in the UV range. For those with visible light sensitivity, a physical agent such as opaque clothing is the only available external photoprotective measure.

REFERENCES

1. Lim, HW, Hawk J. Evaluation of the photosensitive patient. In: Lim HW, Hönigsmann H, Hawk J, eds. Photodermatology. New York: Informa Healthcare, 2007:139–148.
2. Fesq H, Ring J, Abeck D. Management of polymorphous light eruption: clinical course, pathogenesis, diagnosis, and intervention. Am J Clin Dermatol 2003; 4(6):399–406.
3. Naleway AL, Greenlee RT, Melski JW. Characteristics of diagnosed polymorphous light eruption. Photodermatol Photoimmunol Photomed 2006; 22(4):205–207.
4. Hönigsmann H, Hojyo-Tomoka MT. Polymorphous light eruption, hydroa vacciniforme, and actinic prurigo. In: Lim HW, Hönigsmann H, Hawk Jeds. Photodermatology. New York: Informa Healthcare, 2007:149–168.
5. Ortel B, Tanew A, Wolff K, et al. Polymorphous light eruption: action spectrum and photoprotection. J Am Acad Dermatol 1986; 14(5 pt 1):748–753.
6. Lim HW, Hawk J. Photodermatoses. In: Bolognia JL, Jorizzo JL, Rapini RP, eds. Dermatology. 2nd ed. London: Mosby, 2008:1333–1351.
7. Gschnait F, Schwarz T, Ladich I. Treatment of polymorphous light eruption. Arch Dermatol Res 1983; 275(6):379–382.
8. Stege H, Budde M, Grether-Beck S, et al. Sunscreens with high SPF values are not equivalent in protection from UVA induced polymorphous light eruption. Eur J Dermatol 2002; 12:IV–VI.
9. Werth VP, Hönigsmann H. Photoaggravated dermatoses. In: Lim HW, Hönigsmann H, Hawk J, eds. Photodermatology. New York: Informa Healthcare, 2007:251–266.
10. Sanders CJ, Van Weeleden H, Kazzaz GA, et al. Photosensitivity in patients with lupus erythematosus: a clinical and photobiological study of 100 patients using a prolonged phototest protocol. Br J Dermatol 2003; 149(1):131–137.

11. Kochevar IE. Action spectrum and mechanisms of UV radiation-induced injury in lupus erythematosus. J Invest Dermatol 1985; 85(1 suppl):140s–143s.
12. Costner MI, Sontheimer RD. Lupus erythematosus. In: Freedberg IM, Eisen AZ, Wolf K, et al., eds. Fitzpatrick's Dermatology in General Medicine. New York: McGraw-Hill, 2003: 1677–1693.
13. Herzinger T, Plewig G, Rocken M. Use of sunscreens to protect against ultraviolet-induce lupus erythematosus. Arthritis Rheum 2004; 50(9):3045–3046.
14. Stege H, Budde MA, Grether-Beck S, et al. Evaluation of the capacity of sunscreens to photoprotect lupus erythematosus patients by employing the photoprovocation test. Eur J Dermatol 2002; 12:VII–IX.
15. Uetsu N, Miyauchi-Hashimoto H, Okamoto H, et al. The clinical and photobiological characteristic of solar urticaria in 40 patients. Br J Dermatol 2000; 142(1):32–38.
16. Faurschou A, Wulf HC. Synergistic effect of broad-spectrum sunscreens and antihistamines in the control of idiopathic solar urticaria. Arch Dermatol 2008; 144(6):765–769.
17. Peyron JL, Raison-Peyron N, Meynadier J, et al. Prevention of solar urticaria using a broadspectrum sunscreen and determination of solar urticaria protection factor (SUPF). In: Rougier A, Schaefer H, eds. Protection of the Skin Against Ultraviolet Radiations. France: John Libbey Eurotext, 1998:201–205.

7
Sunscreens and Photocarcinogenesis

Gillian M. Murphy
National Photodermatology Unit, Beaumont and Mater Misericordiae Hospitals, Dublin, Ireland

John L. M. Hawk
St. John's Institute of Dermatology, St. Thomas' Hospital, London, U.K.

SYNOPSIS

- Careful sunscreen use can reduce the incidence of new AKs and the numbers of existing AKs.
- A 4.5-year study with an 8-year follow-up showed that sunscreen use can have a prolonged preventive effect against the development of squamous cell carcinoma, and perhaps also a minimal benefit against the development of basal cell carcinoma.
- The role of sunscreen use in melanoma prevention is less clear. However, systematic review of all studies from 1966 to 2003 has shown no evidence for a relationship between sunscreen use and increased melanoma risk.
- UVR filter chemicals may be absorbed systemically to a mild extent, and titanium dioxide and zinc oxide nanoparticles may generate free radicals upon exposure to UVR in vitro. However, no clinical relevance for these observations has been demonstrated. Nevertheless, sunscreen use should probably be restricted in very young infants.

INTRODUCTION

Sunscreens have long been recognized as agents offering effective protection against ultraviolet radiation (UVR)-induced inflammation, or sunburn, and indeed, the so-called sun protection factor (SPF) of such products is a measure of their protective efficacy. This value is in fact an assessment of their combined activity against ultraviolet B (UVB) (280–315 nm) radiation, which produces about 90% of the sunburning effect, and ultraviolet A (UVA) (315–400 nm), which produces only around 10%; the differential

Table 1 **Possible Cutaneous Consequences of Ultraviolet Exposure**

Adverse effects	Beneficial effects
Acute	Acute
Sunburn	Vitamin D formation
Tanning	Immunosuppression (prevents some photodermatoses)
Freckling	
Thickening	
Immunosuppression (facilitates cancer development)	
Folate depletion	
Photodermatoses	
Intermediate	
Mole formation	
Pseudoporphyria	
Onycholysis	
Chronic	
Photoaging	
Cancer	

effects of UVB and UVA are partly due to the variable UVR spectral activity at inducing the cutaneous DNA lesions believed to initiate the response (1). However, sunburn (particularly its most visible and measurable endpoint, erythema) is but one of multiple UVR-induced skin effects, usually detrimental, which are summarized in full in Table 1. Photocarcinogenesis is clearly the most serious of these, and it is therefore extremely important that sunscreens protect against this as well. This chapter now considers in detail whether they do so.

Solar UVB accounts for most of the cutaneous photocarcinogenic response, initially through the cumulative production of mutations following direct DNA absorptive damage to presumably epidermal basal layer keratinocytes or melanocytes. Persistence of these lesions is then apparently facilitated by concomitantly induced skin immunosuppressive change, apparently through variable UVB effects on epidermal DNA and urocanic acid. However, UVA can also be independently carcinogenic, inducing alone to a small extent the same DNA lesions, as well as more profuse secondary, generally free radical-induced DNA damage, following non-DNA UVA absorption elsewhere in the cell. UVA also induces immunosuppressive effects facilitating cancer progression, though again much less efficiently than UVB.

To fully and reliably prevent skin cancer, sunscreens should block both UVA and UVB penetration into the skin, and hence avoid their potentially damaging effects. In addition, the UVR-sunscreen interactions enabling this process should also not cause harm, the UVR preferably being dissipated as minor amounts of heat rather than as free radicals, which may be injurious to the cells in which they occur.

Until some 20 years ago, sunscreens offered good efficacy against UVB but relatively little against UVA. However, particularly in the last 10 years, advances in the chemistry of UV filters have led to the production of multiple UVA absorbers, which even now are able to offer significant protection against the UVA wavelengths, complying with or bettering recent recommendations, available for review on the

Web site http://ec.europa.eu/enterprise/cosmetics/sunscreens/synthesis_doc_06_06.pdf, which state that sunscreen UVA protection should be at least a third of the SPF value as measured by its in vivo protectivity against persisting pigment darkening of the skin. Thus, sunscreen efficacy has greatly improved in recent years, and would now be expected to provide protection against the whole range of cutaneous solar effects, including carcinogenesis, rather than just against sunburn (Table 1). Nevertheless, the true, rather than theoretical, efficacy of these products and their ability to prevent skin cancer now need to be addressed.

The matter may be considered under the following headings:

1. Is there satisfactory evidence that sunscreens can reduce the risk of development of actinic keratoses (AKs), firmly believed to be the earliest detectable forerunners of skin cancer?
2. Is there satisfactory evidence that sunscreens can reduce the risk of development of fully developed and potentially invasive skin cancers, namely squamous cell carcinoma (SCC), basal cell carcinoma (BCC), and malignant melanoma (MM)?
3. Is there satisfactory evidence that sunscreens do not in fact increase the risk of development of skin cancer risk, rather than reducing it?

These questions are now addressed with reference to the published literature.

CLINICAL STUDIES ON SUNSCREEN EFFICACY AGAINST AK DEVELOPMENT

AKs, which demonstrate partial thickness dysplasia of the epidermis and may thus be considered as a form of carcinoma in situ, are widely regarded as the earliest clinical markers of skin cancer risk. They have, therefore, been used as a surrogate for the possible future development of invasive skin cancer, such that several studies have examined whether prospective sunscreen use can reduce their incidence and thus presumably also the incidence of subsequent skin cancer.

Fifty-three patients with AKs were prospectively enrolled into a placebo-controlled, double-blind study over a three-year period, each using an SPF 29 sunscreen constantly over two years; of them, 37 patients were available for evaluation. The rate of appearance of new lesions was significantly reduced in the treatment group compared with control subjects, while those with darker skins also had fewer lesions, as did women and patients with fewer lesions at enrolment. Some non-melanoma skin cancers also appeared during the study period, but their numbers were too small for statistical evaluation (2).

A larger randomized, controlled trial of the effect on AKs of the daily use of a broad-spectrum sunscreen cream of SPF 17 in 588 people aged 40 years or older was conducted in Australia over a six-month period during the summer. The subjects applied either sunscreen or the product base daily to exposed sites. The mean number of AKs increased by 1.0 per subject in the base cream group while decreasing by 0.6 in the sunscreen group (difference, 1.53; 95% confidence interval, 0.81–2.25). The sunscreen group also developed fewer new lesions (rate ratio, 0.62; 95% confidence interval, 0.54–0.71) and more remissions (odds ratio, 1.53; 95% confidence interval, 1.29–1.80) than the base cream group. The amount of sunscreen used was also related to both the development of new lesions and the remission of existing ones with a dose-response relationship (3).

In a final study considering the degree of sunscreen protection offered against the development of AKs, a large, randomized, controlled study was undertaken at a latitude of 26° south in Queensland, Australia, between February 1992 and August 1996. Participants

($n = 1621$; age: 25–74 years) were randomized to the daily use of a high SPF sunscreen (15+) on the head, neck, arms, and hands regularly every morning, or use of their own personal sunscreen as they normally would. They were also randomly assigned to take either 30 mg of β-carotene or placebo each day. The ratio of AK counts in 1994 relative to 1992 was lower in those randomized to trial sunscreen use (1.20; 95% confidence interval, 1.04–1.39) rather than to personal sunscreen (1.57; 1.35–1.84). This 24% reduction was deemed equivalent to the prevention of an average of one additional SCC per person over that time. A reduction in the rate of change of prevalence was also seen in the sunscreen intervention group between 1994 and 1996, but was not statistically significant. No effect on the rate of change of prevalence was seen in the β-carotene arm of the study. Daily trial sunscreen application thus retarded the rate of AK acquisition among adults in a subtropical environment, while β-carotene supplementation made no difference (4).

All these three studies therefore confirm that the use of sunscreens can reduce the incidence of new AKs and the numbers of existing AKs.

CLINICAL STUDIES ON SUNSCREEN EFFICACY AGAINST SKIN CANCER DEVELOPMENT

Squamous Cell and Basal Cell Carcinomas

In the same Australian randomized trial discussed above for AK prevention, additional endpoints after 4.5 years of follow-up were the incidence of BCC and SCC, both in terms of numbers of people treated for newly diagnosed disease and total numbers of tumors occurring. Participants ($n = 1383$) underwent full-skin examination by a dermatologist in the follow-up period, and 250 were found to have developed 758 new skin cancers. There were no significant differences in the incidence of first new cancers between groups randomly assigned daily trial sunscreen or personal sunscreen use [BCC 2588 vs. 2509 per 100,000; rate ratio 1.03 (95% confidence interval, 0.73–1.46); SCC 876 vs. 996 per 100,000; rate ratio 0.88 (0.50–1.56)], but in terms of total numbers of tumors, SCC incidence was significantly lower in the trial sunscreen group [1115 vs. 1832 per 100,000; 0.61 (0.46–0.81)], although there was no effect on the incidence of BCCs. Cutaneous SCC numbers, but not apparently the numbers of people affected, thus seem amenable to reduction through the routine use of sunscreen by adults over 4.5 years. Such results may relate to varying levels of personal care in sunscreen application during the trial. β-Carotene supplementation again had no effect (5).

After cessation of the trial, participants were also followed for a further eight years to evaluate any possible latency of sunscreen preventive effect on the development of BCCs and SCCs. After this prolonged follow-up, BCC tumor rates tended to decrease (by 25%) though not significantly in people formerly randomized to trial sunscreen use compared with those applying personal sunscreen as they wished. By contrast, SCC tumor rates were significantly decreased by almost 40% during the entire follow-up period (rate ratio, 0.62; 95% confidence interval, 0.38–0.99). Regular application of sunscreen thus appears to have a prolonged preventive effect against SCC development, and perhaps also a minimal possible benefit in reducing BCC (6).

Multi-failure survival methods were also used in this study to evaluate the effect of sunscreen application on the time to first and then subsequent BCCs. Three different approaches of time to ordered multiple events were applied and compared, namely through the Andersen-Gill, Wei-Lin-Weissfeld, and Prentice-Williams-Peterson models. Robust variance estimation approaches were used for each model. Trial sunscreen treatment was not associated in the Andersen-Gill model with a reduced time to first BCC occurrence (hazard ratio = 1.04, 95% confidence interval, 0.79–1.45), but the time to subsequent tumors was probably reduced among the trial sunscreen group, although statistical significance was not reached (hazard ratio = 0.82, 0.59–1.15). Similarly, both the Wei-Lin-Weissfeld and the Prentice-Williams-Peterson models revealed trends toward a lower risk of subsequent BCC tumors among the sunscreen intervention group. These results demonstrate the importance of conducting multiple-event analysis for recurring events, as risk factors for a single event may differ from those when the events are repeated (7).

Hunter et al. on the other hand found a higher risk for BCC in women who used sunscreen than in those who did not in a retrospective study (8), this higher risk persisting even after multiple adjustments were made for confounding factors such as skin type and time spent out of doors. However, such studies are difficult to quantify with regard to exact UVR exposure and sunscreen use, and must be regarded with caution.

MALIGNANT MELANOMA

Efforts to assess whether sunscreens reduce the risk of MM have not been fully successful, mostly because this tumor is relatively rare compared with non-melanoma skin cancers, with only a tenth of the incidence of the latter (http://www.ncri.ie/ncri/index.shtml). Thus, clinical trials sufficiently powered to detect possible sunscreen efficacy must inevitably be extremely large to detect any significant change. Nevertheless, several retrospective epidemiological studies have suggested that sunscreen use may increase MM risk, and to study this apparent paradox further, an approximate surrogate and strong predictor for MM development, the development of high melanocytic nevus counts in adults, has been used instead in a number of clinical studies with and without sunscreen use.

One such randomized trial between 1993 and 1996 investigated the efficacy of a broad-spectrum, high-SPF sunscreen against the development of nevi in 458 white Canadian schoolchildren in grades 1 and 4. Three hundred and nine children were available for analysis. Each child's nevi were enumerated at the start and end of the study, and the parents of those randomly assigned to the active treatment ($n = 222$) were given a supply of SPF 30 broad-spectrum sunscreen with directions to apply it to the exposed sites of the child when he/she was expected to be in the sun for 30 minutes or more. Children in the control group ($n = 236$) received no sunscreen and no sun-care advice. Sunscreen group subjects developed fewer nevi than control group children (median counts, 24 vs. 28; $p = 0.048$), although significant interaction was detected with freckling in the sunscreen group, indicating that sunscreen use was more important for children with freckles than those without. Modelling of the data further suggested that freckled children in the sunscreen group developed 30% to 40% fewer nevi than freckled children in the control group. These data indicate that broad-spectrum sunscreens may attenuate the number of nevi occurring in white children, and thus possibly also the risk of MM, especially in those with freckles (9).

Another study examining the number of nevi in six- to seven-year-old European children, according to their reported sunscreen use, has also been conducted. Whole-body and site-specific counts of nevi 2 mm in diameter or larger were performed in 631 children in their first year of primary school in four European cities. Independently, parents were interviewed regarding the sun exposure, sunscreen use, and physical sun protection of their children. After adjustment for sun exposure and host characteristics, (e.g., skin phototype and eye color), the relative risk for high nevus counts on the trunk was 1.68 (95% confidence interval, 1.09–2.59) for the highest level of sunscreen use and 0.59 (0.36–0.97) for the highest level of wearing of clothes in the sun. Thus the sunscreen SPF had no effect on nevus counts despite a high median value of 17.4. Numbers of sunburns were also not associated with nevus count, the highest risk with sunscreen use in fact being among children who had never experienced burning. In white European children, therefore, sunscreen use appeared associated with the development of nevi, probably because it allowed a longer time in the sun with suboptimal product application. The wearing of clothes, however, appeared definitely effective in reducing nevus proliferation. The authors therefore concluded that as high nevus counts are a strong MM predictor, sunscreen use may facilitate MM occurrence by encouraging recreational sun exposure (10).

Benign pigmented nevi are clearly not MM, so definitive conclusions are not possible from these trials, more so because the sunscreen used and behavior of the study participants can clearly lead to variable study outcomes. Therefore, although the second series of results have led to suggestions that sunscreens may in fact increase MM risk, a more balanced view is that if sunscreens are used appropriately from early life and as part of an overall photoprotective package of reduced sun exposure, effective protective clothing, and careful sunscreen use, such problems seem unlikely to occur. However, effective sunscreen use appears to be uncommon, most users appearing to apply less than 50% and often less than 25% of the amount of product needed to provide the listed SPF. Greater care is therefore essential.

It is further well known that blistering sunburning in early life nearly doubles the risk of adult MM. Therefore, reducing childhood sunburning should reduce later MM development. From 2001 to 2004, a cluster-randomized trial of educational intervention to reduce sunburn rates (primary outcome) and improve sun-protection behavior (secondary outcome) was undertaken in Italian schoolchildren. A total of 122 primary schools (grades 2 and 3) were randomized to receive, or not, an intervention consisting of an educational curriculum at school, conducted by trained teachers, which included the showing of a short video and the distribution of booklets to children and their parents. Behavior while in the sun was assessed at baseline and 14 to 16 months afterwards. In a subgroup (44% of the total sample), melanocytic nevi were also counted. Of the 11,230 children enrolled, 8611 completed the study. A total of 1547 children (14%) reported a history of sunburns at baseline. At follow-up, no difference in sunburn episodes was documented between the study groups (odds ratio 0.97, 95% confidence interval 0.84–1.13), and similar sun protection habits were reported. No significant impact of the educational program was therefore documented at one-year follow-up (11). This very large study reproduces smaller studies carried out in a number of European countries, which all similarly conclude that although knowledge may improve, behavior does not seem to alter.

Finally, in a very high-risk group of adult renal transplant recipients, in whom skin cancer incidence is increased by up to 250 times, and all of whom had been repeatedly instructed in photoprotective behavior, male patients working outdoors, especially older ones at highest risk who had already developed skin cancer, were those who used sunscreens least, while low-risk females working indoors used them most (12).

Evidence points toward recreational UVR exposure as being the major risk factor for MM occurrence. A multinational study examined the effect of sun exposure on the risk of multiple primary MMs compared with that of one MM. People ($n = 2023$) with a first primary MM (controls) and people ($n = 1125$) with multiple primary MMs (cases) were enrolled in seven centers in four countries, had their residential history taken to enable estimation of their likely ambient UVR exposure, and were interviewed about their sun exposure. The risk of multiple primary MMs was increased significantly ($p < 0.05$), with an odds ratio of 2.10 for highest ambient UVR irradiance at birth and 10 years of age, 1.85

for beach and waterside activities, 1.57 for vacations in sunnier climates, 1.50 for sunburns, and 1.38 for lifetime recreational sun exposure. However, occupational sun exposure did not increase risk (odds ratio, 1.03 for highest exposure). Thus, recreational exposure at any age increased risk and appeared to add to that from ambient UVR exposure in early life. This study therefore concluded that people who have had an MM can expect to reduce their risk of further tumors by reducing their recreational sun exposure at any age. The same is also probably true for those who have never had an MM (13). Nevertheless, this study suggesting that sunscreen use might be helpful in reducing MM risk is based on sun exposure recall, which may not be fully reliable.

A provocative suggestion has also been made that any, rather than just careless, sunscreen use during exposure may promote skin cancer development. Thus, Garland hypothesized that such use in Queensland led to the steep rise in MM numbers seen there before the rest of Australia, where he suggested sunscreens were promoted later (14). However, Queensland is at a much lower latitude than much of the rest of Australia, so higher rates would be expected there anyway, and the comment was in fact a hypothesis rather than a researched study, so should not necessarily be given significant credence.

A research study leading to a similar possible conclusion, however, was undertaken by Autier et al. as a case-control study with 418 MM cases and 438 healthy controls in France, Belgium, and Germany (15). They considered in particular those who had sunburns in childhood and those who had not and those who were aware of the hazards of UVR exposure and those who were not. They then attempted to correct for these confounding factors and found higher risks for MM in each group for those who used sunscreen. However, the difficulty remained as to whether the corrections employed were appropriate, in that those who had experienced sunburn would indeed have been more at risk of skin cancer, and might also have tended to use less sunscreen, which was why they would tend to burn. Also, MM risk in adult life increases in any case with sunburn in childhood and adolescence, regardless of subsequent sunscreen use. Further, the amount of sunscreen used could clearly not have been reliably assessed retrospectively, and any subjects using sunscreen, presumably often poorly, were more likely to be exposed and at risk than those who were not.

Westerdahl et al. also performed a case-control study on 571 patients with MM and 913 healthy controls (16). All participants were asked about sunburn, hair color, sunbathing habits, and the use of sunscreen. A significantly elevated risk for MM was again associated with regular sunscreen use, despite adjustments with respect to sunburn history, hair color, and other factors. However, again, ensuring that sunscreen users were not those already most at risk of skin cancer was difficult to assess in such a retrospective study.

On the other hand, Holly et al. looked at the profile of 452 women with cutaneous MM in a population-based case-control study. Retrospective histories of sunburning and sunscreen use were compiled, together with other risk factors such as skin type. Ease of sunburning and the number and frequency of sunburns were again strongly associated with MM development, but sunscreen use now showed a decreased MM risk (17). A smaller case-control study carried out in Spain of 105 MM cases and 138 controls again showed that fair-skin type and sunburn increased MM risk, but once more that sunscreen use mitigated it (18). Next, a case-control study in Brazil of 103 MM patients and 206 matched controls, assessing multiple risk factors such as skin color, sunburn, and sunscreen use, showed that frequent sunburns once more increased risk but again that sunscreen use had a protective effect, now apparently correlating with increasing values of the SPF, although only values over SPF 15 showed significant protection (19).

Finally, however, a case-control study of 542 MM cases and 538 controls recruited from 27 Italian centers after multivariate analysis adjusting for age, sex, skin type, sunburns, and freckling showed no correlation at all between sunscreen use and subsequent MM risk (20).

Therefore, from the foregoing section, three studies suggest a protective effect of sunscreens against MM, two an increase in risk by encouraging prolonged sun exposure and one no effect at all. Review of these studies demonstrates variations in study size and design, which are likely to explain these discrepancies (21). More recently, a systematic review of all studies from 1966 to 2003 showed that there was no evidence to support the relationship between sunscreen use and an increased risk of melanoma (22,23).

OVERALL ASSESSMENT OF EFFICACY OF SKIN CANCER PREVENTION BY SUNSCREENS

In 2000, an international group of experts met at the International Agency for Research on Cancer (IARC) in Lyons and conducted a detailed review of the studies then available. They concluded that topical sunscreen use reduced the risk of sunburn and probably prevented SCC development if used mainly during unintentional sun exposure. However, no conclusions could be drawn concerning their efficacy against BCC and MM, although it was felt that there was insufficient evidence to say that sunscreen use increased MM risk. Nevertheless, sunscreen use can permit extended intentional sun exposure, which may almost certainly increase MM risk if the sunscreen is inadequately applied, or if sunscreen with inadequate broad-spectrum (UVB and UVA) coverage is used. The workshop therefore warned against a sole reliance on sunscreens for protection against UVR effects (24,25).

POSSIBLE ADVERSE EFFECTS OF SUNSCREEN PENETRATION INTO HUMAN SKIN

There is considerable evidence that so-called chemical (also known as organic) sunscreens, containing benzophenones, cinnamates, and other non-particulate substances, are partly absorbed into and through human skin. Absorption varies according to body site (26), concentration of the chemical and vehicle (27), and co-use with solvents such as insecticides and insect repellents (28). However, no evidence has been produced to suggest that such absorbed ingredients lead to harm (29), particularly as all have to pass vigorous toxicology testing, either as decreed by the Food and Drug Administration (FDA), which regulates sunscreens as drugs, or else by the European Union (EU), where toxicological testing is also stringent. Despite this, however, concerns have been raised as to whether potential endocrinological, particularly oestrogenic, or even carcinogenic effects may occur. On the other hand, detailed testing has shown no such harmful outcomes (29–32), although it does seem prudent to avoid the use of chemical sunscreens in infants, and perhaps also in those with very widespread skin disease, as the large body surface area to weight ratio of the former, and perhaps the more easily penetrated skin of both, may possibly lead to more significant blood concentrations.

Particulate, or mineral, sunscreens (also known as inorganic or physical sunscreens) such as zinc oxide (ZnO) and titanium dioxide (TiO$_2$), when used as nanoparticles, though often claimed to be inert, instead become highly reactive when UVR irradiated, generating free radicals potentially able to induce important DNA damage, particularly if epidermal basal cells or melanocytes are exposed. However, many studies have shown that not even nanoparticles of ZnO and TiO$_2$ penetrate to the viable epidermis (33,34) nor has any evidence of DNA damage been detected in vivo. Furthermore, such sunscreens have their mineral particles suspended in an organic resin coated with inorganic oxides, making them very photostable. Concerns regarding any potential harm have thus been largely dispelled, particularly as many such preparations are now also marketed with additives such as ascorbic acid (vitamin C), tocopherol (vitamin E), β-carotene, and other antioxidants, which can potentially further negate any free radical effects. The actual benefits of such additives are uncertain, however, having been extrapolated only from in vitro testing, but since it has been definitely shown that mineral sunscreens prevent DNA damage, and block p53 production, their safety in this respect seems assured.

AN OVERALL APPROACH TO EFFECTIVE PHOTOPROTECTION

The protection factor of a sunscreen in vivo is determined by the amount applied (35), and since sunscreens are generally used in an inadequate amount in practice (12,36), even by educated subjects, it is clear that their use alone will very commonly be insufficient for reliable skin cancer protection. Thus, exposed areas of skin are commonly missed, inadequate or uneven amounts of sunscreen are applied, or the sunscreen is applied late, irregularly, or forgotten altogether. Therefore, careful basic behavior when UVR intensity is high, particularly by fair-skinned subjects, such as exposure toward the end of the day, the seeking of shade, the use of clothing cover, and the wearing of hats should therefore be emphasised in addition to sunscreen use as very important aspects of reducing skin cancer risk. Such measures should be applied all year round in tropical areas, from March to October in temperate northern regions, and from October to March in southern climes.

Skin cancer is an increasing problem worldwide for all white-skinned races, with excessive UVR exposure as the major risk factor. All subjects when outdoors should therefore adopt the above overall approach to sun protection. If they do, along with avoiding use of sunbed, known to increase the risk of SCC and MM (37), a further increase, and eventually a decrease, in skin cancer incidence should steadily become evident over the decades to come.

REFERENCES

1. Young AR, Chadwick CA, Harrison GI, et al. The similarity of action spectra for thymine dimers in human epidermis and erythema suggests that DNA is the chromophore for erythema. J Invest Dermatol 1998; 111:982–998.
2. Naylor MF, Boyd A, Smith DW, et al. High sun protection factor sunscreens in the suppression of actinic neoplasia. Arch Dermatol 1995; 131:170–175.
3. Thompson SC, Jolley D, Marks R. Reduction of solar keratoses by regular sunscreen use. N Engl J Med 1993; 329:1147–1151.
4. Darlington S, Williams G, Neale R, et al. A randomized controlled trial to assess sunscreen application and beta carotene supplementation in the prevention of solar keratoses. Arch Dermatol 2003; 139:451–455.
5. Green A, Williams G, Neale R, et al. Daily sunscreen application and betacarotene supplementation in prevention of basal-cell and squamous-cell carcinomas of the skin: a randomised controlled trial. Lancet 1999; 354:723–729.
6. van der Pols JC, Williams GM, Pandeya N, et al. Prolonged prevention of squamous cell carcinoma of the skin by regular sunscreen use. Cancer Epidemiol Biomarkers Prev 2006; 15(12):2546–2548.
7. Pandeya N, Purdie DM, Green A, et al. Repeated occurrence of basal cell carcinoma of the skin and multifailure survival analysis: follow-up data from the Nambour Skin Cancer Prevention Trial. Am J Epidemiol 2005; 161:748–754.

8. Hunter DJ, Colditz GA, Stampfer MJ, et al. Risk factors for basal cell carcinoma in a prospective cohort of women. Ann Epidemiol 1990; 1:13–23.

9. Gallagher RP, Rivers JK, Lee TK, et al. Broad-spectrum sunscreen use and the development of new nevi in white children: randomized controlled trial. JAMA 2000; 283:2955–2960.

10. Autier P, Doré JF, Cattaruzza MS, et al. Sunscreen use, wearing clothes, and number of nevi in 6- to 7-year-old European children. European Organization for Research and Treatment of Cancer Melanoma Cooperative Group. J Natl Cancer Inst 1998; 90:1873–1880.

11. Naldi L, Chatenoud L, Bertuccio P, et al. Oncology Cooperative Group of the Italian Group for Epidemiologic Research in Dermatology (GISED). Improving sun-protection behavior among children: results of a cluster-randomized trial in Italian elementary schools. The "SoleSi SoleNo-GISED" Project. J Invest Dermatol 2007; 127:1871–1877.

12. Moloney FJ, Almarzouqi E, O'Kelly P, et al. Sunscreen use before and after transplantation and assessment of risk factors associated with skin cancer development in renal transplant recipients. Arch Dermatol 2005; 141:978–982.

13. Kricker A, Armstrong BK, Goumas C, et al. Ambient UV, personal sun exposure and risk of multiple primary melanomas. Cancer Causes Control 2007; 18:295–304.

14. Garland C, Garland F, Gorham E. Could sunscreens increase melanoma risk? Am J Public Health 1992; 82:614–615.

15. Autier P, Dore JF, Schifflers E, et al. Melanoma and use of sunscreens: an EORTC case control study in Germany, Belgium and France. The EORTC melanoma cooperative group. Int J Cancer 1995; 61:749–755.

16. Westerdahl J, Ingvar C, Masback A, et al. Sunscreen use and malignant melanoma. Int J Cancer 2000; 87:145–150.

17. Holly EA, Aston DA, Cress RD, et al. Cutaneous melanoma in women. I. Exposure to sunlight, ability to tan, and other risk factors related to ultraviolet light. Am J Epidemiol 1995; 141:923–933.

18. Rodenas JM, Gado-Rodriguez M, Herranz MT, et al. Sun exposure, pigmentary traits, and risk of cutaneous malignant melanoma: a case-control study in a Mediterranean population. Cancer Causes Control 1996; 7:275–283.

19. Bakos L, Wagner M, Bakos RM, et al. Sunburn, sunscreens, and phenotypes: some risk factors for cutaneous melanoma in southern Brazil. Int J Dermatol 2002; 41:557–562.

20. Naldi L, Gallus S, Imberti GL, et al. Sunscreens and cutaneous malignant melanoma: an Italian case-control study. Int J Cancer 2000; 86:879–882.

21. Dennis LK, Beane Freeman LE, Vanbeek MJ. Sunscreen use and the risk for melanoma: a quantitative review. Ann Intern Med 2003; 139:966–978.

22. Huncharek M, Kupelnick B. Use of topical sunscreens and the risk of malignant melanoma; a meta analysis of 9067 patients from 11 case-control studies. Am J Public Health 2002; 92:1173–1177.

23. Vainio H, Bianchini F. Cancer-preventive effects of sunscreens are uncertain. Scand J Work Environ Health 2000; 26:529–531.

24. Vainio H, Bianchini F. eds. IARC Handbook of Cancer Prevention Sunscreens. Vol. 5. Lyon: IARC Press, 2001.

25. Benson HA, Sarveiya V, Risk S, et al. Influence of anatomical site and topical formulation on skin penetration of sunscreens. Ther Clin Risk Manag 2005; 1:209–218.

26. Chatelain E, Gabard B, Surber C. Skin penetration and sun protection factor of five UV filters: effect of the vehicle. Skin Pharmacol Appl Skin Physiol 2003; 16:28–35.

27. Kasichayanula S, House JD, Wang T, et al. Percutaneous characterization of the insect repellent DEET and the sunscreen oxybenzone from topical skin application. Toxicol Appl Pharmacol 2007; 223:187–194.

28. Nohynek GJ, Schaefer H. Benefit and risk of organic ultraviolet filters. Regul Toxicol Pharmacol 2001; 33:285–299.

29. Janjua NR, Kongshoj B, Andersson AM, et al. Sunscreens in human plasma and urine after repeated whole-body topical application. J Eur Acad Dermatol Venereol 2008; 22:456–461.

30. Janjua NR, Kongshoj B, Petersen JH, et al. Sunscreens and thyroid function in humans after short-term whole-body topical application: a single-blinded study. Br J Dermatol 2007; 156:1080–1082.

31. Janjua NR, Mogensen B, Andersson AM, et al. Systemic absorption of the sunscreens benzophenone-3, octyl-methoxycinnamate, and 3-(4-methyl-benzylidene) camphor after whole-body topical application and reproductive hormone levels in humans. J Invest Dermatol 2004; 123:57–61.

32. Cross SE, Innes B, Roberts MS, et al. Human skin penetration of sunscreen nanoparticles: in-vitro assessment of a novel micronized zinc oxide formulation. Skin Pharmacol Physiol 2007; 20:148–154.

33. Lademann J, Weigmann H, Rickmeyer C, et al. Penetration of titanium dioxide microparticles in a sunscreen formulation into the horny layer and the follicular orifice. Skin Pharmacol Appl Skin Physiol 1999; 12:247–256.

34. Faurschou A, Wulf HC. The relation between sun protection factor and amount of suncreen applied in vivo. Br J Dermatol 2007; 156:716–719.

35. Azurdia RM, Pagliaro JA, Diffey BL, et al. Sunscreen application by photosensitive patients is inadequate for protection. Br J Dermatol 1999; 140:255–258.

36. International Agency for Research on Cancer Working Group on artificial ultraviolet (UV) light and skin cancer. The association of use of sunbeds with cutaneous malignant melanoma and other skin cancers: a systematic review. Int J Cancer 2006; 120:1116–1122.

37. International Agency for Research on Cancer Working Group on artificial ultraviolet (UV) light and skin cancer. The association of use of sunbeds with cutaneous malignant melanoma and other skin cancers: a systematic review. Int J Cancer 2007; 120(5):1116–1122.

8
Sunscreens, Photoimmunosuppression, and Photoaging

Gary M. Halliday
Discipline of Dermatology, Dermatology Research Laboratories, University of Sydney, Sydney, New South Wales, Australia

Herbert Hönigsmann
Department of Dermatology, Medical University of Vienna, Vienna, Austria

SYNOPSIS

- Aging of the skin consists of intrinsic aging and extrinsic aging or photoaging.
- Suberythemogenic doses of UV are sufficient to cause photoaging and immunosuppression. UVA has a major role in photoaging and immunosuppression. Therefore, sunscreen protection is less effective against immunosuppression than against sunburn.
- DNA photolesions, urocanic acid, NO, ROS, PGE_2, IL-10, and PAF are all involved in immunosuppression.
- Photoaging is triggered by receptor-initiated signaling, mitochondrial DNA mutations, protein oxidation, and telomere-based DNA damage responses.
- Protection against photoaging and immunosuppression consists of seeking shade and using sunscreens and photoprotective clothing. DNA repair enzymes and dietary botanicals show promise as protective agents.

INTRODUCTION

The immune system is essential for maintaining good health, as it destroys the majority of cells that develop abnormal or cancerous properties in addition to infectious agents, including viruses, bacteria, and parasites. Only tumor cells that fail to be eliminated by the immune system develop into a clinical cancer, and even then, they are controlled by the immune system, and sometimes even regress (1). As the skin is our external barrier, it is exposed to environmental insults in addition to receiving direct exposure to high levels of potentially infectious agents. It therefore needs a very effective immune system to deal with these health hazards. Ultraviolet radiation (UVR) in sunlight is probably the most dangerous environmental insult that the immune system of humans is exposed to. It suppresses immunity at exposure levels that are only 0.25 to 0.5 of those required to cause sunburn. It is therefore very important for sunscreens to provide a high level of protection to the immune system. A key challenge is how to protect the immune system from UVR without detracting from the beneficial effects of sunlight such as vitamin D production. Sunscreens do protect the immune system of humans from UV, but not as effectively as they prevent sunburn. This is probably due to UVA- in addition to UVB-suppressing skin immunity, while sunburn is largely due to UVB, and sunscreens provide a higher level of protection from UVB than UVA. Also, probably for the same reason, the sun protection factor (SPF), which is based on sunburn as a biological endpoint, does not predict how well a sunscreen protects the immune system.

Like the immune system, skin aging is a complex phenomenon that is controlled by both environmental factors and the genetic makeup of the individual. It consists of two different progressive processes that ultimately determine the skin appearance. Chronological or intrinsic aging affects both unexposed and UVR-exposed skin. In unexposed skin such as buttocks, abdomen, or upper inner arm, the changes are not too dramatic and are characterized by dryness, laxity, fine wrinkles, and skin atrophy. Extrinsic aging is the result of harmful environmental factors, mainly chronic repeated exposure to sunlight or UVR from artificial sources, hence it is more accurately termed "photoaging." It contributes to a premature aging phenotype even in younger individuals. As opposed to common beliefs, suberythemogenic doses suffice to induce chronic skin damage, both photoaging and immunosuppression. Whereas the action spectrum for UVR-induced tanning and erythema are almost identical and mostly attributable to UVB, indirect evidence suggests that UVA has a greater role in long-term sun damage and photoaging (2). Clinical characteristics comprise fine and coarse wrinkling, sagging, roughness, dryness, laxity, and pigmentary changes, and irregular mottled pigmentation, often associated with a leathery texture of the skin. Many of the functions of skin that decline with age show an accelerated decline in photoaged skin. Photoaging affects fair-skinned subjects (skin phototype I or II) most severely. There is also an increased risk of benign and malignant neoplasms on photoaged skin.

SKIN IMMUNITY

The immune system is broadly divided into two arms called cellular and humoral. Cellular refers to effector T lymphocytes migrating into the skin to destroy their target; humoral refers to B lymphocytes remaining in a lymphoid organ where they secrete antibody that reaches the skin via the blood to bind the target, leading to its destruction by activating effector mechanisms such as complement or phagocytosis. In both cases, skin immunity is dependent upon immune events that occur locally in the skin as well as activation of lymphocytes in secondary lymphoid organs, primarily skin-draining lymph nodes. Thus, skin immunity is not isolated to the skin but is dependent on events in internal organs of the body.

The epidermis and dermis both contain hematopoietic-derived dendritic antigen-presenting cells (DCs). In the epidermis, these are named "Langerhans cells" (LC) after Paul Langerhans who was the first to describe these cells (3,4). Upon sensing a signal suggesting that an immune response should be activated, such as cytokines from stressed keratinocytes that may be harboring an infection or undergoing malignant transformation, or pattern-recognition molecules from infectious agents binding to toll-like receptors in

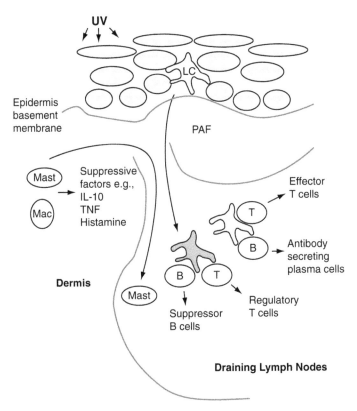

Figure 1 Immune system of the skin is suppressed by UV radiation. The immune system of the skin includes keratinocytes in the epidermis (*shaded circles, becoming oblong as they differentiate and move to surface of skin*) in addition to LC. LC take up antigen in the epidermis and migrate via dermal lymphatics to draining lymph nodes. Here, they present the antigen to T and B lymphocytes that develop into T effector and antibody-secreting plasma cells, respectively. T cells then migrate from the lymph nodes to the skin to destroy the antigen. UV radiation causes keratinocytes to produce immunosuppressive cytokines such as TNF and damages LC so that their numbers are depleted from the epidermis. UV also causes suppressor macrophages (Mac) to infiltrate the dermis where they secrete immunosuppressive factors such as IL-10. UV also activates mast cells to produce immunosuppressive factors, including histamine, and migrate to the draining lymph nodes. The combination of damaged LC and mast cells migrating to the lymph node, and other factors produced in response to UV radiation such as PAF, activates suppressor B and regulatory T cells that cause immunosuppression. See text for details and references. *Abbreviations*: LC, Langerhans cells; TNF, tumor necrosis factor; IL, interleukin; PAF, platelet-activating factor.

the skin, the DCs migrate to draining lymph nodes (5,6). If the DCs phagocytosed antigen while in the skin, they can then activate antigen-specific T and B lymphocytes in the draining lymph node, inducing effector immunity (Fig. 1). If DCs are not activated in the manner described above, then they activate regulatory T cells that suppress immunity (7). These cellular events are controlled by a large range of cytokines and other factors that are secreted by keratinocytes and other cells of the skin or immune system.

UVR-Induced Immunosuppression: Molecular and Cellular Mechanisms

UV can suppress immunity to antigen exposure at the locally irradiated site (local immunosuppression) and also to an antigen at a skin site distal to the irradiated site (systemic immunosuppression). Additionally, UV can suppress both the induction of primary immunity (response to first encounter with antigen) and reactivation of memory immunity (response to second encounter with antigen). It can therefore suppress many facets of the immune response. There is good evidence that UV is important for suppressing protective immunity to both cancers (8) and infectious agents (9). Considering how finely tuned the immune system is so that autoimmunity is not induced while protective immunity to tumors and infectious agents is activated, it is not surprising that UV, which extensively disrupts skin function, interferes with this process. Additionally, the immune system is regulated at multiple levels; there are many steps at which immunity is potentially susceptible to interference by UVR.

Several chromophores absorb UV, resulting in immunosuppression. DNA is a primary chromophore in which UV causes the formation of cyclobutane pyrimidine dimer (CPD) photolesions that can lead to immunosuppression (Fig. 2) in mice (10) and humans (11). It is unclear why these photolesions in DNA lead to immunosuppression. It is possible that they disrupt transcription of key genes or that their repair may use such large amounts of cellular energy that the cells are unable to mediate immune defence. This is consistent with our recent finding that nicotinamide, the precursor for NAD+, which is essential for ATP production, protects humans from UV immunosuppression (12). *Trans*-urocanic acid, which is found in the epidermis, isomerizes to *cis*-urocanic acid upon absorption of UV and contributes to UV immunosuppression (13,14). Recent evidence indicates that it may do this by binding to the serotonin receptor (15).

UVR also activates nitric oxide (NO) synthase, leading to increased NO production. Reactive oxygen species (ROS) are also produced following UV absorption by a large range of incompletely characterized chromophores (16). ROS and NO can interact to form long-lived reactive nitrogen species (Fig. 2). At low doses, these molecules contribute to signaling and activation of cells, while at higher doses they cause oxidative damage to lipids, proteins, and DNA, resulting in stress or damage to the cell, and at even higher doses they can kill the cells (17). ROS and NO contribute to UV-induced

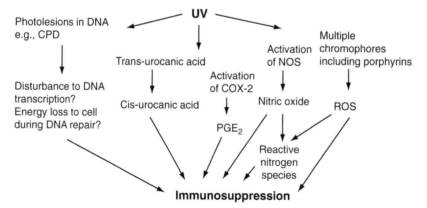

Figure 2 UV radiation is absorbed by chromophores in the skin and activates immunosuppressive mechanisms. UV is absorbed by DNA in skin cells, causing the formation of CPD, and by trans-urocanic acid, which isomerizes to the suppressive *cis* form. UV is also absorbed by a range of incompletely characterized chromophores resulting in the formation of ROS. It also activates the enzymes COX-2 and NOS, leading to production of PGs such as PGE_2 and NO, respectively. All of these events lead to immunosuppression. See text for details and references. *Abbreviations*: CPD, cyclobutane pyrimidine dimers; ROS, reactive oxygen species; COX-2, cyclooxygenase-2; NO, nitric oxide; NOS, nitric oxide synthase; PG, prostaglandin.

immunosuppression in both humans and mice (18–20), although whether this is due to redox signaling or oxidative damage is not known. Other key factors that contribute to UV immunosuppression include prostaglandin E_2 (PGE_2) produced from activated cyclo-oxygenase-2 (COX-2), interleukin (IL)-10 (21), and the phospholipid mediator platelet-activating factor (PAF) (22).

Considering that UV disrupts such a large number of molecular pathways leading to suppression of both primary and memory immunity, it is not surprising that many different immune cellular defects have been identified following UV exposure. UV reduces the number of LC in the skin, impairing the induction of immunity to an antigen applied locally to the irradiated skin (Fig. 1). UV causes damaged LC to migrate to draining lymph nodes where they have impaired ability to induce immunity (23–25). UV also causes mast cells to migrate from the skin to draining lymph nodes (26,27) and an influx of macrophages into the skin (28), both of which contribute to UV-induced immunosuppression. These alterations to LC, macrophages, and mast cells lead to a decrease in antigen-induced expansion of T effector and memory lymphocytes (29), thereby decreasing the magnitude of the immune response. This is accompanied by activation of both T (30) and B lymphocytes (31), which suppress immunity. Thus, UV causes a large number of major disturbances to cells of the skin immune system, including inhibition of antigen-presenting cells, T effector and memory cells, and also activation of T and B cells with immunosuppressive properties. This results in UV being a potent immunosuppressant.

Immunosuppression is Caused by Lower Doses of UVR Than are Required to Cause Sunburn

A key feature of UV-induced immunosuppression, which is important for sunscreen protection, is that it is caused by low doses of sunlight. Contact hypersensitivity (CS) is a skin immune response to contact allergens applied topically to the surface of the skin. UV that simulates the solar spectrum (solar-simulated UV, ssUV) has been shown to suppress primary immunity in light-skinned Caucasian humans at doses as low as 0.25 to 0.5 of the dose required to cause sunburn (32). SsUV doses about half of what is required to cause barely detectable sunburn in humans with skin types 1 to IV have also been shown to suppress the reactivation of memory immunity (33,34). Thus, for sunscreens to protect the immune system from the same dose of sunlight as they protect from sunburn, they would need to provide at least twice the protective capacity for immunosuppression as sunburn. Unfortunately, the level of protection of sunscreens for immunosuppression is substantially lower than that for sunburn.

PHOTOAGING: MOLECULAR AND CELLULAR MECHANISMS

Photoaging affects various layers of the skin with major damage seen in the connective tissue of the dermis. It is triggered by receptor-initiated signaling, mitochondrial damage, protein oxidation, and telomere-based DNA damage responses. Photodamaged skin displays variable epidermal thickness, dermal elastosis, decreased and or fragmented collagen, increased matrix-metalloproteinases (MMP), and inflammatory infiltrates (35,36).

In addition to being important for UVR-induced immunosuppression, ROS play a major role in photoaging and induce changes in gene expression pathways related to collagen degradation and elastin accumulation. There is evidence that singlet oxygen as generated by UVA irradiation results in the common deletion mutation of mitochondrial

DNA. Additionally, most likely through disruption of oxidative phosphorylation, it increases the overall ROS load, subsequently activating the transcription of MMP-encoding genes. Elevated MMPs degrade dermal collagen and elastin in skin. Most recently, Yarosh et al. reported that unirradiated fibroblasts increase MMP production and digest collagen when exposed to cell culture media from irradiated keratinocytes. Enhanced DNA repair in the keratinocytes ameliorates this response. This suggests that soluble factors induced by DNA damage in UVR-exposed epidermal keratinocytes signal collagen degradation by fibroblasts in the dermis (37).

The major role of ROS in aging is well accepted. The highest turnover of ROS occurs in the mitochondria (38), and it is estimated that 1% to 4% of oxygen uptake into the cell is turned into ROS (39). From rodent studies, the impact of mitochondria and mutations of the mitochondrial genome on aging is now generally accepted (40,41).

The same is true for UVR-induced skin aging where several groups could demonstrate the involvement of ROS-induced mitochondrial DNA mutations in the pathogenesis of photoaging (42–46). The frequency of mutations of mitochondrial DNA is 20 times that of nuclear DNA (44). The fact that mitochondria are the loci with the highest ROS production in the cell and also the loci of energy production through the respiratory chain strengthens the link between energy metabolism and aging in general and UVR-induced skin aging in particular (47). Topical and systemic antioxidants have been shown to supplement the photoprotective effects of sunscreen (48). Therapeutic interventions that decrease the formation of ROS and increase the cellular antioxidant enzyme levels and activities could restore homeostatic balances within the cell.

Recent evidence also suggests that signaling via transforming growth factor-β (TGF-β) may also play an important role in the pathophysiology of photoaging. TGF-β regulates cell differentiation, growth, and repair. In the epidermis, it exerts a negative effect on cell growth, whereas in the dermis it induces synthesis of procollagen and fibronectin. Recent studies have identified a correlation between TGF-β expression and age-related skin changes, in particular, solar elastosis (49–51).

Shortening of telomere lengths has been suggested to represent a molecular clock that signals replicative senescence. So far, telomere length has not been systematically studied in chronically irradiated cell cultures. However, there is evidence that oxidative stress results in telomere shortening, which triggers a p53-dependent cell cycle arrest (52). Both intrinsic skin aging and photoaging are postulated to disrupt the telomere loop and initiate DNA damage signaling through the p53 tumor suppressor protein (53).

PROTECTION FROM IMMUNOSUPPRESSION AND PHOTOAGING

Avoidance of sun exposure, sun-protective clothing, and regular use of sunscreens prevent progression of photoaging and photoimmunosuppression. Peak times for UV exposure are between 10 a.m. and 4 p.m., and sun avoidance should be encouraged during this time. Sunscreens are the first line of defense against UV irradiation. Many UV filters have been developed in recent years that combine sufficient UVB and UVA protection and are safe and cosmetically acceptable. However, preventive measures alone minimally reverse existing changes, although regression of actinic keratoses is well documented after prolonged periods of sunscreen application (54). New strategies may further improve currently used photoprotective measures. The addition of repair enzymes and/or antioxidants enhances the skin's recovery from UV-induced DNA damage. Several botanical agents, mainly vitamins and polyphenols, have been shown to influence signal transduction pathways leading to photoprotective effects (55).

Photoprotective Clothing

Clothing, hats, and sunglasses that protect from sun exposure must be part of a package of sensible protection. Photoprotective clothing is rated using the UV protection factor (UPF), which is defined as the amount of radiation filtered through a sample of fabric. A UPF of 40 to 50 provides excellent UV protection, transmitting less than 2.6% of effective UVR (56). Summer clothing characteristically has a UPF of 10 or higher and thus provides protection equivalent to that of an SPF 30 sunscreen in normal use (57).

A variety of different methods and standards exist for labeling UV-protective textiles, but none are mandatory for manufacturers. Assessment of UV transmission measured by spectrophotometric methods seems to be more suitable than in vivo methods. To fulfill the protective properties advocated by the Australian/New Zealand standard, the UPF must be greater than 15 (58), whereas UPF should be greater than 40 and average UVA transmission lower than 5% according to the European Committee for Standardization (59,60). A UPF of 40 or more was also recommended as sufficient for extreme exposures in every geographical location and as being adequate to resist against UPF-decreasing effects (e.g., stretch, wetness) (61). Recommendations exist, but there is no mandatory standard for photoprotective clothing in the United States at present (62).

Sunscreen Protection of the Immune System

The level of protection provided by a sunscreen is usually reported as an SPF. This is a ratio of the lowest dose of sunlight that causes sunburn with and without sunscreen protection. Therefore, it provides a guide to the fold change in sunlight dose that causes sunburn with sunscreen protection, rather than the absolute dose of sunlight that is reduced by the sunscreen. A similar concept, an immune protection factor (IPF), based on the same principles of a ratio of minimum immunosuppressive dose with and without sunscreen protection was first proposed by Bestak and colleagues (63) in murine studies, but has been widely adopted in human studies by a number of groups. The first report of this in humans found one sunscreen to have a lower IPF than SPF, while another sunscreen protected similarly from these biological endpoints (64).

Since then, a number of in vivo studies in humans by different research groups who have quantitated the level of immunoprotection provided by sunscreens have mostly come to similar conclusions that sunscreens protect the human immune system from ssUV, but in most cases not as effectively as they prevent sunburn. The technical differences in these studies, such as protocol of irradiation and immune endpoint have been contrasted in a consensus paper (65).

Using ssUV suppression of memory CS to nickel as an immune endpoint in humans, IPF has been compared to SPF and UVA protection factors (determined from UVA-induced minimal persistent pigment darkening) for six commercially available sunscreens. While IPF significantly correlated with UVA protection factors, immune protection was not related to SPF. Additionally, two measures of the breadth of spectrum protection, both determined from the absorption spectrum of the sunscreens, showed that the sunscreen breadth of absorption that extended into the UVA waveband significantly correlated with immune protective capacity (66). This indicates that the SPF does not predict the level of protection to the immune system and that UVA protection is important for a sunscreen to provide a high level of protection to the immune system. In these studies, the IPF of the sunscreens ranged from 18% to 131% of the SPF, but were mostly below the SPF.

Protection against systemic suppression of recall delayed-type hypersensitivity (DTH) to a range of antigens injected into the skin has also been found to be dependent on

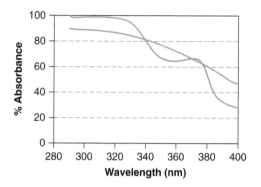

Figure 3 Absorption spectra of two modern commercially available sunscreens. Currently available sunscreens provide good broad-spectrum protection across the entire UV range, but absorb UVB better than UVA, with absorption decreasing as visible light is approached.

the ability of a sunscreen to protect from UVA (67). In another study, the level of protection of nickel recall CS was related to the sunscreen offering broad-spectrum protection (68). A further study of ssUV suppression of the induction of primary CS in humans found that the IPF was only about half the SPF of the sunscreen, and it was concluded that this was due to the poor UVA absorption by the sunscreen (69). This is consistent with two other studies in humans that found sunscreens with high UVA absorption to be substantially more protective than sunscreens with low UVA protection at preventing UV suppression of the induction of CS to dinitrochlorobenzene (70,71). A number of studies in mice have also found that sunscreens protect from UV-induced immunosuppression, but not as effectively as they prevent sunburn (72,73), and that good UVA absorption is important for a sunscreen to protect the immune system from UV (63,74).

The ability of sunscreens to prevent a particular biological response, in this case immunosuppression, is dependent on the wavebands of UV that cause the response, in relation to the absorption spectrum of the sunscreen. Even modern broad-spectrum sunscreens absorb UVB better than UVA (Fig. 3). They are generally less effective against long-wavelength UVA that is approaching the boundary with visible light (400 nm). A sunscreen that absorbed strongly in the long UVA waveband would also be likely to absorb visible light, unless a chemical filter with a sharp cutoff at 400 nm could be developed that also had other suitable characteristics for use in a sunscreen. A sunscreen filter with an absorption spectrum extending into the visible light range would be opaque, hence it would reduce sunscreen use by large proportions of the population; therefore, the inability of UVA filters to provide excellent protection at the long UVA spectrum, especially at 380 to 400 nm range, is probably unavoidable at present.

Sunburn is largely caused by UVB, with UVA only making a small contribution to this effect (75), and therefore UVA absorption only has a small effect on the SPF of a sunscreen. This contrasts with the immune system, as it is sensitive to both UVB and UVA. UVA suppresses reactivation of memory immunity to nickel (33) and reactivation of memory DTH responses in humans (67). UVA also suppresses the local induction of primary CS in humans (76). Interactions between these wavebands are evidenced by the observation that in humans UVA augments UVB-induced immunosuppression by a greater extent than either waveband alone would do (34,77). UVA has also been shown to suppress reactivation of memory DTH (74) and the induction of primary systemic CS (78) and primary local CS (79) in mice. However, other studies have reported UVA to be immunoprotective in mice (80), and this is likely to be dependent on UVA dose and mouse strain (78).

Thus, in summary, sunscreens are protective against UV-induced immunosuppression in humans, but not as effectively as against sunburn. This is probably due to UVA being highly immunosuppressive in humans and in some murine studies and sunscreens absorbing UVA less effectively than UVB.

Protection of UV-Induced Changes to Cellular and Molecular Aspects of the Immune System by Sunscreens

Sunscreens inhibit UVR from depleting LCs from the epidermis (81). The mixed lymphocyte reaction, where LCs from the skin stimulate proliferation of allogeneic lymphocytes in vitro, has been used to show that sunscreens also protect LC function from the effects of UV (82,83). Sunscreens also reduce UV-induced migration of suppressor macrophages into the skin (84).

Sunscreens prevent UV from increasing production of cytokines such as tumor necrosis factor (TNF) that are associated with immunosuppression (85). They also reduce UVA-induced free radical formation, but only by about 50%, which is considerably less protection than the SPF of the sunscreens (86). Sunscreens have also been shown to prevent photoisomerization of urocanic acid to the suppressive *cis* form in human skin (87,88).

Thus, sunscreens reduce many of the cellular and molecular changes that lead to photoimmunosuppression, although a lack of comprehensive dose-response studies make it difficult to determine the level of protection afforded by sunscreens in most cases. However, these data are consistent with sunscreens providing some level of immunoprotection.

Protection of Photoaging by Sunscreens

In animal studies, sunscreens have been shown to prevent photodamage and allow for its repair (89,90). Although direct clinical evidence is lacking, indirect evidence that sunscreen use can lead to repair of photodamage comes from numerous clinical trials in which sunscreens are used in both control and treatment arms (54).

Since UVA also has an important role in photoaging as well as photoimmunosuppression, the UVB-SPF alone may be a poor guide to the ability of a sunscreen to protect against photoaging. Sunscreens with greater UVA-blocking or -absorbing ability may be more effective at protecting against photodamage (91,92). The new regulations for sunscreen labeling within the European Union (93), which demand a UVA protection factor of at least one-third that of the UVB-SPF, will certainly help to improve protection. These regulations are expected to find worldwide acceptance.

Protection by DNA Damage Repair Enzymes

Because photoaging and photoimmunosuppression are due, at least in part, to UVR-induced DNA damage (as discussed above), enhancing cellular DNA repair capacity would likely reduce photodamage. Indeed, the enzyme T4 endonuclease V (T4N5), derived from a bacteriophage, recognizes CPD, the main DNA photolesions induced by UVB, and initiates repair by enhancing their cleavage (94). Encapsulating the enzyme in liposomes facilitates its delivery into the skin. Probably, through enhancing repair of DNA damage, T4N5 also decreases the synthesis and release of immunosuppressive cytokines like TNF and IL-10 (95) and reduces UVR-induced immunosuppression in humans (11). The delivery of enzymes that repair DNA damage or oligonucleotides that enhance the endogenous capacity for DNA damage repair may prove to be a valuable means of achieving protection against UV irradiation and decrease the incidence of chronic damage, including photoaging.

Systemic Protection

A new protective strategy has emerged from observations that oxidative stress plays a major role in the induction of photoaging and photoimmunosuppression. A large number of antioxidants have been found to exhibit protective effects against the different ROS involved in photoaging (96). The data suggesting these protective effects against ROS-induced photoaging derive mainly from in vitro studies (38). Thus, antioxidants may play an important role in the prevention of aging (38). It is unknown as to which antioxidants are the best and whether the topical or the oral route or combinations of both are most effective.

Dietary botanicals are of particular interest as some have been shown to inhibit UV-induced immune suppression and photocarcinogenesis. These chemopreventive agents reduce UVB-induced immunosuppression and photocarcinogenesis through the induction of immunoregulatory cytokines such as IL-12. This cytokine regulates DNA repair and stimulates cytotoxic T cells within tumors. Botanicals are of potential use as adjuncts with sunscreens in the prevention of photocarcinogenesis (97) and have been shown to be effective at protecting the immune system in clinical trials in humans (98).

Recently, orally administered *Polypodium leucotomos* (PL) (Heliocare®) was shown to decrease the incidence of phototoxicity in subjects receiving psoralen-UVA photochemotherapy (PUVA) treatment and in normal healthy subjects (99). PL extract is derived from a fern in Central America and has demonstrated potent antioxidant activity. It has been used in Mayan folk medicine as a remedy against rheumatic pain. Taken orally, it provides for an SPF of about 3. UV-exposed keratinocytes and fibroblasts treated with PL have also exhibited significantly improved membrane integrity, reduced lipid peroxidation, enhanced elastin expression, and inhibited MMP-1 expression (100). A preliminary study illustrated that PL treatment helped to ameliorate and to partially inhibit some of the histological damage associated with photoaging of skin (101). Thus, PL may be an additional measure to protect against photoaging in combination with topical sunscreens (102).

Another dietary substance of protective potential is silymarin, a naturally occurring polyphenolic flavonoid derived from the seeds of the milk thistle plant *Silybum marianu*. In animal studies, it has been shown to exhibit antioxidant, anti-inflammatory, and immunomodulatory properties that could contribute to preventing skin cancer as well as photoaging. It is bioavailable in skin and other tissues after systemic administration (103). Green tea polyphenols, administered topically or orally, have been shown to downregulate UV-induced erythema in humans, and photocarcinogenesis in mice. Rigorous clinical studies are clearly needed to validate the significance of these findings in the human setting.

CONCLUSIONS

The experimental evidence clearly shows that sunscreens currently available commercially do protect from photoimmunosuppression and photoaging. However, for two different reasons, they do not protect from immunosuppression to the same extent as they protect from sunburn. UVR suppresses immunity at lower doses than are required to cause sunburn. Therefore, even if sunscreens protect the skin against sunburn, immunosuppression could still occur. Furthermore, most sunscreens studied have a lower IPF than SPF. The reason for this appears to be quite straightforward and is due to the differences in action spectra for sunburn and immunosuppression. While sunburn is primarily due to UVB, with UVA only making a small contribution, UVA makes a large contribution to both immunosuppression and photoaging in humans. While modern broad-spectrum sunscreens do provide some level of protection right up to the long UVA waveband, they absorb UVB much more efficiently than UVA. This relatively poor absorption of UVA does not reduce the ability of sunscreens to provide high-level protection from sunburn, but does reduce their ability to provide high-level protection to the immune system and against photoaging. For these reasons, the SPF of a sunscreen does not predict how well the sunscreen protects the immune system, but a broad-spectrum sunscreen is more effective than the one with poor UVA absorption. The addition of biologically active ingredients to sunscreen filters that prevent key steps in UV immunosuppression and photoaging is likely to improve immunoprotection. Likely candidates include ROS scavengers or inhibitors and botanicals.

While photoaging has been considered in the past mainly to be a cosmetic problem, it is increasingly clear that prevention of photoaging, photodamage, and photoimmunosuppression may prevent the development of precancerous and cancerous skin lesions.

The use of photoprotective measures to prevent signs of photoaging is gaining increasing public interest, with many cosmetic products for daily use now containing sunscreens. The regular use of sunscreens should be encouraged, combined with so-called sunsmart behavior during the summer months or when on vacation in places with sunny climates. The daily use of products providing a full protection throughout the UV spectrum is beneficial to reduce skin damage contributing to premature skin aging (91). The only known defenses against photoaging beyond sun avoidance are the use of sunscreens and/or UV-protective clothes to block or reduce the amount of UV reaching the skin and perhaps the administration of DNA repair enzymes and antioxidant supplementation.

REFERENCES

1. Halliday GM, Patel A, Hunt MJ, et al. Spontaneous regression of human melanoma/nonmelanoma skin cancer: Association with infiltrating CD4+ T cells. World J Surg 1995; 19 (3):352–358.
2. Lim HW, Naylor M, Honigsmann H, et al. American Academy of Dermatology consensus conference on UVA protection of sunscreens: Summary and recommendations. J Am Acad Dermatol 2001; 44(3):505–508.
3. Stoitzner P, Tripp CH, Eberhart A, et al. Langerhans cells cross-present antigen derived from skin. Proc Natl Acad Sci U S A 2006; 103(20):7783–7788.
4. Granstein RD, Matsui MS. UV radiation-induced immunosuppression and skin cancer. Cutis 2004; 74:4–9.
5. Cumberbatch M, Dearman RJ, Griffiths CEM, et al. Langerhans cell migration. Clin Exp Dermatol 2000; 25(5):413–418.
6. Ebner S, Ehammer Z, Holzmann S, et al. Expression of C-type lectin receptors by subsets of dendritic cells in human skin. Int Immunol 2004; 16(6):877–887.
7. Heath WR, Carbone FR. Cross-presentation, dendritic cells, tolerance and immunity. Ann Rev Immunol 2001; 19:47–64.
8. Kripke ML. Immunologic unresponsiveness induced by UV radiation. Immunol Rev 1984; 80:87–102.
9. Norval M. The effect of ultraviolet radiation on human viral infections. Photochem Photobiol 2006; 82(6):1495–1504.
10. Kripke ML, Cox PA, Alas LG, et al. Pyrimidine dimers in DNA initiate systemic immunosuppression in UV-irradiated mice. Proc Natl Acad Sci U S A 1992; 89(16):7516–7520.

11. Kuchel JM, Barnetson RS, Halliday GM. Cyclobutane pyrimidine dimer formation is a molecular trigger for solar-simulated ultraviolet radiation-induced suppression of memory immunity in humans. Photochem Photobiol Sci 2005; 4(8):577–582.

12. Damian DL, Patterson CRS, Stapelberg M, et al. UV radiation-induced immunosuppression is greater in men and prevented by topical nicotinamide. J Invest Dermatol 2008; 128:447–454.

13. Noonan FP, De Fabo EC. Immunosuppression by Ultraviolet B Radiation: Initiation by Urocanic Acid. Immunol Today 1992; 13(7):250–254.

14. Norval M, Gibbs NK, Gilmour J. The role of urocanic acid in UV-induced immunosuppression—recent advances (1992–1994). Photochem Photobiol 1995; 62(2):209–217.

15. Walterscheid JP, Nghiem DX, Kazimi N, et al. Cis-urocanic acid, a sunlight-induced immunosuppressive factor, activates immune suppression via the 5-HT2A receptor. Proc Natl Acad Sci U S A 2006; 103(46):17420–17425.

16. Halliday GM. Inflammation, gene mutation and photoimmunosuppression in response to UVR-induced oxidative damage contributes to photocarcinogenesis. Mutat Res; Fundam Mol Mech Mutagen 2005; 571:107–120.

17. Rigas B, Sun Y. Induction of oxidative stress as a mechanism of action of chemopreventive agents against cancer. Br J Cancer 2008; 98(7):1157–1160.

18. Kuchel JM, Barnetson RS, Halliday GM. Nitric oxide appears to be a mediator of solar-simulated ultraviolet radiation-induced immunosuppression in humans. J Invest Dermatol 2003; 121(3):587–593.

19. Yuen KS, Halliday GM. Alpha-tocopherol, an inhibitor of epidermal lipid peroxidation, prevents ultraviolet radiation from suppressing the skin immune system. Photochem Photobiol 1997; 65(3):587–592.

20. Yuen KS, Nearn MR, Halliday GM. Nitric oxide-mediated depletion of Langerhans cells from the epidermis may be involved in UVA radiation-induced immunosuppression. Nitric Oxide 2002; 6(3):313–318.

21. Ullrich SE. Photoimmune suppression and photocarcinogenesis. Front Biosci 2002; 7:D684–D703.

22. Walterscheid JP, Ullrich SE, Nghiem DX. Platelet-activating factor, a molecular sensor for cellular damage, activates systemic immune suppression. J Exp Med 2002; 195(2):171–179.

23. Bergstresser PR, Toews GB, Streilein JW. Natural and perturbed distributions of Langerhans cells: responses to ultraviolet light, heterotopic skin grafting, and dinitrofluorobenzene sensitization. J Invest Dermatol 1980; 75(1):73–77.

24. Moodycliffe AM, Kimber I, Norval M. The effect of ultraviolet-B irradiation and urocanic acid isomers on dendritic cell migration. Immunology 1992; 77(3):394–399.

25. Vink AA, Moodycliffe AM, Shreedhar V, et al. The inhibition of antigen-presenting activity of dendritic cells resulting from UV irradiation of murine skin is restored by in vitro photorepair of cyclobutane pyrimidine dimers. Proc Natl Acad Sci U S A 1997; 94(10):5255–5260.

26. Byrne SN, Limon-Flores AY, Ullrich SE. Mast cell migration from the skin to the draining lymph nodes upon ultraviolet irradiation represents a key step in the induction of immune suppression. J Immunol 2008; 180(7):4648–4655.

27. Hart PH, Grimbaldeston MA, Swift GJ, et al. Dermal mast cells determine susceptibility to ultraviolet B-induced systemic suppression of contact hypersensitivity responses in mice. J Exp Med 1998; 187(12):2045–2053.

28. Hammerberg C, Duraiswamy N, Cooper KD. Active induction of unresponsiveness (tolerance) to DNFB by in vivo ultraviolet-exposed epidermal cells is dependent upon infiltrating class II MHC(+) CD11b(bright) monocytic/macrophagic cells. J Immunol 1994; 153(11):4915–4924.

29. Rana S, Byrne SN, Macdonald LJ, et al. Ultraviolet B suppresses immunity by inhibiting effector and memory T cells. Am J Pathol 2008; 172(4):993–1004.

30. Schwarz T. 25 years of UV-induced immunosuppression mediated by T cells—from disregarded T suppressor cells to highly respected regulatory T cells. Photochem Photobiol 2008; 84(1):10–18.

31. Byrne SN, Halliday GM. B cells activated in lymph nodes in response to ultraviolet irradiation or by interleukin-10 inhibit dendritic cell induction of immunity. J Invest Dermatol 2005; 124 (3):570–578.

32. Kelly DA, Young AR, McGregor JM, et al. Sensitivity to sunburn is associated with susceptibility to ultraviolet radiation-induced suppression of cutaneous cell-mediated immunity. J Exp Med 2000; 191(3):561–566.

33. Damian DL, Barnetson RS, Halliday GM. Low-dose UVA and UVB have different time courses for suppression of contact hypersensitivity to a recall antigen in humans. J Invest Dermatol 1999; 112(6):939–944.

34. Poon TSC, Barnetson RSC, Halliday GM. Sunlight-induced immunosuppression in humans is initially because of UVB, then UVA, followed by interactive effects. J Invest Dermatol 2005; 125(4):840–846.

35. Yaar M, Gilchrest BA. Photoageing: mechanism, prevention and therapy. Br J Dermatol 2007; 157(5):874–887.

36. Fisher GJ, Varani J, Voorhees JJ. Looking older. Fibroblast collapse and therapeutic implications. Arch Dermatol 2008; 144:666–672.

37. Yarosh D, Dong K, Smiles K. UV-induced degradation of collagen I is mediated by soluble factors released from keratinocytes. Photochem Photobiol 2008; 84(1):67–68.

38. Berneburg M, Plettenberg H, Krutmann J. Photoaging of human skin. Photodermatol Photoimmunol Photomed 2000; 16(6):239–244.

39. Barzilai A, Rotman G, Shiloh Y. ATM deficiency and oxidative stress: a new dimension of defective response to DNA damage. DNA Repair (Amst) 2002; 1(1):3–25.

40. Trifunovic A, Wredenberg A, Falkenberg M, et al. Premature ageing in mice expressing defective mitochondrial DNA polymerase. Nature 2004; 429(6990):417–423.

41. Yasui H, Sakurai H. Age-dependent generation of reactive oxygen species in the skin of live hairless rats exposed to UVA light. Exp Dermatol 2003; 12(5):655–661.

42. Birch-Machin MA, Tindall M, Turner R, et al. Mitochondrial DNA deletions in human skin reflect photo rather than chronologic aging. J Invest Dermatol 1998; 110(2):149–152.

43. Berneburg M, Gattermann N, Stege H, et al. Chronically ultraviolet-exposed human skin shows a higher mutation frequency of mitochondrial DNA as compared to unexposed skin and the hematopoietic system. Photochem Photobiol 1997; 66(2):271–275.

44. Berneburg M, Grether-Beck S, Kurten V, et al. Singlet oxygen mediates the UVA-induced generation of the photoaging-associated mitochondrial common deletion. J Biol Chem 1999; 274(22):15345–15349.

45. Berneburg M, Plettenberg H, Medve-Konig K, et al. Induction of the photoaging-associated mitochondrial common deletion in vivo in normal human skin. J Invest Dermatol 2004; 122 (5):1277–1283.

46. Berneburg M, Gremmel T, Kurten V, et al. Creatine supplementation normalizes mutagenesis of mitochondrial DNA as well as functional consequences. J Invest Dermatol 2005; 125 (2):213–220.

47. Berneburg M, Trelles M, Friguet B, et al. How best to halt and/or revert UV-induced skin ageing: strategies, facts and fiction. Exp Dermatol 2008; 17(3):228–240.

48. Edlich RF, Winters KL, Lim HW, et al. Photoprotection by sunscreens with topical antioxidants and systemic antioxidants to reduce sun exposure. J Long Term Eff Med Implants 2004; 14(4):317–340.

49. Yin L, Morita A, Tsuji T. The crucial role of TGF-beta in the age-related alterations induced by ultraviolet A irradiation. J Invest Dermatol 2003; 120(4):703–705.

50. Quan TH, He TY, Kang S, et al. Solar ultraviolet irradiation reduces collagen in photoaged human skin by blocking transforming growth factor-beta type II receptor/Smad signaling. Am J Pathol 2004; 165(3):741–751.

51. Tsoureli-Nikita E, Watson RE, Griffiths CE. Photoageing: the darker side of the sun. Photochem Photobiol Sci 2006; 5(2):160–164.

52. Saretzki G, Sitte N, Merkel U, et al. Telomere shortening triggers a p53-dependent cell cycle arrest via accumulation of G-rich single stranded DNA fragments. Oncogene 1999; 18 (37):5148–5158.

53. Kosmadaki MG, Gilchrest BA. The role of telomeres in skin aging/photoaging. Micron 2004; 35(3):155–159.

54. Darlington S, Williams G, Neale R, et al. A randomized controlled trial to assess sunscreen application and beta carotene supplementation in the prevention of solar keratoses. Arch Dermatol 2003; 139(4):451–455.

55. Verschooten L, Claerhout S, Van Laethem A, Agostinis P, Garmyn M. New strategies of photoprotection. Photochem Photobiol 2006; 82(4):1016–1023.

56. Morison WL. Photoprotection by clothing. Dermatol Ther 2003; 16(1):16–22.

57. Diffey BL. Sun protection with clothing. Br J Dermatol 2001; 144(3):449–450.

58. Georgouras KE, Stanford DG, Pailthorpe MT. Sun protective clothing in Australia and the Australian/New Zealand standard: an overview. Australas J Dermatol 1997; 38(suppl 1):S79–S82.

59. CEN-The European Committee for Standardization. Fabrics-solar UV protective properties-classification and marking of apparel. Stassart, Brussels: CEN, 1999:PrEN 13758.

60. Lautenschlager S, Wulf HC, Pittelkow MR. Photoprotection. Lancet 2007; 370(9586):528–537.

61. Laperre J, Gambichler T. Sun protection offered by fabrics: on the relation between effective doses based on different action spectra. Photodermatol Photoimmunol Photomed 2003; 19 (1):11–16.

62. Hatch KL. American standards for UV-protective textiles. Recent Results Cancer Res 2002; 160:42–47.

63. Bestak R, Barnetson RSC, Nearn MR, et al. Sunscreen protection of contact hypersensitivity responses from chronic solar-simulated ultraviolet irradiation correlates with the absorption spectrum of the sunscreen. J Invest Dermatol 1995; 105(3):345–351.

64. Damian DL, Barnetson RS, Halliday GM. Measurement of in vivo sunscreen immune protection factors in humans. Photochem Photobiol 1999; 70(6):910–915.

65. Fourtanier A, Moyal D, Maccario J, et al. Measurement of sunscreen immune protection factors in humans: A consensus paper. J Invest Dermatol 2005; 125(3):403–409.

66. Poon TSC, Barnetson RS, Halliday GM. Prevention of immunosuppression by sunscreens in humans is unrelated to protection from erythema and dependent on protection from ultraviolet A in the face of constant ultraviolet B protection. J Invest Dermatol 2003; 121(1):184–190.

67. Moyal DD, Fourtanier AM. Broad-spectrum sunscreens provide better protection from the suppression of the elicitation phase of delayed-type hypersensitivity response in humans. J Invest Dermatol 2001; 117(5):1186–1192.

68. Damian DL, Halliday GM, Barnetson RS. Broad-spectrum sunscreens provide greater protection against ultraviolet-radiation-induced suppression of contact hypersensitivity to a recall antigen in humans. J Invest Dermatol 1997; 109(2):146–151.

69. Kelly DA, Seed PT, Young AR, et al. A commercial sunscreen's protection against ultraviolet radiation- induced immunosuppression is more than 50% lower than protection against sunburn in humans. J Invest Dermatol 2003; 120(1):65–71.

70. Wolf P, Hoffmann C, Quehenberger F, et al. Immune protection factors of chemical sunscreens measured in the local contact hypersensitivity model in humans. J Invest Dermatol 2003; 121(5):1080–1087.

71. Baron ED, Fourtanier A, Compan D, et al. High ultraviolet A protection affords greater immune protection confirming that ultraviolet A contributes to photoimmunosuppression in humans. J Invest Dermatol 2003; 121(4):869–875.

72. Reeve VE, Bosnic M, Boehm-Wilcox C, et al. Differential protection by two sunscreens from UV radiation-induced immunosuppression. J Invest Dermatol 1991; 97:624–628.

73. Wolf P, Donawho CK, Kripke ML. Analysis of the protective effect of different sunscreens on ultraviolet radiation-induced local and systemic suppression of contact hypersensitivity and inflammatory responses in mice. J Invest Dermatol 1993; 100(3):254–259.

74. Nghiem DX, Kazimi N, Clydesdale G, et al. Ultraviolet A radiation suppresses an established immune response: Implications for sunscreen design. J Invest Dermatol 2001; 117(5):1193–1199.

75. McKinlay AF, Diffey BL. A reference action spectrum for ultraviolet induced erythema in human skin. CIE J 1987; 6:17–22.

76. LeVee GJ, Oberhelman L, Anderson T, et al. UVA II exposure of human skin results in decreased immunization capacity, increased induction of tolerance and a unique pattern of epidermal antigen-presenting cell alteration. Photochem Photobiol 1997; 65(4):622–629.

77. Kuchel JM, Barnetson RSC, Halliday GM. Ultraviolet A augments solar-simulated ultraviolet radiation-induced local suppression of recall responses in humans. J Invest Dermatol 2002; 118(6):1032–1037.

78. Byrne SN, Spinks N, Halliday GM. Ultraviolet A irradiation of C57BL/6 mice suppresses systemic contact hypersensitivity or enhances secondary immunity depending on dose. J Invest Dermatol 2002; 119(4):858–864.

79. Bestak R, Halliday GM. Chronic low-dose UVA irradiation induces local suppression of contact hypersensitivity, Langerhans cell depletion and suppressor cell activation in C3H/HeJ mice. Photochem Photobiol 1996; 64(6):969–974.

80. Reeve VE, Bosnic M, Boehm-Wilcox C, et al. Ultraviolet A radiation (320–400 nm) protects hairless mice from immunosuppression induced by ultraviolet B radiation (280–320 nm) or cis-urocanic acid. Int Arch Allergy Immunol 1998; 115(4):316–322.

81. Ho KKL, Halliday GM, Barnetson RS. Sunscreens protect epidermal Langerhans cells and Thy-1+ cells but not local contact sensitization from the effects of ultraviolet light. J Invest Dermatol 1992; 98(5):720–724.

82. Davenport V, Morris JF, Chu AC. Immunologic protection afforded by sunscreens *in vitro*. J Invest Dermatol 1997; 108(6):859–863.

83. Mommaas AM, van Praag MC, Bouwes Bavinck JN, et al. Analysis of the protective effect of topical sunscreens on the UVB-radiation-induced suppression of the mixed-lymphocyte reaction. J Invest Dermatol 1990; 95(3):313–316.

84. Hurks HMH, Vandermolen RG, Outluiting C, et al. Differential effects of sunscreens on UVB-induced immunomodulation in humans. J Invest Dermatol 1997; 109(6):699–703.

85. Hofmann-Wellenhof R, Smolle J, Roschger A, et al. Sunburn cell formation, dendritic cell migration, and immunomodulatory factor production after solar-simulated irradiation of sunscreen-treated human skin explants in vitro. J Invest Dermatol 2004; 123(4):781–787.

86. Haywood R, Wardman P, Sanders R, et al. Sunscreens inadequately protect against ultraviolet-A-induced free radicals in skin: Implications for skin aging and melanoma? J Invest Dermatol 2003; 121(4):862–868.

87. van der Molen RG, Out-Luiting C, Driller H, et al. Broad-spectrum sunscreens offer protection against urocanic acid photoisomerization by artificial ultraviolet radiation in human skin. J Invest Dermatol 2000; 115(3):421–426.

88. Olivarius FD, Wulf HC, Crosby J, et al. Sunscreen protection against cis-urocanic acid production in human skin. Acta Derm Venereol 1999; 79(6):426–430.

89. Kligman LH, Akin FJ, Kligman AM. Prevention of ultraviolet damage to the dermis of hairless mice by sunscreens. J Invest Dermatol 1982; 78(2):181–189.

90. Kligman LH, Akin FJ, Kligman AM. Sunscreens promote repair of ultraviolet radiation-induced dermal damage. J Invest Dermatol 1983; 81(2):98–102.

91. Seite S, Colige A, Piquemal-Vivenot P, et al. A full-UV spectrum absorbing daily use cream protects human skin against biological changes occurring in photoaging. Photodermatol Photoimmunol Photomed 2000; 16(4):147–155.

92. Takeuchi T, Uitto J, Bernstein EF. A novel in vivo model for evaluating agents that protect against ultraviolet A-induced photoaging. J Invest Dermatol 1998; 110(4):343–347.

93. European Commission's Recommendation of 22 September 2006 on the efficacy of sunscreen products and the claims made relating thereto. Document C 2006; 4089.

94. Yarosh D, Alas LG, Yee V, et al. Pyrimidine dimer removal enhanced by DNA repair liposomes reduces the incidence of UV skin cancer in mice. Cancer Res 1992; 52(15):4227–4231.

95. Wolf P, Maier H, Mullegger RR, et al. Topical treatment with liposomes containing T4 endonuclease V protects human skin in vivo from ultraviolet-induced upregulation of interleukin-10 and tumor necrosis factor-alpha. J Invest Dermatol 2000; 114(1):149–156.

96. Lawrence N. New and emerging treatments for photoaging. Dermatol Clin 2000; 18(1):99–112.

97. Katiyar SK. UV-induced immune suppression and photocarcinogenesis: chemoprevention by dietary botanical agents. Cancer Lett 2007; 255(1):1–11.

98. Friedmann AC, Halliday GM, Barnetson RS, et al. The topical isoflavonoid NV-07 alpha reduces solar-simulated UV-induced suppression of Mantoux reactions in humans. Photochem Photobiol 2004; 80(3):416–421.
99. Middelkamp-Hup MA, Pathak MA, Parrado C, et al. Oral Polypodium leucotomos extract decreases ultraviolet-induced damage of human skin. J Am Acad Dermatol 2004; 51(6):910–918.
100. Philips N, Smith J, Keller T, et al. Predominant effects of Polypodium leucotomos on membrane integrity, lipid peroxidation, and expression of elastin and matrix metalloproteinase-1 in ultraviolet radiation exposed fibroblasts, and keratinocytes. J Dermatol Sci 2003; 32(1):1–9.
101. Alcaraz MV, Pathak MA, Rius F, et al. An extract of Polypodium leucotomos appears to minimize certain photoaging changes in a hairless albino mouse animal model. A pilot study. Photodermatol Photoimmunol Photomed 1999; 15(3–4):120–126.
102. Gonzalez S, Alonso-Lebrero JL, Del Rio R, et al. Polypodium leucotomos extract: a nutraceutical with photoprotective properties. Drugs Today 2007; 43(7):475–485.
103. Baliga MS, Katiyar SK. Chemoprevention of photocarcinogenesis by selected dietary botanicals. Photochem Photobiol Sci. 2006; 5(2):243–253.

9
Effect of Photoprotection on Vitamin D and Health

Heike Bischoff-Ferrari
Centre on Aging and Mobility, University of Zurich, Zurich, Switzerland

Henry W. Lim
Department of Dermatology, Henry Ford Hospital, Detroit, Michigan, U.S.A.

SYNOPSIS

- There are only three sources of vitamin D: sunlight, diet (fatty fish, cod liver oil, egg yolk), and vitamin D supplement. Vitamin D_2 is less potent than D_3 in maintaining serum 25(OH)D levels.
- 700 to 1000 IU of vitamin D_3 per day may bring 50% of younger and older adults up to 75 to 100 nmol/L of serum 25(OH)D, a range that has been associated with optimal health, as assessed by bone health, muscle strength, fall prevention, prevention of hypertension, control of diabetes, risk of colorectal and breast cancers, and mortality from cancer (especially GI tract cancer).
- Individuals who practice rigorous photoprotection, those who stay/work mostly indoor, those with dark skin, and those who are obese are at risk to have less than adequate 25(OH)D levels. However, those living in sunny climate have also been shown to have low serum 25(OH)D levels.
- Balanced diet and vitamin D_3 supplement (1000 IU daily for adults at risk of vitamin D insufficiency), together with photoprotection, are the most appropriate approach to obtaining the beneficial effects of vitamin D and maintaining our cutaneous health.

METABOLISM OF VITAMIN D

Pre-Vitamin D_3 Production by the Skin

The two natural sources of vitamin D for humans are the sun and nutrition, with the sun being the major source. In human skin, pre-vitamin D_3 is produced photochemically from a cholesterol precursor, 7-dehydrocholesterol, which has a structure that resembles that of steroid hormones with a cyclopentanoperhydrophenanthrene ring. Most of pre-vitamin D_3 and vitamin D_3 (cholecalciferol) is manufactured in the lower epidermal layers of the skin, specifically in the stratum basale and stratum spinosum.

The maximal action spectrum for the synthesis of pre-vitamin D_3 from 7-dehydrocholesterol is at 300 ± 5 nm; both the intensity and the quality of UVB irradiation determine the amount of pre-vitamin D_3 produced. Accordingly, winter sunlight exposure may be largely insufficient in reaching the stratum basale and spinosum for the photocemical conversion of 7-dehydrocholesterol into pre-vitamin D_3, resulting in little or no vitamin D produced during winter months. On the other hand, unprotected skin will produce maximal vitamin D_3 in the summer months (1).

Another determinant of the quantity of vitamin D_3 produced in the skin is its concentration of melanin (i.e., skin pigmentation) (1). Melanin, produced by melanocytes located primarily in the stratum basale, is a neutral-density filter that absorbs UVB; the concentration of melanin determines the amount of UVB that can penetrate the 7-dehydrocholesterol containing lower epidermal region. In dark skin with high melanin content, the amount of vitamin D_3 synthesized per UVB exposure unit is reduced. Several studies have documented the pronounced variation in serum 25-hydroxyvitamin D [25(OH)D] levels by race/ethnicity, with the lowest levels documented in U.S. black individuals of all ages compared with their white counterparts (2–4). Consistently, a higher degree of tanning reduces the amount of vitamin D production in the skin per unit time spent in the sun due to increased melanin production (5). However, it is important to note that melanin does not change the amount of vitamin D that can be produced; rather the exposure time needed for vitamin D production is increased in individuals with darker skin pigmentation (6). Because of the higher minimal erythema doses to UVB (MED-B) in individuals with dark skin, it may take three to six times longer exposure for these individuals to produce the same amount of pre-vitamin D_3 compared with individuals with fair skin (6).

Additionally, the amount of UVB exposure time individuals require to produce a given amount of vitamin D depends on their distance from the equator. Individuals living at latitudes distant from the equator with prolonged winters will be exposed to less intense doses of UVB compared with those living closer to the equator; therefore, they produce less vitamin D despite the abundant availability of 7-dihydrocholesterol in their skin.

A key factor that affects the availability of 7-dihydroxyvitamin $(OH)_2$ D for pre-vitamin D_3 production is age. Compared with skin obtained from young individuals, skin from older persons may produce up to four times less pre-vitamin D_3 (7).

Dietary Sources of Vitamin D and Current Recommendations

Natural dietary sources of vitamin D are rare; significant amounts are primarily found in fatty fish, such as salmon, mackerel, and herring, with 240 to 1300 IU vitamin D_3 per serving (3 oz, or 85 grams), cod liver oil, and egg yolk. Thus, in some countries as the United States, milk has been fortified with vitamin D, which typically provides 100 IU per 8 oz glass. Notably, unless fatty fish and fortified milk products are consumed on a daily basis, diet alone is clearly an insufficient strategy to meet up-to-date recommendations of at least 800 IU vitamin D per day for fall and fracture prevention among older individuals (8,9) (Fig. 1). Furthermore, for those with lactose intolerance, fortified milk products are not an option.

The 1997 U.S. Dietary Reference Intake (DRI) recommendations for adequate intake of vitamin D for infants, children, and adults are listed on Table 1. With the development of the literature since 1997 suggesting that fall and fracture reduction, as well as general health benefits of vitamin D occur at higher 25(OH) D levels and higher intakes than defined by the 1997 DRIs, an update is being discussed by many experts.

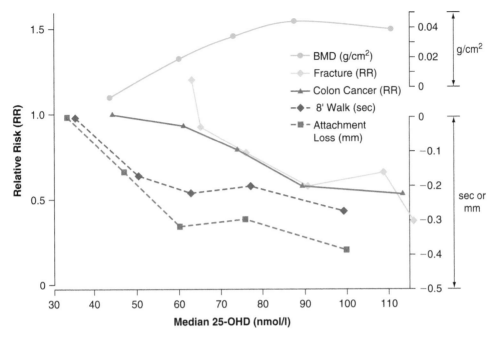

Figure 1 Solid lines relate to left axis, dashed lines relate to variables on right axis. The outcomes depicted as RRs are fracture risk [data from meta-analysis of RCTs (22)] and colon cancer [data from the Nurses Health Study (91)]. For BMD, the example of older Caucasian was chosen [data from NHANES III (3)] and the unit is displayed in the upper part of the right side y-axis. For lower extremity, we chose the 8 ft walk (8'walk) test results from NHANES III discussed in this chapter (47) and the unit is seconds, as shown on the lower half of the right side y-axis. Attachment loss is based on data discussed in this chapter (70) and is given in mm units for older men, as displayed on the lower half of the right side y-axis. On the basis of this summary of all outcomes, the desirable serum 25(OH)D level to be achieved for optimal health is at least about 75 nmol/L and best 90 to 100 nmol/L. *Source*: Adapted from Ref. 9.

Table 1 1997 U.S. Dietary Reference Intake (DRIs) Recommendations For Adequate Intake Of Vitamin D[a]

Age group	Recommendation (per day)
Children and adults up to 50-yr old	200 IU
Adults, 51–70-yr old	400 IU
Adults >70-yr old	600–800 IU

[a]1997 recommendation: Safe tolerable upper intake level (UL): 25 µg (1000 IU) per day for infants up to 12 months of age, and 50 µg (2000 IU) per day for children, adults, pregnant, and lactating women.

New data also suggest that the 1997-defined safe tolerable upper intake level of 50 µg/day (2000 IU) may be safely increased to 250 µg/day (10,000 IU) vitamin D per day (10).

Directly relevant to clinical practice, new data suggest that certain subgroups of the population, such as individuals with severe vitamin D deficiency of less than 12 ng/mL 25(OH)D (or 30 nmol/L) and obese individuals, will need higher vitamin D intakes to reach desirable 25(OH)D levels (11,12). Also, healthy adult individuals living above 30° latitude will need more than 200 to 600 IU vitamin D during winter months to reach desirable 25(OH)D levels of 75 to 100 nmol/L (9). Because of seasonal fluctuations of 25(OH)D levels (13), some individuals may be in the desirable range during summer months. However, these levels will not sustain during the winter months even in sunny latitudes (14,15). Furthermore, several studies suggest that many older persons will not achieve optimal serum 25(OH)D levels during summer months, suggesting that vitamin D supplementation should be independent of season in older persons (15–17).

As a 2007 example of an updated recommendation, the Canadian Cancer Society recommends that adults should consider taking vitamin D supplementation of 25 μg per day (1000 IU) a day during fall and winter (18). Furthermore, according to the Canadian Cancer Society, adults at higher risk of having lower vitamin D levels should consider taking vitamin D supplementation of 25 μg per day (1000 IU) all year round. This includes older people, people with dark skin, those who do not go outside often, and those who wear clothing that covers most of their skin (18). The Canadian recommendation is supported by several experts in the field of vitamin D (8,9,12,19,20).

25(OH)D and 1,25(OH)$_2$D

Both vitamin D_3 produced by the skin and vitamin D (D_3 or D_2) from dietary sources or supplements are hydroxylated by the liver to 25(OH)D, which is a largely unrestricted step (21). The metabolite 25(OH)D is the major circulating metabolite of vitamin D; its serum concentration has become the clinically accepted marker of vitamin D nutritional state (9,21). Although 25(OH)D needs further hydroxylation by the kidney to 1,25(OH)$_2$D, the so-called active metabolite, it is 25(OH)D that has been correlated with important endpoints such as fractures (22), function (23), diabetes (24), cancer (25), and blood pressure (26). We have learned in recent years that not only the kidney carries the 1-alpha-hydroxylase enzyme for 1,25(OH)$_2$D hydroxylation, but many other tissues (27), which may explain why the substrate 25(OH)D might better reflect the biologic effects of vitamin D.

What Dose of Vitamin D3 is Needed to Achieve Adequate 25(OH)D Levels, and What Levels are Considered Safe?

Studies suggest that 700 to 1000 IU of vitamin D per day may bring 50% of younger and older adults up to 75 to 100 nmol/L of serum 25(OH)D (28–30). Thus, to bring most older adults to the desirable range of 75 to 100 nmol/L, vitamin D doses higher than 700 to 1000 IU would be needed. The current intake recommendation for older persons (Table 1, 600 IU per day) may bring most individuals to 50 to 60 nmol/L, but not to 75 to 100 nmol/ L (3). In studies in young adults, intakes of as high as 4000 IU to 10,000 IU are known to be safe (31,32), and 4000 IU daily may bring 88% of healthy young men and women to at least 75 nmol/L of 25(OH)D (32). Heaney and colleagues, in a study of healthy men, estimated that 1000 IU vitamin D_3 per day are needed during winter months in Nebraska to maintain a late summer starting level of 70 nmol/L; in those with baseline 25(OH)D levels between 20 and 40 nmol/L, they may require a daily dose of 2200 IU vitamin D to reach and maintain 80 nmol/L level (12,31).

If 75 nmol/L of 25(OH)D were the minimum target level of a revised DRI, the new DRI should meet the requirements of 97% of the population (33). On the basis of a dose–response calculation proposed by Dr. Heaney of about 1.0 nmol/(1 μg day) at the lower end of the distribution and 0.6 nmol/(1 μg day) at the upper end (12), a daily oral dose of 2000 IU (50 μg/day), the safe upper intake limit as defined by the National Academy of Science (34), may shift the Third National Health and Nutrition Examination Survey (NHANES III) distribution so that only about 10% to 15% of individuals were below

75 nmol/L. This may result in a 35 nmol/L shift in already replete individuals from between 75 to 140 nmol/L (NHANES III distribution) to 110 to 175 nmol/L, which are levels observed in healthy outdoor workers (i.e. farmers: 135 nmol/L (35) and lifeguards: 163 nmol/L (36)). Notably, enhancing 25(OH)D levels to about 80 nmol/L will increase calcium absorption by up to 65% (37). Thus, calcium recommendations may need downward adjustment with a higher DRI for vitamin D; calcium intakes of 800 mg per day, rather than the current recommend daily value of 1000 mg, may be sufficient in a vitamin D–replete state (38). One study on the relative importance of vitamin D and calcium suggested that calcium supplementation above 800 mg per day may only improve calcium metabolism in individuals with low 25(OH)D levels (38).

Vitamin D toxicity can cause nausea, vomiting, poor appetite, constipation, weakness, and weight loss; it can also cause hypercalcemia, resulting in cardiac arrthymia, and calcinosis. As a first sign of toxicity, only serum 25(OH)D levels of above 220 nmol/L have been associated with hypercalcemia (39,40). Accordingly, the upper end of the acceptable range should probably not exceed 200 nmol/L (80 ng/mL).

Vitamin D_2 or Vitamin D_3

Supplemental vitamin D is sold in two forms, D2 (ergocalciferol) derived from plants and D3 (cholecalciferol), the physiologic form. D2 is less potent than D3 in maintaining 25(OH)D levels as a high intermittent or daily regimen, as suggested by two direct comparison trials (11,36), although this was challenged by a recent trial showing similar potency of daily D2 and daily D3 (37). However, because primary anti-fracture evidence is documented with daily 700 to 800 IU D3 (22), and because there is no anti-fracture evidence from classically randomized trials with D2 (41), there is no obvious advantage of vitamin D_2 over D_3 today.

VITAMIN D AND HEALTH

The Vitamin D Receptor (VDR) Knock-Out Mouse Model and its Perspectives in Vitamin D Effects on General Health

Perspectives from the VDR knock-out mouse model lend support to the close relationship between vitamin D and multiple health outcomes (42). Mice lacking the VDR have not only impaired bone formation (43), but also have small and atrophic muscle fibers (44), suffer from hypertension and cardiac hypertrophy (45,46), and have impaired insulin secretory capacities (47). These key abnormalities reflect symptoms observed in humans with vitamin D deficiency: men and women with 25(OH)D levels below 12 to 15 ng/mL (below 30–40 nmol/L) are at increased risk for low bone density (3), fractures (22), decreased lower extremity function and strength (23,48), and increased risk for incident hypertension (26,49) and type II diabetes (24). Consistently, the wide distribution of the VDR in all human organ systems plus the presence of the enzyme 1-alpha-hydroxylase in many tissues (27) suggest that the role of vitamin D may be beyond its established endocrine function balancing calcium uptake and bone health.

Benefit of a Higher 25(OH)D Serum Concentration on Bone Health

The association between serum 25(OH)D and hip bone mineral density (BMD) among humans was addressed among 13,432 individuals of NHANES III, including both younger (20–49 years) and older (50+ years) individuals, with different ethnic racial backgrounds were examined by some of the authors (3). Compared with subjects in the lowest quintile of 25(OH)D, those in the highest quintile had higher mean BMD by 4.1% in younger whites (test for trend; $p < 0.0001$), by 4.8% in older whites ($p < 0.0001$), by 1.8% in younger Mexican Americans ($p = 0.004$), by 3.6% in older Mexican Americans ($p = 0.01$), by 1.2% in younger blacks ($p = 0.08$) and by 2.5% in older blacks ($p = 0.03$). In the regression analysis, higher serum 25(OH)D levels were associated with higher BMD throughout the reference range of 22.5 to 94 nmol/L in all subgroups. In younger whites and Mexican Americans, higher 25(OH)D was associated with higher BMD even beyond 100 nmol/L. Consistent with the data from NHANES III, recent observational studies suggest that the association between 25(OH)D and BMD may be less in black individuals (50) and generally in individuals with darker skin tones (50,51), which may be explained, in part, by their smaller variation in 25(OH)D serum levels lacking the higher-end distribution of 25(OH)D levels observed in the white U.S. population (3,50).

A dose-response relationship between higher 25(OH)D serum levels and antifracture efficacy was suggested by a meta-analyses of high-quality double-blind primary prevention trials including older white individuals in the United States and Europe (22). The association was significant for both hip and any nonvertebral fracture based on meta-regression analyses, and remained significant after cross-calibration of the different assays to the widely used DiaSorin assay (52). Optimal fracture prevention appeared to occur in trials with achieved mean 25(OH)D levels of approximately 75 to 100 nmol/L. This level was reached only in trials that gave 700 to 800 IU cholecalciferol, and the pooled result from these trials resulted in a reduction of hip fractures by 26% (pooled RR = 0.74; 95% CI [0.61,0.88]) and any nonvertebral fracture by 23% (pooled RR = 0.77; 95% CI [0.68,0.87]) compared with calcium or placebo.

Benefit of a Higher 25(OH)D Serum Concentration on Muscle and Falling

The vitamin D effect on muscle adds a unique benefit to fracture prevention strategies beyond bone density, which is especially important in older individuals, and in the prevention of hip and nonvertebral fractures (22,53). The primary and highly prevalent risk factor of fractures in older individuals is muscle weakness and falling, which is why fall reduction should be an integral part of fracture prevention in the elderly (53–55).

Four lines of evidence support a role of vitamin D in muscle health. First, proximal muscle weakness is a prominent feature of the clinical syndrome of vitamin D deficiency (56,57). Second, The VDR is expressed in human muscle tissue (58) and vitamin D bound to its nuclear receptor in muscle tissue may promote de novo protein synthesis (56,59) and a relative increase in the diameter and number of type II muscle fibers (59). Third, several observational studies point towards a positive association between 25(OH)D and muscle strength or lower extremity function in older persons (23,60,61). Finally, in several double-blind randomized controlled trials, vitamin D supplementation increased muscle strength (62) and balance (63) and reduced the risk of falling in community-dwelling individuals unselected (64) or selected for a previous fall (65), as well as in institutionalized individuals (62,66,67). Fall reduction with vitamin D appears to depend on dose based on data from one multiple-dose trial (66) and a meta-analyses of high-quality trials with effects seen at higher intake of at least 700 IU, but not below (53).

A dose–response relationship between vitamin D status and muscle health was examined in NHANES III including 4100 ambulatory adults aged 60 years and older (23). Muscle function was assessed by the 8-ft walk test and sit-to-stand test (68,69). In both tests, performance speed continued to increase throughout the reference range of 25(OH) D (22.5–94 nmol/L) with most improvement starting at 25(OH)D levels of 60 nmol/L and optimal improvement occurring in 25(OH)D levels in the range of 75 to 100 nmol. Similar results were found in a Dutch cohort of older individuals (70).

Benefit of a Higher 25(OH)D Serum Concentration on Cardiovascular Health

In two small randomized controlled trials (RCTs), vitamin D supplementation reduced blood pressure in hypertensive subjects (71) and elderly community-dwelling women (72). In the latter trial, within two months, supplementation with vitamin D (800 IU/day) plus calcium (1200 mg/day) led to a decrease in systolic BP by 13 mmHg ($p = 0.02$), a decrease in diastolic BP by 6 mmHg ($p = 0.10$), and a decrease in heart rate by 4 bpm (beats/min) ($p = 0.02$) compared with calcium alone (1200 mg/day). Similarly, in a randomized controlled trial by Krause and colleagues, UVB irradiation significantly lowered systolic BP by 6 mmHg [-14;-1] and diastolic BP by 6 mmHg [-12;-2] within six weeks when compared with UVA irradiation (71). In the UVB group 25(OH)D levels increased from 58 to 151 nmol/L, while there was no increase in the UVA group.

With respect to optimal serum levels of 25(OH)D, there is evidence from two large prospective cohort studies among men and women that the serum level of 25(OH)D that confers the maximum benefit in regard to prevention of incident hypertension is 75 nmol/L or higher, with a significant trend between higher baseline 25(OH)D serum levels and lower risk of hypertension over a four-year follow-up (26). The difference in risk comparing individuals at the lower end of 37.5 nmol/L or less with those at the higher end of at least 75 nmol/L was 2.7-fold among women and 6.1-fold among men (26). Consistently, another large epidemiological study showed a significant relation between serum 25(OH)D concentrations and systolic, diastolic, and pulse pressure among the total adult population of NHANES III; the lowest pressure levels was observed at 25(OH)D levels above 85.7 nmol/L (49).

Mechanistically, going back to the mice lacking the VDR, Li and colleagues found that renin and angiotensin II expression was increased in these mice, leading to vasoconstriction (73). In humans, the stimulation of the renin angiotensin system has been associated with hypertension, myocardial infarction, and stroke (74,75).

Contributing to the cardiovascular benefit of vitamin D, several studies suggest a potential anti-atherosclerotic activity of vitamin D. In vascular smooth muscle, several studies have documented the presence of the VDR (76,77), and vitro studies have found that 1,25(OH)$_2$D antagonizes the mitogenic effect of epidermal growth factor on mesangial cell growth (78,79). Epidemiologically, a potential antiarteriosclerotic effect of vitamin D is supported by recent findings within NHANES 2001 to 2004, where across quartiles of 25(OH)D, from lowest to highest, the prevalence of peripheral arterial disease was 8.1%, 5.4%, 4.9%, and 3.7% (p trend <0.001) (80). After multivariable adjustment for demographics, comorbidities, physical activity level, and laboratory measures, the prevalence ratio of peripheral arterial disease for the lowest, compared with the highest, 25(OH)D quartile (<17.8 and ≥29.2 ng/mL, respectively) was 1.80 (95% CI 1.19, 2.74). For each 10 ng/mL (25 nmol/L) decrease in 25(OH)D level, the prevalence ratio of peripheral arterial disease increased by 35% (95% CI 15, 59%).

Benefit of a Higher 25(OH)D Serum Concentration on Diabetes

Type 1 Diabetes

High doses of 1,25(OH)$_2$D prevent insulitis and the onset of type 1 diabetes in VDR(-I-) mice (81) and nonobese diabetic-prone mice (NOD) (82), while dietary correction of hypocalemia alone does not. Furthermore, in NOD mice, vitamin D deficiency appears to accelerate type 1 diabetes (83), which mechanistically, may be explained by altered T-lymphocyte reponse (84).

Consistently, epidemiologic data suggest that vitamin D intake in early life may reduce the risk of type 1 diabetes in later life (85–87). Risk reduction was 26% with cod liver oil (85), 33% with general vitamin D supplementation (86), and 78% with 2000 IU per day vitamin D supplementation (87). These observations point to the importance of preventing vitamin D deficiency in early childhood. Whether a higher intake of vitamin D during pregnancy affects the diabetes risk of the offspring is less clear, however, in one study, lower levels of anti-islet cell antibodies were found in children of mothers with a higher food-derived intake of vitamin D during the third trimester of pregnancy (88).

Type 2 Diabetes

Laboratory studies among humans and large epidemiologic studies support a benefit of serum 25(OH)D concentrations on insulin sensitivity. In one study of 126 healthy adults, there was a positive correlation between 25(OH)D serum concentrations and insulin sensitivity as measured with hyperglycemic clamp ($r = 0.25$) (89), and in a study of 142 Dutch men aged 70 to 88 years, 25(OH)D serum concentrations were inversely correlated with serum insulin levels ($r = -0.18$ to -0.23) and glucose concentrations ($r = -0.26$) during an oral glucose tolerance test (90). In the NHANES III survey, including adults aged 20 years and older, for 25(OH)D levels of 81 nmol/L or higher compared with 43.9 nmol/L or lower, the OR was 0.25 (95% CI 0.11–0.60) among whites and 0.17 (95% CI 0.08–0.37) among Mexican Americans, without a difference observed among African-Americans (24). Furthermore, in the same cohort, serum 25(OH)D concentrations were inversely associated with insulin resistance [assessed by homeostasis model assessement of insulin resistant (HOMA-IR) method], with best levels observed in the top quartile of 25(OH)D of 81 nmol/L or higher (91).

In intervention studies, vitamin D supplementation increased insulin secretion among a small group of 10 patients with type II diabetes (92), whereas in another study of 35 type II diabetes patients, there was no change in insulin secretion with 1,25(OH)$_2$D treatment (93). In a larger three-year randomized controlled trial among 445 older individuals aged 65 years and older treated with either 700 IU vitamin D$_3$ plus 500 mg calcium or placebo, there was significant effect modification by baseline fasting glucose (94). Among participants with impaired fasting glucose at baseline, those who took combined calcium-vitamin D supplements had a lower rise in fasting blood glucose at three years compared with those on placebo ($p = 0.04$) and a lower increase in HOMA-insulin resistance ($p = 0.03$). As this study combined vitamin D with calcium, the effect may have been caused by either of the substances—vitamin D or calcium (95).

Benefit of a Higher 25(OH)D Serum Concentration on Cancer Risk and Mortality from Cancer

Most studies that have examined circulating 25(OH)D levels and subsequent risk of colorectal cancer or adenoma, the cancer precursor, have found a lower risk associated with higher 25(OH)D levels (96–103), with few exceptions (104). Furthermore, when the relationships between colorectal cancer and dietary or supplementary vitamin D have been investigated in cohort studies of men (105,106) and women (98,99,107–109) or both sexes (110,111), and in case-control studies (112–119), the majority of studies suggested inverse associations of vitamin D intake with colon or rectal cancer, or both (105–108,111,113,115,117,118). Most importantly, all the studies of colorectal cancer that took into account supplementary vitamin D reported an inverse association (106–108,111,118–120). Finally, after supplementation with vitamin D, circulating 25(OH)D levels are inversely associated with the size of the proliferative compartment in the colorectal mucosa in humans (121), and both 1,25(OH)$_2$D and 25(OH)D reduce proliferation and increase differentiation in vitro for colorectal cancer cells (122–125).

A recent meta-analysis of observational studies that reported risk of colorectal cancer by quantiles of 25(OH)D documented a significant dose–response relationship with a lower risk among individuals with higher 25(OH)D serum concentrations (p trend < 0.0001) (126). According to the pooled analysis, individuals with serum 25(OH)D of approximately 92.5 nmol/L (median of the top quintile) had a 50% lower risk of colorectal cancer than those with serum <15 nmol/L in the lowest quintile (126). Thus, consistent with an earlier review (9) and supported by a 2004 NIH (National Institute of Health) sponsored symposium on the role of vitamin D in cancer chemoprevention and treatment (12,127,128), optimal colorectal cancer prevention may be associated with serum 25(OH)D concentrations close to 90 nmol/L.

Finally, lending further support to the vitamin D-cancer hypothesis, an increment of 25 nmol/L in predicted 25(OH)D level was associated with a 17% reduction in total cancer incidence, a 29% reduction in total cancer mortality, and a 45% reduction in digestive-system cancer mortality in a comprehensive prospective analysis from a large male U.S. cohort (Health Professionals Follow-Up Study) (25). However, in a study of almost 17,000 participants in NHANES III, total cancer mortality was unrelated to baseline vitamin D status, although colorectal cancer mortality was inversely related to serum 25(OH)D level (129).

Vitamin D may also reduce breast cancer risk in women. A recent meta-analysis of observational studies that reported risk of breast cancer by quantiles of 25(OH)D documented a significant dose–response relationship with a lower risk among women with higher 25(OH)D serum concentrations (p trend < 0.001). According to the pooled analysis, women with serum 25(OH)D of approximately 120 nmol/L (median of the top quintile) had a 50% lower risk of breast cancer than those with serum <32 nmol/L in the lowest quintile (130).

For breast cancer, there is a phenotype from the mouse model lacking the VDR. These mice exhibit enhanced proliferation of mammary glands (131), and show increased proliferation response to exogeneously administered estrogen and progesterone (131). A calcium diet in these mice may normalize their estrogen levels and fertility (132), while the abnormal mammary phenotype is retained. In humans, breast cancer cells express the VDR (133) and 1,25(OH)$_2$D$_3$ suppresses growth of these cells, while promoting their differentiation (134).

Other Potential Benefits a Higher 25(OH)D Serum Concentration

Dental Health

Today, one RCT tested the benefit of vitamin D (700 IU/day) plus calcium (500 mg/day) supplementation compared with placebo with regard to tooth loss in healthy older individuals aged 65 years and older. Over a three-year treatment period, vitamin D plus calcium reduced tooth loss by 60% (OR = 0.4; 95% CI [0.2, 0.9]), while serum 25(OH)D levels increased from 71 nmol/L to 112 nmol/L in the treatment group (135). This effect is supported by two epidemiologic studies showing a significant inverse association between higher 25-hydrocyvitamin D levels and periodontal (136) disease and gingivitis (137). Periodontal disease and gingivitis are the leading causes of tooth loss, particularly in older persons (138–141), and tooth loss is an important determinant of nutrient intake and quality of life (142–144).

Osteoarthritis and Rheumatoid Arthritis

Osteoarthritis (OA) is the leading cause of disability in later age (145), and disability due to OA includes pain (146), muscle weakness (147), impaired function (13,14), falls (148–150), and fractures (149–152). Factors that have been associated with knee pain in OA are subchondral bone alterations (153,154), muscle weakness (155–158), and vitamin D deficiency (159). Two independent epidemiological studies demonstrated an inverse association of vitamin D and the risk for radiographic OA of the hip and knee. In the Framingham cohort study, risk of radiographic knee OA progression increased three- to fourfold for participants in the middle and lower tertile of both vitamin D intake (OR for lowest vs. highest tertile = 4.0, 95% CI, 1.4,11.6) and serum level (OR = 2.9, 95% CI, 1.0–8.2) (160). Low-serum vitamin D concentrations also predicted incident radiographic knee OA defined as loss of joint space (OR = 2.3, 95% CI, 0.9,5.5). In the Study of Osteoporotic Fractures, women in the lowest tertile of 25(OH)D levels were found to have an increased risk for development of hip OA defined as space narrowing (OR = 2.5, 95% CI, 1.1,5.3) at the hip joint and radiographic progression of disease (continuous measure of disease progression: $\beta = -0.1$, 95% CI, $-0.2, -0.02$) (161). The benefits of higher vitamin D intake or serum level in individuals with OA may be explained by the benefits of vitamin D on bone density (3,30,162,163), muscle strength (58,62,164,165), and function (60,62). In addition, some evidence suggests a direct cartilage effect of vitamin D by regulating less mature chondrocytes and promoting their maturation (166,167). Additionally, cartilage cell-line findings of OA patients indicate that the VDRs redevelop in the presence of vitamin D (168).

For rheumatoid arthritis (RA), in the Iowa Women's Health Study, greater total intake of vitamin D was inversely associated with risk of RA (RR = 0.67; 95% CI 0.44–1.0) (169). In another study of Italian individuals with RA, higher serum 25(OH)D levels were inversely correlated with disease activity [assessed by Disease Activity Score-28 joint count (DAS28)] during summer time (correlation coefficient = -0.57; $p < 0.0001$) (170). The documented benefit of vitamin D on disease activity may be due to the potential immunomodulatory effects of vitamin D. Activated T and B lymphocytes, macrophages, and monocytes carry the VDR (171,172), and a positive correlation has been found between interleukin levels (IL-1, IL-2) and $1,25(OH)_2D/25(OH)D$ ratio in synovial fluid of patients with RA (173).

Immune-Modulatory and Anti-inflammatory Effects

The immune-modulatory and anti-inflammatory effects of vitamin D are further supported by studies that suggest that a low 25(OH)D status is associated with a higher incidence in tuberculosis (174) and multiple sclerosis (175). For tuberculosis, recent data show a link between toll-like receptors and vitamin D-mediated innate immunity, and suggest that lower 25(OH)D levels in black individuals may contribute to their susceptibility to microbial infection (176).

PHOTOPROTECTION, SKIN COLOR, AND VITAMIN D

Sun Exposure and Serum Vitamin D Levels

As expected from a vitamin that is synthesized upon UVB exposure in epidermal keratinocytes, serum vitamin D levels correlated with sun exposure. As early as 1981, in a study done in Dundee, Scotland, it was reported that serum 25(OH)D levels among outdoor workers, with a mean age of 41 years, peaked at 80 nmol/L in November, while those of indoor workers, with a mean age of 32 years, 50 nmol/L in October. Since the peak of UV radiation was in July, the maximum serum levels occurring a few months later was attributed to the storage of vitamin D, a fat-soluble vitamin (177). In vitro, it has been demonstrated that skin from 77- and 82-year-old subjects had less capacity to synthesize vitamin D_3 compared with skin from 8- and 18-year-old subjects (7). This is reflected in a study of 912 men and women, all older than 65 years, over a 56 weeks period. The 25(OH) D levels fell with advancing age; while the levels were higher in the summer than winter, the values equalized (to about 10 ng/mL, or 25 nmol/L) by the age of 95 years (178).

More recent studies suggested that incidental sun exposure alone, even in geographic locations with abundant sunlight, may not be sufficient to achieve adequate vitamin D status (defined as 75 nmol/L, or 30 ng/mL) in a large portion of the studied population. Serum 25(OH)D levels in 30 premenopausal and 60 postmenopausal women were assessed in Santiago, Chile, a location that has mild Mediterranean-like climate. These women were otherwise healthy and fully ambulatory. Twenty seven percent of premenopausal women and sixty percent of postmenopausal subjects, had levels less than 50 nmol/L (or 20 ng/mL) (179). An analysis of published data on vitamin D status of postmenopausal women in Eastern Asia showed that using serum 25(OH)D level of 75 nmol/L (or 30 ng/mL) as cut-off, the prevalence of vitamin D insufficiency was 47% in Thailand, 49% in Malaysia, 90% in Japan and 92% in South Korea; using a lower cut-off level of 30 nmol/L (12 ng/mL), the prevalence was 21% in China and 57% in South Korea (180). Dietary deficiency, lifestyle choices, cultural customs, and aging were suggested by the authors as potential contributory factors to these findings.

Another study evaluated the serum 25(OH)D levels in 92 healthy natives (67 men, 28 women) residing in Kashmir Valley, northern India, for at least five years. The age range of the subjects was between 18 and 40 years (181). In spite of abundant sunlight, 49 of the 64 men, and 27 or the 28 women, for a total of 83% of subjects studied, had inadequate serum level of less than 50 nmol/L (or 20 ng/mL). Similarly, an evaluation of vitamin D status of 126 healthy ambulatory adults (18–87 years) in southeast Queensland, Australia, at the end of the winter showed 43% of the subjects had serum 25(OH)D level of less than 50 nmol/L; of note, in Queensland, winter is characterized by sunny climate. Levels were higher in those who spent more time in the sun, while the following factors were associated with lower levels: obesity, black hair, dark skin, or brown eyes (182).

Serum 25(OH)D levels in healthy, ambulatory volunteers (119 males and 82 females) living in Christchurch, New Zealand, were evaluated (183). The age range was 18–83 years, with a median of 45 years. When 75 nmol/L (30 ng/mL) was used as the cut-off, the results showed that 88% had vitamin D insufficiency at the end of summer (February) and all had insufficiency at the end of winter (June/July). Similar results were observed in a study done in Honolulu, Hawaii (184): Serum 25(OH)D was measured in 93 healthy adults, with self-reported sun exposure of 28.9 ± 1.5 hours per week. Levels of less than 75 nmol/L (or 30 ng/mL) were observed in 51% of the subjects.

Therefore, while sun exposure is associated with increase serum vitamin D levels, emerging data from many parts of the world show that living in sunny climate can still be associated with vitamin D insufficiency.

Photoprotection and Serum Vitamin D Levels

Conflicting data have been generated on the association of photoprotection and vitamin D status. In laboratory settings, application of sunscreen with an SPF8 significantly suppressed the increase in 25(OH)D levels following exposure to one minimal erythema dose of simulated sunlight (185). However, in a randomized, double-blind control trial of

113 healthy adults (>40 years), comparing the daily use of a broad-spectrum sunscreen (SPF17) versus placebo cream over a summer period showed no difference in the increase of serum 25(OH)D (186). A study of eight xeroderma pigmentosum patientswho practiced rigorous photoprotection, followed for six years, showed a mean serum 25(OH)D levels of 17.8 ± 1.5 ng/mL; they were associated with normal calcium, ionized calcium, and parathyroid hormone levels (187). A study of 24 sunscreen (SPF15) users and 19 controls over two years showed a significantly higher 25(OH)D levels in the summer of the second year in the nonsunscreen user group and significantly lower levels in the winter in the sunscreen group (188); however, the lower levels of serum vitamin D did not cause secondary hyperparathyroidism, or an increment in bone biological markers.

More recent studies also confirmed photoprotection resulted in decreased serum vitamin D levels. A study of 50 patients in Dublin, Ireland, with photosensitive lupus erythematosus who practiced good photoprotection showed that 64% of them had 25(OH)D levels of less than 80 nmol/L, and 4% had levels less than 25 nmol/L (or 10 ng/mL) (189). Evaluation of 25(OH)D levels among 36 internal medicine residents in Portland, Oregon, showed that 26% had levels <50 nmol/L (20 ng/mL) in the fall and 47% in the spring (190).

In summary, it is increasingly clear that photoprotection, or lack of outdoor activity, is associated with lower vitamin D levels. However, although data are limited, these lower levels have not been associated with secondary hyperparathyroidism, or detectable alteration in metabolism of bone.

Skin Types and Serum Vitamin D Levels

Several studies have shown that serum vitamin D levels are correlated with skin types. An evaluation of 25(OH)D levels in the US population demonstrated a mean level of 80 nmol/mL in whites, 60 nmol/L in Mexicans, and 50 nmol/L in African Americans (3). Among individuals older than 60 years, 67% of whites and 88% of African Americans had levels less than 80 nmol/L. Another study evaluated levels in Asians in the United Kingdom showed that 20% to 34% of children had levels less than 25 nmol/L, and 50% to 60% of adults had levels less than 12.5 nmol/L (191).

SUMMARY AND RECOMMENDATIONS

Data from many epidemiologic studies have now shown that serum 25(OH)D levels of 75 to 100 nmol/L are associated with optimal health, as assessed by bone health, muscle strength, fall prevention, prevention of hypertension, control of diabetes, risk of colorectal and breast cancers, and mortality from cancer (especially GI tract cancer). Other benefits associated with adequate levels of serum 25(OH)D include dental health, osteo- and rheumatoid arthritis, risk of tuberculosis, and risk of multiple sclerosis. Most of the studies used the physiologic form of vitamin D, which is vitamin D_3. Although data are conflicting, D2 probably is less potent than D_3 in maintaining 25(OH)D levels. Studies have shown that 700 to 1000 IU of vitamin D_3 per day may bring 50% of younger and older adults up to 75 to 100 nmol/L of 25(OH)D, strongly suggesting that the current U.S. Dietary Reference Intake (DRIs) recommendations for adequate daily intake of vitamin D (ranging from 200 IU for infants, to 600 IU/day for individuals older than 70 years) are probably too low.

Individuals who practice rigorous photoprotection, those who stay/work mostly indoor, and those with dark skin are at risk to have less-than-adequate 25(OH)D levels. However, data from many parts of the world showed that those living in sunny climate may still have low serum vitamin D levels. Furthermore, because vitamin D is a fat-soluble vitamin, obesity is also associated with low level of serum vitamin D.

Chronic sun exposure has been well established to be associated with photoaging and photocarcinogenesis (see Chapter 6). Therefore, to achieve and maintain optimum serum 25(OH)D levels of 75 to 100 nmol/L, a balanced diet and vitamin D supplement are the most appropriate ways of achieving this goal. It should be noted that unless fatty fish (the most common natural dietary source) and fortified milk products are consumed on a daily basis, diet alone is insufficient to achieve the optimum serum level. For individuals with lactose intolerance, fortified milk products are not an option. Current data indicate that for individuals at risk of vitamin D insufficiency, vitamin D_3 supplement at 1000 IU per day for adults is an appropriate amount to achieve optimum serum vitamin D level. Aside from the 1997 U.S. Dietary Reference Intake (DRIs) recommendation of 200 IU of vitamin D for infants and children, no rigorous study has been done to reevaluate this recommendation.

By practicing photoprotection, together with balanced diet and vitamin D supplement, one should be able to maintain our cutaneous health, as well as getting the beneficial effects of vitamin D.

REFERENCES

1. Chen TC, Chimeh F, Lu Z, et al. Factors that influence the cutaneous synthesis and dietary sources of vitamin D. Arch Biochem Biophys 2007; 460(2):213–217.
2. Harris SS, Dawson-Hughes B. Seasonal changes in plasma 25-hydroxyvitamin D concentrations of young American black and white women. Am J Clin Nutr 1998; 67(6):1232–1236.
3. Bischoff-Ferrari HA, Dietrich T, Orav EJ, et al. Positive association between 25-hydroxy vitamin D levels and bone mineral density: a population-based study of younger and older adults. Am J Med 2004; 116(9):634–639.
4. Bodnar LM, Catov JM, Wisner KL, et al. Racial and seasonal differences in 25-hydroxyvitamin D detected in maternal sera frozen for over 40 years. Br J Nutr 2008; 23:1–7.
5. Rockell JE, Skeaff CM, Williams SM, et al. Association between quantitative measures of skin color and plasma 25-hydroxyvitamin D. Osteoporos Int 2008; 12:12.
6. Lo CW, Paris PW, Holick MF. Indian and Pakistani immigrants have the same capacity as Caucasians to produce vitamin D in response to ultraviolet irradiation. Am J Clin Nutr 1986; 44(5):683–685.
7. MacLaughlin J, Holick MF. Aging decreases the capacity of human skin to produce vitamin D3. J Clin Invest 1985; 76(4):1536–1538.
8. Dawson-Hughes B, Heaney RP, Holick MF, et al. Estimates of optimal vitamin D status. Osteoporos Int 2005; 16(7):713–716. Epub 2005 Mar 18.
9. Bischoff-Ferrari HA, Giovannucci E, Willett WC, et al. Estimation of optimal serum concentrations of 25-hydroxyvitamin D for multiple health outcomes. Am J Clin Nutr 2006; 84(1):18–28.
10. Hathcock JN, Shao A, Vieth R, et al. Risk assessment for vitamin D. Am J Clin Nutr 2007; 85 (1):6–18.
11. Heaney RP. Barriers to optimizing vitamin D3 intake for the elderly. J Nutr 2006; 136 (4):1123–1125.
12. Heaney RP. The Vitamin D requirement in health and disease. J Steroid Biochem Mol Biol 2005; 15:15.
13. Dawson-Hughes B, Harris SS, Dallal GE. Plasma calcidiol, season, and serum parathyroid hormone concentrations in healthy elderly men and women. Am J Clin Nutr 1997; 65(1):67–71.
14. Grant WB, Holick MF. Benefits and requirements of vitamin D for optimal health: a review. Altern Med Rev 2005; 10(2):94–111.
15. McKenna MJ. Differences in vitamin D status between countries in young adults and the elderly. Am J Med 1992; 93(1):69–77.

16. Theiler R, Stahelin HB, Kranzlin M, et al. Influence of physical mobility and season on 25-hydroxyvitamin D-parathyroid hormone interaction and bone remodelling in the elderly. Eur J Endocrinol 2000; 143(5):673–679.

17. Holick MF. Environmental factors that influence the cutaneous production of vitamin D. Am J Clin Nutr 1995; 61(suppl):638S–645S.

18. Canadian Cancer Society. Available at: http://www.cancer.ca, 2007.

19. Vieth R. Why the optimal requirement for Vitamin D3 is probably much higher than what is officially recommended for adults. J Steroid Biochem Mol Biol 2004; 89–90(1–5):575–579.

20. Holick MF. Vitamin D: importance in the prevention of cancers, type 1 diabetes, heart disease, and osteoporosis. Am J Clin Nutr 2004; 79(3):362–371.

21. Norman AW. Sunlight, season, skin pigmentation, vitamin D, and 25-hydroxyvitamin D: integral components of the vitamin D endocrine system. Am J Clin Nutr 1998; 67(6):1108–1110.

22. Bischoff-Ferrari HA, Willett WC, Wong JB, et al. Fracture prevention with vitamin D supplementation: a meta-analysis of randomized controlled trials. JAMA 2005; 293(18):2257–2264.

23. Bischoff-Ferrari HA, Dietrich T, Orav EJ, et al. Higher 25-hydroxyvitamin D concentrations are associated with better lower-extremity function in both active and inactive persons aged >=60 y. Am J Clin Nutr 2004; 80(3):752–758.

24. Scragg R, Sowers M, Bell C. Serum 25-hydroxyvitamin D, diabetes, and ethnicity in the Third National Health and Nutrition Examination Survey. Diabetes Care 2004; 27(12):2813–2818.

25. Giovannucci E, Liu Y, Rimm EB, et al. Prospective study of predictors of vitamin D status and cancer incidence and mortality in men. J Natl Cancer Inst 2006; 98(7):451–459.

26. Forman JP, Giovannucci E, Holmes MD, et al. Plasma 25-hydroxyvitamin D levels and risk of incident hypertension. Hypertension 2007; 19:19.

27. Zehnder D, Bland R, Williams MC, et al. Extrarenal expression of 25-hydroxyvitamin d(3)-1 alpha-hydroxylase. J Clin Endocrinol Metab 2001; 86(2):888–894.

28. Tangpricha V, Pearce EN, Chen TC, et al. Vitamin D insufficiency among free-living healthy young adults. Am J Med 2002; 112:659–662.

29. Barger-Lux MJ, Heaney RP, Dowell S, et al. Vitamin D and its major metabolites: serum levels after graded oral dosing in healthy men. Osteoporos Int 1998; 8(3):222–230.

30. Dawson-Hughes B. Impact of vitamin D and calcium on bone and mineral metabolism in older adults. In: Holick MF, ed. Biologic Effects of Light 2001. Boston, MA: Kluwer Academic Publishers, 2002:175–183.

31. Heaney RP, Davies KM, Chen TC, et al. Human serum 25-hydroxycholecalciferol response to extended oral dosing with cholecalciferol. Am J Clin Nutr 2003; 77(1):204–210.

32. Vieth R, Chan PC, MacFarlane GD. Efficacy and safety of vitamin D3 intake exceeding the lowest observed adverse effect level. Am J Clin Nutr 2001; 73(2):288–294.

33. Yates AA. Process and development of dietary reference intakes: basis, need, and application of recommended dietary allowances. Nutr Rev 1998; 56(4 Pt 2):S5–S9.

34. Intakes ScotSEoDR (Standard Committee on the Scientific Evaluation of Dietary Reference). Dietary Reference Intakes: Calcium, Phosphorus, Magnesium, Vitamin D, and Fluoride. Washington, D.C.: National Academy Press, 1997.

35. Haddock L, Corcino J, Vazquez MD. 25(OH)D serum levels in the normal Puerto Rican population and in subjects with tropical sprue and paratyroid disease. P R Health Sci J 1982; 1:85–91.

36. Haddad JG, Chyu KJ. Competitive protein-binding radioassay for 25-hydroxycholecalciferol. J Clin Endocrinol Metab 1971; 33(6):992–995.

37. Heaney RP, Dowell MS, Hale CA, et al. Calcium absorption varies within the reference range for serum 25-hydroxyvitamin D. J Am Coll Nutr 2003; 22(2):142–146.

38. Steingrimsdottir L, Gunnarsson O, Indridason OS, et al. Relationship between serum parathyroid hormone levels, vitamin D sufficiency, and calcium intake. JAMA 2005; 294 (18):2336–2341.

39. Gertner JM, Domenech M. 25-Hydroxyvitamin D levels in patients treated with high-dosage ergo- and cholecalciferol. J Clin Pathol 1977; 30(2):144–150.

40. Vieth R. Vitamin D supplementation, 25-hydroxyvitamin D concentrations, and safety. Am J Clin Nutr 1999; 69(5):842–856.

41. Bischoff-Ferrari HA. How to select the doses of vitamin D in the management of osteoporosis. Osteoporos Int 2007; 18(4):401–407.

42. Bouillon R, Bischoff-Ferrari H, Willett W. Vitamin D and health: perspectives from mice and man. J Bone Miner Res 2008; 28:28.

43. Li YC, Amling M, Pirro AE, et al. Normalization of mineral ion homeostasis by dietary means prevents hyperparathyroidism, rickets, and osteomalacia, but not alopecia in vitamin D receptor-ablated mice. Endocrinology 1998; 139(10):4391–4396.

44. Endo I, Inoue D, Mitsui T, et al. Deletion of vitamin D receptor gene in mice results in abnormal skeletal muscle development with deregulated expression of myoregulatory transcription factors. Endocrinology 2003; 144(12):5138–5144. Epub 2003 Aug 13.

45. Li YC. Vitamin D regulation of the renin-angiotensin system. J Cell Biochem 2003; 88 (2):327–331.

46. Li YC, Qiao G, Uskokovic M, et al. Vitamin D: a negative endocrine regulator of the renin-angiotensin system and blood pressure. J Steroid Biochem Mol Biol 2004; 89–90(1–5):387–392.

47. Zeitz U, Weber K, Soegiarto DW, et al. Impaired insulin secretory capacity in mice lacking a functional vitamin D receptor. Faseb J 2003; 17(3):509–511.

48. Wicherts IS, van Schoor NM, Boeke AJ, et al. Vitamin D status predicts physical performance and its decline in older persons. J Clin Endocrinol Metab 2007; 6:6.

49. Scragg R, Sowers M, Bell C. Serum 25-hydroxyvitamin D, ethnicity, and blood pressure in the Third National Health and Nutrition Examination Survey. Am J Hypertens 2007; 20(7):713–719.

50. Hannan MT, Litman HJ, Araujo AB, et al. Serum 25-hydroxyvitamin D and bone mineral density in a racially and ethnically diverse group of men. J Clin Endocrinol Metab 2008; 93(1):40–46.

51. Hosseinpanah F, Rambod M, Hossein-Nejad A, et al. Association between vitamin D and bone mineral density in Iranian postmenopausal women. J Bone Miner Metab 2008; 26(1):86–92.

52. Lips P, Chapuy MC, Dawson-Hughes B, et al. An international comparison of serum 25-hydroxyvitamin D measurements. Osteoporos Int 1999; 9(5):394–397.

53. Bischoff-Ferrari HA, Dawson-Hughes B, Willett CW, et al. Effect of vitamin D on falls: a meta-analysis. JAMA 2004; 291(16):1999–2006.

54. Tinetti ME, Williams CS. Falls, injuries due to falls, and the risk of admission to a nursing home. N Engl J Med 1997; 337(18):1279–1284.

55. Bischoff-Ferrari HA. Fracture epidemiology in the elderly. In: Duque G, Kiel DP, eds. Osteoporosis in Older Persons Pathophysiology and Therapeutic Approach. Godalming, UK: Springer-Verlag London Limited, 2008.

56. Boland R. Role of vitamin D in skeletal muscle function. Endocr Rev 1986; 7:434–447.

57. Glerup H, Mikkelsen K, Poulsen L, et al. Hypovitaminosis D myopathy without biochemical signs of osteomalacic bone involvement. Calcif Tissue Int 2000; 66(6):419–424.

58. Bischoff-Ferrari HA, Borchers M, Gudat F, et al. Vitamin D receptor expression in human muscle tissue decreases with age. J Bone Miner Res 2004; 19(2):265–269.

59. Sorensen OH, Lund B, Saltin B, et al. Myopathy in bone loss of ageing: improvement by treatment with 1 alpha-hydroxycholecalciferol and calcium. Clin Sci (Colch) 1979; 56(2):157–161.

60. Mowe M, Haug E, Bohmer T. Low serum calcidiol concentration in older adults with reduced muscular function. J Am Geriatr Soc 1999; 47(2):220–226.

61. Dhesi JK, Bearne LM, Moniz C, et al. Neuromuscular and psychomotor function in elderly subjects who fall and the relationship with vitamin D status. J Bone Miner Res 2002; 17(5):891–897.

62. Bischoff HA, Stahelin HB, Dick W, et al. Effects of vitamin D and calcium supplementation on falls: a randomized controlled trial. J Bone Miner Res 2003; 18(2):343–351.

63. Pfeifer M, Begerow B, Minne HW, et al. Effects of a short-term vitamin D and calcium supplementation on body sway and secondary hyperparathyroidism in elderly women. J Bone Miner Res 2000; 15(6):1113–1118.

64. Bischoff-Ferrari HA, Orav EJ, Dawson-Hughes B. Effect of cholecalciferol plus calcium on falling in ambulatory older men and women: a 3-year randomized controlled trial. Arch Intern Med 2006; 166(4):424–430.

65. Prince RL, Austin N, Devine A, et al. Effects of ergocalciferol added to calcium on the risk of falls in elderly high-risk women. Arch Intern Med 2008; 168(1):103–108.

66. Broe KE, Chen TC, Weinberg J, et al. A higher dose of vitamin d reduces the risk of falls in nursing home residents: a randomized, multiple-dose study. J Am Geriatr Soc 2007; 55 (2):234–239.

67. Flicker L, MacInnis RJ, Stein MS, et al. Should older people in residential care receive vitamin D to prevent falls? Results of a randomized trial. J Am Geriatr Soc 2005; 53(11): 1881–1888.

68. Guralnik JM, Ferrucci L, Simonsick EM, et al. Lower-extremity function in persons over the age of 70 years as a predictor of subsequent disability. N Engl J Med 1995; 332(9):556–561.

69. Seeman TE, Charpentier PA, Berkman LF, et al. Predicting changes in physical performance in a high-functioning elderly cohort: MacArthur studies of successful aging. J Gerontol 1994; 49(3):M97–M108.

70. Wicherts IS, Schoor Van NM, Boeke AJP, et al. Vitamin D deficiency and neuromuscular performance in the Longitudinal Ading Study Amsterdam (LASA). J Back Musculoskeletal Rehabil 2005; 20(suppl 1):S35, abstract 1134.

71. Krause R, Buhring M, Hopfenmuller W, et al. Ultraviolet B and blood pressure. Lancet 1998; 352(9129):709–710.

72. Pfeifer M, Begerow B, Minne HW, et al. Effects of a short-term vitamin D(3) and calcium supplementation on blood pressure and parathyroid hormone levels in elderly women. J Clin Endocrinol Metab 2001; 86(4):1633–1637.

73. Li YC, Kong J, Wei M, et al. 1,25-Dihydroxyvitamin D(3) is a negative endocrine regulator of the renin-angiotensin system. J Clin Invest 2002; 110(2):229–238.

74. Laragh JH. Renin-angiotensin-aldosterone system for blood pressure and electrolyte homeostasis and its involvement in hypertension, in congestive heart failure and in associated cardiovascular damage (myocardial infarction and stroke). J Hum Hypertens 1995; 9(6):385–390.

75. Fujita T. Symposium on the etiology of hypertension–summarizing studies in 20th century. 5. Renin-angiotensin system and hypertension. Intern Med 2001; 40(2):156–158.

76. Koh E, Morimoto S, Fukuo K, et al. 1,25-Dihydroxyvitamin D3 binds specifically to rat vascular smooth muscle cells and stimulates their proliferation in vitro. Life Sci 1988; 42 (2):215–223.

77. Merke J, Hofmann W, Goldschmidt D, et al. Demonstration of 1,25(OH)2 vitamin D3 receptors and actions in vascular smooth muscle cells in vitro. Calcif Tissue Int 1987; 41(2):112–114.

78. Hariharan S, Hong SY, Hsu A, et al. Effect of 1,25-dihydroxyvitamin D3 on mesangial cell proliferation. J Lab Clin Med 1991; 117(5):423–429.

79. Mitsuhashi T, Morris RC Jr., Ives HE. 1,25-dihydroxyvitamin D3 modulates growth of vascular smooth muscle cells. J Clin Invest 1991; 87(6):1889–1895.

80. Melamed ML, Muntner P, Michos ED, et al. Serum 25-Hydroxyvitamin D Levels and the Prevalence of Peripheral Arterial Disease. Results from NHANES 2001 to 2004. Arterioscler Thromb Vasc Biol 2008; 16:16.

81. Gysemans C, van Etten E, Overbergh L, et al. Unaltered diabetes presentation in NOD mice lacking the vitamin D receptor. Diabetes 2008; 57(1):269–275.

82. Mathieu C, Laureys J, Sobis H, et al. 1,25-Dihydroxyvitamin D3 prevents insulitis in NOD mice. Diabetes 1992; 41(11):1491–1495.

83. Giulietti A, Gysemans C, Stoffels K, et al. Vitamin D deficiency in early life accelerates Type 1 diabetes in non-obese diabetic mice. Diabetologia 2004; 47(3):451–462.

84. Gregori S, Giarratana N, Smiroldo S, et al. A 1alpha,25-dihydroxyvitamin D(3) analog enhances regulatory T-cells and arrests autoimmune diabetes in NOD mice. Diabetes 2002; 51 (5):1367–1374.

85. Stene LC, Joner G. Use of cod liver oil during the first year of life is associated with lower risk of childhood-onset type 1 diabetes: a large, population-based, case-control study. Am J Clin Nutr 2003; 78(6):1128–1134.

86. Vitamin D supplement in early childhood and risk for Type I (insulin-dependent) diabetes mellitus. The EURODIAB Substudy 2 Study Group. Diabetologia 1999; 42(1):51–54.

87. Hypponen E, Laara E, Reunanen A, et al. Intake of vitamin D and risk of type 1 diabetes: a birth-cohort study. Lancet 2001; 358(9292):1500–1503.

88. Fronczak CM, Baron AE, Chase HP, et al. In utero dietary exposures and risk of islet autoimmunity in children. Diabetes Care 2003; 26(12):3237–3242.

89. Chiu KC, Chu A, Go VL, et al. Hypovitaminosis D is associated with insulin resistance and beta cell dysfunction. Am J Clin Nutr 2004; 79(5):820–825.

90. Baynes KC, Boucher BJ, Feskens EJ, et al. glucose tolerance and insulinaemia in elderly men. Diabetologia 1997; 40(3):344–347.

91. Chonchol M, Scragg R. 25-Hydroxyvitamin D, insulin resistance, and kidney function in the Third National Health and Nutrition Examination Survey. Kidney Int 2007; 71(2):134–139.

92. Borissova AM, Tankova T, Kirilov G, et al. The effect of vitamin D3 on insulin secretion and peripheral insulin sensitivity in type 2 diabetic patients. Int J Clin Pract 2003; 57(4):258–261.

93. Orwoll E, Riddle M, Prince M. Effects of vitamin D on insulin and glucagon secretion in non-insulin-dependent diabetes mellitus. Am J Clin Nutr 1994; 59(5):1083–1087.

94. Pittas AG, Harris SS, Stark PC, et al. The effects of calcium and vitamin D supplementation on blood glucose and markers of inflammation in nondiabetic adults. Diabetes Care 2007; 30 (4):980–986.

95. Pittas AG, Dawson-Hughes B, Li T, et al. Vitamin D and calcium intake in relation to type 2 diabetes in women. Diabetes Care 2006; 29(3):650–656.

96. Garland CF, Comstock GW, Garland FC, et al. Serum 25-hydroxyvitamin D and colon cancer: eight-year prospective study. Lancet 1989; 2:1176–1178.

97. Tangrea J, Helzlsouer K, Pietinen P, et al. Serum levels of vitamin D metabolites and the subsequent risk of colon and rectal cancer in Finnish men. Cancer Causes Control 1997; 8:615–625.

98. Feskanich D, Ma J, Fuchs CS, et al. Plasma vitamin d metabolites and risk of colorectal cancer in women. Cancer Epidemiol Biomarkers Prev 2004; 13(9):1502–1508.

99. Levine AJ, Harper JM, Ervin CM, et al. Serum 25-hydroxyvitamin D, dietary calcium in take, and distal colorectal adenoma risk. NutrCancer 2001; 39:35–41.

100. Peters U, McGlynn KA, Chatterjee N, et al. Vitamin D, calcium, and vitamin D receptor polymorphism in colorectal adenomas. Cancer Epidemiol Biomarkers Prev 2001; 10:1267–1274.

101. Platz EA, Hankinson SE, Hollis BW, et al. Plasma 1,25-dihydroxy-and 25-hydroxyvitamin D and adenomatous polyps of the distal colorectum. Cancer Epidemiol Biomarkers Prev 2000; 9:1059–1065.

102. Grau MV, Baron JA, Sandler RS, et al. Vitamin D, calcium supplementation, and colorectal adenomas: results of a randomized trail. J Natl Cancer Inst 2003; 95:1765–1771.

103. Slattery ML, Neuhausen SL, Hoffman M, et al. Dietary calcium, vitamin D, VDR genotypes and colorectal cancer. Int J Cancer 2004; 111(5):750–756.

104. Braun MM, Helzlsouer KJ, Hollis BW, et al. Prostate cancer and prediagnostic levels of serum vitamin D metabolites (Maryland, United States). Cancer Causes Control 1995; 6:235–239.

105. Garland C, Shekelle RB, Barrett-Conner E, et al. Dietary vitamin D and calcium and risk of colorectal cancer: a 19-year prospective study in men. Lancet 1985; 1:307–309.

106. Kearney J, Giovannucci E, Rimm EB, et al. Calcium, vitamin D and dairy foods and the occurrence of colon cancer in men. Am J Epidemiol 1996; 143:907–917.

107. Bostick RM, Potter JD, Sellers TA, et al. Relation of calcium, vitamin D, and dairy food intake to incidence of colon cancer in older women. Am J Epidemiol 1993; 137:1302–1317.

108. Martinez ME, Giovannucci EL, Colditz GA, et al. Calcium, vitamin D, and the occurrence of colorectal cancer among women. J Natl Cancer Inst 1996; 88:1375–1382.

109. Lin J, Zhang SM, Cook NR, et al. Intakes of calcium and vitamin D and risk of colorectal cancer in women. Am J Epidemiol 2005; 161(8):755–764.

110. Jarvinen R, Knekt P, Hakulinen T, et al. Prospective study on milk products, calcium and cancers of the colon and rectum. Eur J Clin Nutr 2001; 55:1000–1007.

111. McCullough ML, Robertson AS, Rodriguez C, et al. Calcium, vitamin D, dairy products, and risk of colorectal cancer in the cancer prevention study II nutrition cohort (United States). Cancer Causes Control 2003; 14:1–12.

112. Heilbrun LK, Nomura A, Hankin JH, et al. Dietary vitamin D and calcium and risk of colorectal cancer (letter). Lancet 1985; 1(8434):925.

113. Benito E, Stiggelbout A, Bosch FX, et al. Nutritional factors in colorectal cancer risk: a case-control study in Majorca. Int J Cancer 1991; 49:161–167.

114. Peters RK, Pike MC, Garabrandt D, et al. Diet and colon cancer in Los Angeles County, California. Cancer Causes Control 1992; 3:457–473.

115. Ferraroni M, La Vecchia C, D'Avanzo B, et al. Selected micronutrient intake and the risk of colorectal cancer. Br J Cancer 1994; 70:1150–1155.

116. Boutron MC, Faivre J, Marteau P, et al. Calcium, phosphorus, vitamin D, dairy products and colorectal carcinogenesis: a French case-control study. Br J Cancer 1996; 74:145–151.

117. Pritchard RS, A. BJ, Gerhardsson de Verdier M. Dietary calcium, vitamin D, and the risk of colorectal cancer in Stockholm, Sweden. Cancer Epidemiol Biomarkers Prev 1996; 5:897–900.

118. Marcus PM, Newcomb PA. The association of calcium and vitamin D, and colon and rectal cancer in Wisconsin women. Int J Epidemiol 1998; 27:788–793.

119. Kampman E, Slattery ML, Caan B, et al. Calcium, vitamin D, sunshine exposures, dairy products and colon cancer risk (United States). Cancer Causes Control 2000; 11:459–466.

120. Zheng W, Anderson KE, Kushi LH, et al. A prospective cohort study of intake of calcium, vitamin D, and other micronutrients in relation to incidence of rectal cancer among postmenopausal women. Cancer Epidemiol Biomarkers Prev 1998; 7:221–225.

121. Holt PR, Arber N, Halmos B, et al. Colonic epithelial cell proliferation decreases with increasing levels of serum 25-hydroxy vitamin D. Cancer Epidemiol Biomarkers Prev 2002; 11:113–119.

122. Meggouh F, Lointier P, Saez S. Sex steroid and 1,25-dihydroxyvitamin D3 receptors in human colorectal adenocarcinoma and normal mucosa. Cancer Res 1991; 51(4):1227–1233.

123. Giuliano AR, Franceschi RT, Wood RJ. Characterization of the vitamin D receptor from the Caco-2 human colon carcinoma cell line: effect of cellular differentiation. Arch Biochem Biophys 1991; 285(2):261–269.

124. Vandewalle B, Adenis A, Hornez L, et al. 1,25-dihydroxyvitamin D3 receptors in normal and malignant human colorectal tissues. Cancer Lett 1994; 86(1):67–73.

125. Zhao X, Feldman D. Regulation of vitamin D receptor abundance and responsiveness during differentiation of HT-29 human colon cancer cells. Endocrinology 1993; 132(4):1808–1814.

126. Gorham ED, Garland CF, Garland FC, et al. Optimal vitamin D status for colorectal cancer prevention: a quantitative meta analysis. Am J Prev Med 2007; 32(3):210–216.

127. The Vitamin D Workshop 2004. J Steroid Biochem Mol Biol 2005; 97(1–2):1–2. Epub 2005 Oct 20.

128. Bouillon R, Moody T, Sporn M, et al. NIH deltanoids meeting on Vitamin D and cancer. Conclusion and strategic options. J Steroid Biochem Mol Biol 2005; 97(1–2):3–5. Epub 2005 Jul 25.

129. Freedman DM, Looker AC, Chang SC, et al. Prospective study of serum vitamin D and cancer mortality in the United States. J Natl Cancer Inst 2007; 99:1594–602.

130. Garland CF, Gorham ED, Mohr SB, et al. Vitamin D and prevention of breast cancer: pooled analysis. J Steroid Biochem Mol Biol 2007; 103(3–5):708–711.

131. Zinser GM, Welsh J. Vitamin D receptor status alters mammary gland morphology and tumorigenesis in MMTV-neu mice. Carcinogenesis 2004; 25(12):2361–2372.

132. Johnson LE, DeLuca HF. Vitamin D receptor null mutant mice fed high levels of calcium are fertile. J Nutr 2001; 131(6):1787–1791.

133. Eisman JA, Suva LJ, Sher E, et al. Frequency of 1,25-dihydroxyvitamin D3 receptor in human breast cancer. Cancer Res 1981; 41(12 Pt 1):5121–5124.

134. Colston KW, Berger U, Coombes RC. Possible role for vitamin D in controlling breast cancer cell proliferation. Lancet 1989; 1(8631):188–191.

135. Krall EA, Wehler C, Garcia RI, et al. Calcium and vitamin D supplements reduce tooth loss in the elderly. Am J Med 2001; 111(6):452–456.

136. Dietrich T, Joshipura KJ, Dawson-Hughes B, et al. Association between serum concentrations of 25-hydroxyvitamin D3 and periodontal disease in the US population. Am J Clin Nutr 2004; 80(1):108–113.

137. Dietrich T, Nunn M, Dawson-Hughes B, et al. Association between serum concentrations of 25-hydroxyvitamin D and gingival inflammation. Am J Clin Nutr 2005; 82(3):575–580.

138. Ong G. Periodontal reasons for tooth loss in an Asian population. J Clin Periodontol 1996; 23:307–309.

139. Phipps KR, Stevens VJ. Relative contribution of caries and periodontal disease in adult tooth loss for an HMO dental population. J Public Health Dent 1995; 55:250–252.

140. Stabholz A, Babayof I, Mersel A, et al. The reasons for tooth loss in geriatric patients attending two surgical clinics in Jerusalem, Israel. Gerodontology 1997; 14:83–88.

141. Warren JJ, Watkins CA, Cowen HJ, et al. Tooth loss in the very old: 13–15-year incidence among elderly Iowans. Community Dent Oral Epidemiol 2002; 30:29–37.

142. Ritchie CS, Joshipura K, Hung HC, et al. Nutrition as a mediator in the relation between oral and systemic disease: associations between specific measures of adult oral health and nutrition outcomes. Crit Rev Oral Biol Med 2002; 13:291–300.

143. Marshall TA, Warren JJ, Hand JS, et al. Oral health, nutrient intake and dietary quality in the very old. J Am Dent Assoc 2002; 133(10):1369–1379.

144. Norlen P, Steen B, Birkhed D, et al. On the relations between dietary habits, nutrients, and oral health in women at the age of retirement. Acta Odontol Scand 1993; 51(5):277–284.

145. Guccione AA, Felson DT, Anderson JJ, et al. The effects of specific medical conditions on the functional limitations of elders in the Framingham Study. Am J Public Health 1994; 84 (3):351–358.

146. Felson DT, Zhang Y, Hannan MT, et al. The incidence and natural history of knee osteoarthritis in the elderly. The Framingham Osteoarthritis Study. Arthritis Rheum 1995; 38 (10):1500–1505.

147. Slemenda C, Brandt KD, Heilman DK, et al. Quadriceps weakness and osteoarthritis of the knee. Ann Intern Med 1997; 127(2):97–104.

148. Stewart A, Black AJ. Bone mineral density in osteoarthritis. Curr Opin Rheumatol 2000; 12 (5):464–467.

149. Arden NK, Nevitt MC, Lane NE, et al. Osteoarthritis and risk of falls, rates of bone loss, and osteoporotic fractures. Study of Osteoporotic Fractures Research Group. Arthritis Rheum 1999; 42(7):1378–1385.

150. Arden NK, Griffiths GO, Hart DJ, et al. The association between osteoarthritis and osteoporotic fracture: the Chingford Study. Br J Rheumatol 1996; 35(12):1299–1304.

151. Glowacki J, Hurwitz S, Thornhill TS, et al. Osteoporosis and vitamin-D deficiency among postmenopausal women with osteoarthritis undergoing total hip arthroplasty. J Bone Joint Surg Am 2003; 85-A(12):2371–2377.

152. Arden NK, Crozier S, Smith H, et al. Knee pain, knee osteoarthritis, and the risk of fracture. Arthritis Rheum 2006; 55(4):610–615.

153. Felson DT, Chaisson CE, Hill CL, et al. The association of bone marrow lesions with pain in knee osteoarthritis. Ann Intern Med 2001; 134(7):541–549.

154. Felson DT, McLaughlin S, Goggins J, et al. Bone marrow edema and its relation to progression of knee osteoarthritis. Ann Intern Med 2003; 139(5 Pt 1):330–336.

155. Rasch A, Dalen N, Berg HE. Test methods to detect hip and knee muscle weakness and gait disturbance in patients with hip osteoarthritis. Arch Phys Med Rehabil 2005; 86(12):2371–2376.

156. Baker K, McAlindon T. Exercise for knee osteoarthritis. Curr Opin Rheumatol 2000; 12 (5):456–463.

157. Baker KR, Nelson ME, Felson DT, et al. The efficacy of home based progressive strength training in older adults with knee osteoarthritis: a randomized controlled trial. J Rheumatol 2001; 28(7):1655–1665.

158. Bischoff HA, Roos EM. Effectiveness and safety of strengthening, aerobic, and coordination exercises for patients with osteoarthritis. Curr Opin Rheumatol 2003; 15(2):141–144.

159. Baker K, Zhang YQ, Goggins J, et al. Hypovitaminosis D and its association with muscle strength, pain and physical function in knee osteoarthritis: a 30-month longitudinal, observational study. Arthritis Rheum 2004; 50:S656–657.

160. McAlindon TE, Felson DT, Zhang Y, et al. Relation of dietary intake and serum levels of vitamin D to progression of osteoarthritis of the knee among participants in the Framingham Study. Ann Intern Med 1996; 125(5):353–359.

161. Lane NE, Gore LR, Cummings SR, et al. Serum vitamin D levels and incident changes of radiographic hip osteoarthritis: a longitudinal study. Study of Osteoporotic Fractures Research Group. Arthritis Rheum 1999; 42(5):854–860.

162. Dawson-Hughes B, Harris SS, Krall EA, et al. Effect of calcium and vitamin D supplementation on bone density in men and women 65 years of age or older. N Engl J Med 1997; 337(10):670–676.

163. Ooms ME, Roos JC, Bezemer PD, et al. Prevention of bone loss by vitamin D supplementation in elderly women: a randomized double-blind trial. J Clin Endocrinol Metab 1995; 80 (4):1052–1058.

164. Birge SJ, Haddad JG. 25-hydroxycholecalciferol stimulation of muscle metabolism. J Clin Invest 1975; 56(5):1100–1107.

165. Bischoff HA, Stahelin HB, Urscheler N, et al. Muscle strength in the elderly: its relation to vitamin D metabolites. Arch Phys Med Rehabil 1999; 80(1):54–58.

166. Boyan BD, Sylvia VL, Dean DD, et al. Differential regulation of growth plate chondrocytes by 1alpha, 25-(OH)(2)D(3) and 24R,25-(OH)(2)D(3) involves cell-maturation-specific membrane-receptor-activated phospholipid metabolism. Crit Rev Oral Biol Med 2002; 13(2):143–154.

167. Boyan BD, Sylvia VL, Dean DD, et al. 24,25-(OH)(2)D(3) regulates cartilage and bone via autocrine and endocrine mechanisms. Steroids 2001; 66(3–5):363–374.

168. Bhalla AK, Wojno WC, Goldring MB. Human articular chondrocytes acquire 1,25-(OH)2 vitamin D-3 receptors in culture. Biochim Biophys Acta 1987; 931(1):26–32.

169. Merlino LA, Curtis J, Mikuls TR, et al. Vitamin D intake is inversely associated with rheumatoid arthritis: results from the Iowa Women's Health Study. Arthritis Rheum 2004; 50 (1):72–77.

170. Cutolo M, Otsa K, Laas K, et al. Circannual vitamin d serum levels and disease activity in rheumatoid arthritis: Northern versus Southern Europe. Clin Exp Rheumatol 2006; 24(6):702–704.

171. Tsoukas CD, Provvedini DM, Manolagas SC. 1,25-dihydroxyvitamin D3: a novel immunoregulatory hormone. Science 1984; 224(4656):1438–1440.

172. Mathieu C, van Etten E, Decallonne B, et al. Vitamin D and 1,25-dihydroxyvitamin D3 as modulators in the immune system. J Steroid Biochem Mol Biol 2004; 89–90(1–5):449–452.

173. Inaba M, Yukioka K, Furumitsu Y, et al. Positive correlation between levels of IL-1 or IL-2 and 1,25(OH)2D/25-OH-D ratio in synovial fluid of patients with rheumatoid arthritis. Life Sci 1997; 61(10):977–985.

174. Nnoaham KE, Clarke A. Low serum vitamin D levels and tuberculosis: a systematic review and meta-analysis. Int J Epidemiol 2008; 37(1):113–119.

175. Munger KL, Levin LI, Hollis BW, et al. Serum 25-hydroxyvitamin D levels and risk of multiple sclerosis. JAMA 2006; 296(23):2832–2838.

176. Liu PT, Stenger S, Li H, et al. Toll-like receptor triggering of a vitamin D-mediated human antimicrobial response. Science 2006; 311(5768):1770–1773.

177. Devgun MS, Paterson CR, Johnson BE, et al. Vitamin D nutrition in relation to season and occupation. Am J Clin Nutr 1981; 34:1501–1504.

178. Dattani JT, Exton-Smith AN, Stephen JM. Vitamin D status of the elderly in relation to age and exposure to sunlight. Hum Nutr Clin Nutr 1984; 38(2):131–137.

179. GonzÄlez G, Alvarado JN, Rojas A, et al. High prevalence of vitamin D deficiency in Chilean healthy postmenopausal women with normal sun exposure: additional evidence for a worldwide concern. Menopause 2007; 14(3 Pt 1):455–461.

180. Lim SK, Kung AW, Sompongse S, et al. Vitamin D inadequacy in postmenopausal women in Eastern Asia. Curr Med Res Opin 2008; 24(1):99–106.

181. Zargar AH, Ahmad S, Masoodi SR, et al. Vitamin D status in apparently healthy adults in Kashmir Valley of Indian subcontinent. Postgrad Med J 2007; 83(985):713–716.

182. Kimlin M, Harrison S, Nowak M, et al. Does a high UV environment ensure adequate vitamin D status? J Photochem Photobiol B 2007; 89(2–3):139–147.

183. Livesey J, Elder P, Ellis MJ, et al. Seasonal variation in vitamin D levels in the Canterbury, New Zealand population in relation to available UV radiation. N Z Med J 2007; 120(1262): U2733.

184. Binkley N, Novotny R, Krueger D, et al. Low vitamin D status despite abundant sun exposure. J Clin Endocrinol Metab 2007; 92(6):2130–2135.

185. Holick MF. McCollum Award Lecture, 1994: vitamin D–new horizons for the 21st century. Am J Clin Nutr 1994; 60(4):619–630.

186. Marks R, Foley PA, Jolley D, et al. The effect of regular sunscreen use on vitamin D levels in an Australian population. Results of a randomized controlled trial. Arch Dermatol 1995; 131 (4):415–421.

187. Sollitto RB, Kraemer KH, DiGiovanna JJ. Normal vitamin D levels can be maintained despite rigorous photoprotection: six years' experience with xeroderma pigmentosum. J Am Acad Dermatol 1997; 37(6):942–947.

188. Farrerons J, Barnadas M, Rodríguez J, et al. Clinically prescribed sunscreen (sun protection factor 15) does not decrease serum vitamin D concentration sufficiently either to induce changes in parathyroid function or in metabolic markers. Br J Dermatol 1998; 139(3):422–427.

189. Cusack C, Murray B, Murphy, GM. Photoprotective behaviour and sunscreen use: the effect on vitamin D levels in cutaneous lupus erythematosus. Br J Dermatol 2007; 157(suppl 1):3–4.

190. Haney EM, Stadler D, Bliziotes MM. Vitamin D insufficiency in internal medicine residents. Calcif Tissue Int 2005; 76(1):11–16.

191. Young, AR, and Walker, SL. UV radiation, vitamin D and human health: an unfolding controversy introduction. Photochem Photobiol 2005; 81:1243–1245.

10

Systemic Effects of Topically Applied Sunscreen Ingredients

J. Frank Nash

Central Product Safety, The Procter & Gamble Company, Sharon Woods Technical Center, Cincinnati, Ohio, U.S.A.

SYNOPSIS

- The safety evaluation of UV filters is a structured process consisting of hazard and exposure assessments, the results of which are integrated to estimate human health risk.
- The dermal penetration of a UV filter is the "gate" through which systemic toxicity testing is routinely deemed necessary or unnecessary.
- There is no evidence that the inorganic UV filters, titanium dioxide and zinc oxide, penetrate beyond the stratum corneum of normal, undamaged skin regardless of particle size.
- Whereas organic sunscreens have been found to penetrate skin and have been measured in the blood and urine of human subjects, the systemic exposure is limited.
- A favorable human safety profile exists for commonly used organic and inorganic UV filters.

INTRODUCTION

Sunscreens contain ultraviolet (UV) filters, which absorb solar UV, thereby protecting the skin. Ideally, the UV filters should remain on the surface or in the upper layers of the stratum corneum to maximize product efficacy. For example, with oil/water emulsions, attempts are made to do this by using different materials in the vehicle such as film-forming polymers to maximize coverage and to keep the UV filters on the surface of the skin (1). Despite such efforts and as with any topically applied product, the possibility of absorption into and through the skin exists. If a topically applied ingredient enters the circulatory system, there is a need to understand potential systemic toxicity.

Although the skin penetration of most common UV filters is considered limited (2,3), some of them have been detected in blood and urine samples of humans after topical application of sunscreen products (4–6). Not surprisingly, as detection limits decrease with advanced, more sensitive analytical methods and the field of biomonitoring expands, reports of systemic absorption of UV filters will likely increase (7,8). The presence of a chemical does not by itself translate into adverse health effects. The process leading from exposure through biological effects is multifactorial and requires a careful assessment of each factor to be able to draw credible conclusions. Modern risk assessment practices provide a way to evaluate these various factors in a comprehensive way to address chemical safety concerns. Human risk assessment is defined as "the systematic scientific characterization of potential adverse health effects resulting from human exposures to hazardous agents or situations" (9). This means that a potential toxicity attributed to a chemical or hazardous agent requires information on its inherent toxicological properties and presence (i.e., exposure). Without both of these, i.e., hazard + exposure, the extrapolation from detection in the body to health-related toxicity is, at best, speculative.

There is a structured approach for evaluating the systemic toxicity of chemicals such as UV filters. The standard tests used to establish safety of UV filters and, for that matter, other cosmetic ingredients will be presented. Examples of systemic evaluation of inorganic and organic UV filters will be considered. For common UV filters used in most sunscreen products, systemic effects are minimal largely due to the rather poor dermal penetration. Nonetheless, as with any chemical, safety must be established on a case-by-case basis.

HUMAN SAFETY EVALUATION

The human safety evaluation of any chemical, including UV filters, consists of hazard and exposure assessments, the results of which are integrated to estimate human health risk. The hazard assessment includes in vitro and in vivo toxicological studies. In vitro studies include standard genotoxicity testing, e.g., Ames bacteria mutation assay, and a growing list of alternatives to animal testing. The in vivo studies comprise acute and repeated test material administration measuring any number of toxicological endpoints, often with the focus on systemic effects. In addition, in vitro and/or in vivo dermal penetration studies are conducted to estimate systemic bioavailability of the test material. Finally, given the functional nature of sunscreens, studies with concurrent UV exposure, i.e., photo-toxicology assessment, are often conducted. These may include in vitro photogenotoxicity and phototoxicity studies and in vivo photoirritation, photoallergenicity, and photo co-carcinogenicity studies. Exposure is typically determined using results from historic or empirically derived studies of habits and practices, which include application frequency, "dose," and duration of use.

Hazard Identification

The determination of the intrinsic toxicity of an ingredient or product is called hazard identification. Since, according to the dictum "the dose makes the poison," all materials will have some demonstrable toxicity.

The first step in the process of hazard identification is the chemical/physical characterization of the material, a list of which is presented in Table 1. This has always been a critical starting point in toxicology but has taken on a new level of importance with the concerns surrounding nanotechnology. Such descriptive information may be predictive of a toxicological event based on chemical alerts or class effects. For example,

Table 1 Chemical and Physical Properties of a Test Material

Specification	Description
Chemical identity	Molecular formula/components
Physical form	Gas, liquid, solid (particle size)
Molecular weight	Given in Daltons
Purity	Quality
Characterization of impurities	For polymers, it is imperative to know the monomer
Solubility	Water, organic solvent
Oil/water partition coefficient	n-Octanol/water
Absorption (UV/visible)	Wavelengths and efficiency
Additional information	Color, smell, flash point, etc.

Abbreviation: UV, ultraviolet.

the benzophenone "family" of UV filters, i.e., benzophenone-2, -3, -4, etc., has many of the same toxicological properties because of their structural similarities (10). As such, robust physical/chemical data may allow identification of features critical to assessing potential toxicity and obviate the need for redundant hazard-based testing. These, of course, are generalizations, and all materials must be evaluated on an individual basis. Suffice it to say that the chemical and physical description of the test material is a critically important first step in hazard identification.

Beyond descriptive information, there are experimental data, which are considered in the hazard identification of a test material. Table 2 provides a list of hazard-type toxicity data and the Organization for Economic Co-operation and Development (OECD) test or guideline for each that is often used as a check for completeness of knowledge. For cosmetic ingredients

Table 2 List of Toxicological Tests Used for Hazard Identification

Toxicological test	OECD test/guideline
Acute toxicity	420: Acute oral toxicity—fixed-dose method (updated guideline, adopted December 20, 2001);
	423: Acute oral toxicity—acute toxic class method (updated guideline, adopted December 20, 2001);
	425: Acute oral toxicity; up-and-down procedure (updated guideline, adopted December 20, 2001)
Irritation and corrosivity	404: Acute dermal irritation/corrosion (updated guideline, adopted April 24, 2002);
	405: Acute eye irritation/corrosion (updated guideline, adopted April 24, 2002);
	430: In vitro skin corrosion: TER test (original guideline, adopted April 13, 2004);
	431: In vitro skin corrosion: human skin model test (original guideline, adopted April 13, 2004)
Skin sensitization	429: Skin sensitization: local lymph node assay (updated guideline, adopted April 24, 2002)
Dermal/percutaneous absorption	427: Skin absorption: in vivo method (original guideline, adopted April 13, 2004);
	428: Skin absorption: in vitro method (original guideline, adopted April 13, 2004)

(Continued)

Table 2 List of Toxicological Tests Used for Hazard Identification (*Continued*)

Toxicological test	OECD test/guideline
Repeat-dose toxicity	407: Repeated dose 28-day oral toxicity study in rodents (updated guideline, adopted July 27, 1995); 408: Repeated dose 90-day oral toxicity study in rodents (updated guideline, adopted September 21, 1998); 409: Repeated-dose 90-day oral toxicity study in non-rodents (updated guideline, adopted September 21, 1998); 410: Repeated dose dermal toxicity: 21/28-day study (original guideline, adopted May 12, 1981); 411: Subchronic dermal toxicity: 90-day study (original guideline, adopted May 12, 1981); 412: Repeated-dose inhalation toxicity: 28-day or 14-day study (original guideline, adopted May 12, 1981); 413: Subchronic inhalation toxicity: 90-day study (original guideline, adopted May 12, 1981)
Mutagenicity/genotoxicity	471: Bacterial reverse mutation test (updated guideline, adopted July 21, 1977); 473: In vitro mammalian chromosomal aberration test (updated guideline July 21, 1977)
Carcinogenicity	451: Carcinogenicity studies (original guideline, adopted May 12, 1981); 452: Chronic toxicity studies (original guideline, adopted May 12, 1981); 453: Combined chronic toxicity/carcinogenicity studies (original guideline, adopted May 12, 1981)
Reproductive toxicity	414: Prenatal developmental toxicity study (updated guideline, adopted January 22, 2001); 415: One-generation reproductive toxicity study (original guideline, adopted May 26, 1983); 416: Two-generation reproductive toxicity study (updated guideline, adopted January 22, 2001)
Toxicokinetics studies	417: Toxicokinetics (updated guideline, adopted April 4, 1984)
Phototoxicity	432: In vitro 3T3 NRU phototoxicity test (original guideline, adopted April 13, 2004)

Abbreviations: OECD, Organization for Economic Co-operation; TER, transcutaneous electrical resistance; NRU, neutral red uptake.

and products, it is rare for all studies listed in Table 2 to have been conducted. On the other hand, cosmetic-drug ingredients, such as UV filters, often have a more complete data set. Finally, for pharmaceutical drug products, such toxicological studies are conducted together with clinical safety testing and "targeted" toxicological evaluations.

The most common health-related toxicities for topically applied sunscreens are "site-of-action" or skin-related allergic reactions and irritation (11–13). It may not be surprising that target tissue–related adverse events are most frequent. For example, some frequently used hazard-based sites of contact studies are (*i*) acute and repeat-dose skin irritation/corrosion, (*ii*) contact sensitization, (*iii*) phototoxicity, and (*iv*) human data, such as human repeat insult patch test (RIPT), cumulative irritation, photoallergenicity, and photoirritation. For these endpoint tests, the emphasis today and in the future is for validated, in vitro tests. This is true for the other study types listed in Table 2, but the challenges of designing such alternative test methods may not be possible, i.e., carcinogenicity or chronic toxicity testing.

Dermal Penetration

Beyond target tissue, i.e., skin, toxicity, the most critical assessment of a UV filter is skin penetration. This is the "gate" through which systemic toxicity testing is routinely deemed necessary or unnecessary. The evaluation of dermal penetration is done using in silico physical/chemical or in vitro/in vivo experimental models or both. In general, such evaluations are done using "healthy," undamaged skin, although more recently the need to consider application of sunscreens on damaged skin has been raised. For reference, the structure of skin is presented in Figure 1. A UV filter that makes its way into the circulation must traverse the stratum corneum and epidermis into the capillaries located in the dermis. This journey, up to 100 μm through a diverse heterogeneous tissue, is nothing short of extraordinary, which explains why the skin is such an effective barrier to the constant and diverse environmental insults. Moreover, this helps explain why systemic availability of UV filters is limited.

In silico mathematical models of dermal penetration are useful predictors of "flux" or the rate of transfer of a test material or chemical through the skin. Many of the parameters defined in Table 1, such as oil/water partition coefficient, are used in predicting the degree of skin penetration using in silico models. This approach is useful as a starting point to estimate penetration of new chemical entities (14). Also, such "starting point" estimations are important when considering dose selection for other hazard-based

Human Skin (forearm) 50x

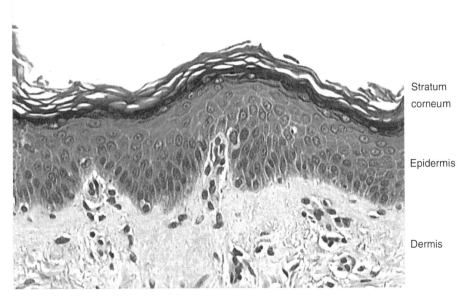

Stratum corneum

Epidermis

Dermis

Figure 1 Histological section of normal human skin. The thickness of the stratum corneum is highly variable depending on the location, e.g., soles of the feet versus facial skin. The epidermis is, generally speaking, 6 to 10 cell layers with a thickness of 50 to 100 μm.

studies. As with any model, there are limitations to the calculated predictions of skin penetration (15).

The experimental determination of skin penetration is accomplished using in vitro methods (16,17). Undamaged skin samples may be obtained from human donors: frozen cadaver or fresh, e.g., breast reduction, or animal, e.g., porcine, rat, etc., sources. The epidermal surface is exposed to air and the dermal portion bathed in a receptor fluid in which the test material is soluble. The UV filter in a simple vehicle or sunscreen product is applied to the epidermal surface at an infinite or finite dose. In general, such studies are conducted over a six-hour or longer time period with multiple samples taken from the receptor fluid and analyzed for the test material. The data obtained in these studies can be used for several purposes including the calculation of the systemic exposure dose.

The use of intact, undamaged skin as a means of assessing dermal penetration has been questioned (18,19). In the case of sunscreens, the concern is based on hypothetical use of products on, for example sunburnt or otherwise damaged skin. Whereas this concern seems to make sense, it is exceedingly difficult and impractical to experimentally model in a reproducible way. For example, damage is subjective, and even if it is quantitated, the extent and impact on human risk assessment are filled with endless possible interpretations. Moreover, the question maybe misplaced. For example, it is logical to assume that damaged skin will result in greater penetration of a test material. Thus, the question is not whether penetration is enhanced, but where does the test material distribute once it is systemically available. This, of course, is a question of distribution, which is better addressed in classical pharmacokinetic studies following intravenous administration. Therefore, rather than model damaged skin and quantify penetration, it may be preferable to conduct pharmacokinetic studies and measure distribution of the test material and continue to determine skin penetration using the existing undamaged skin models.

In most instances, radiolabeled test material is used to provide a signal to follow dermal penetration. These data provide a general picture of the penetration of parent compound and any metabolites or radiolabel that might be transferred to endogenous molecules, e.g., ^{3}H exchange with water. Using quantitative "cold" chemistry is more specific but is analytically challenging and may not provide the limits of detection necessary to assess meaningful exposure.

Beyond the in vitro dermal penetration methods, there are in vivo animal and human pharmacokinetic/toxicokinetic studies. For pharmaceuticals, such studies are done routinely. However, it is relatively rare that full-scale absorption, distribution, metabolism, and excretion (ADME) studies are conducted for UV filters. Such studies are reserved for materials that are believed to penetrate the skin and whose systemic fate needs to be characterized.

In summary, assessment of dermal penetration is critical in the process to assess risk from topically applied products. In the absence of dermal penetration, testing of a UV filter for toxicological endpoints beyond the site of contact may be unwarranted. There are many approaches used to estimate dermal penetration of UV filters. Demonstration of dermal penetration for a UV filter increases the potential for systemic toxicity and the need for a more detailed toxicological evaluation.

Exposure Assessment

For sunscreens, the exposure assessment is essential for determining human health risk. As stated and in general, exposure is limited to site of contact, i.e., skin, since the dermal penetration of the majority of UV filters is limited. Table 3 presents components of an exposure assessment that are needed for sunscreen products. Aside from product type, form, and function, much of the exposure assessment is empirically derived (20). Data

Table 3 Considerations Related to an Exposure Assessment

Exposure assessment	Example
Dose	Body weight (mg/kg) and surface area (mg/cm^2)
Frequency	Number of times product applied in a single day
Site of application	Face/hands versus full body
Duration	Intermittent or repeat daily
Concentration	Percent of raw material
Dermal penetration	For systemic dose
Product type	Recreational versus face cream/moisturizer versus cosmetic, e.g., lipstick
Product form	Aerosol versus emulsion or cream
Function	Protection against high UV dose associated with sweating, swimming, toweling, etc., versus low, intermittent UV dose

from studies of habits and practices and from consumer use are included in the exposure assessment (21,22). Collectively, these data are used to calculate human exposure, which in the formal risk assessment is used to calculate a margin of exposure (MoE) or margin of safety (MoS).

Estimation of Human Risk

As stated, risk assessment is a structured discipline. As such, a brief overview of the risk assessment process will be provided. In considering risk, the first step is identifying the critical effect, which is defined as an adverse effect that occurs in the most sensitive species as the dose increases. Using the critical effect, a point-of-departure (POD) is established. This is the point from which the dose-response data for a material is extrapolated to determine an effect level associated with exposure. The POD is an empirical or an estimated dose of a test material that can be interpolated from the range of observed responses. Most commonly, the POD is obtained in a toxicity study. Examples of such PODs include a NOAEL, defined as the dose (level) that is associated with no observable adverse effect, i.e., toxicologically insignificant, in treated animals; and, a benchmark dose (BMD) defined as an estimated dose of a substance associated with a specified low incidence of risk of a health effect, or the dose associated with a specified measure or change of a biological effect. The BMD is generally considered the equivalent of a NOAEL for the purposes of a risk assessment.

In considering risk, areas of uncertainty involved in the estimation of an acceptable exposure for humans are identified on the basis of the data from the critical toxicology study. For each area of extrapolation or uncertainty that is identified, an uncertainty factor (UF) is assigned. Some UFs are intraspecies (human to human) and interspecies (human to animal) on a scale of 1 to 10. UFs are multiplied together to determine a total UF, usually 100×.

The ultimate step of the quantitative risk assessment process is to characterize the risk associated with estimated human exposure to a material or product. There are two approaches to characterizing this risk: MoE and MoS. The MoE is the ratio of the POD to the estimated human exposure and is expressed as follows:

$$MoE = \frac{POD\ (mg/kg/day)}{Human\ exposure\ (mg/kg/day)}.$$

MoE provides information as to how an estimated human exposure relates to a POD for a defined adverse effect. It does not define whether a particular exposure is expected to be safe. The acceptability of an MoE is determined relative to the uncertainty estimate associated with the POD. For example, if an MoE is 120 and the UFs are 100, then the estimated human exposure is considered to be acceptable.

The MoS is first calculated by dividing the POD by the UFs as estimated by an analysis of the uncertainty associated with the POD. This reference dose (RfD) is defined as "an estimate of daily exposure to the human population that is likely to be without an appreciable risk of deleterious non-cancer effects during a lifetime" and is calculated as follows:

$$RfD(mg/kg/day) = \frac{POE(mg/kg/day)}{Total\ UF}$$

The MoS is the quotient of the RfD divided by the estimated human exposure or

$$MoS = \frac{RfD\ (mg/kg/day)}{Human\ exposure\ (mg/kg/day)}.$$

If the MoS is greater than one, then the estimated human exposure is considered to be acceptable.

Summary of Human Safety Evaluation

The most commonly used UV filters have been evaluated for toxicological effects (23,24). These hazard evaluations have focused on site-of-contact effects, i.e., dermal toxicity, together with functional events, i.e., phototoxicological assessment, and in many cases, repeat dose toxicity studies. The evaluation of dermal penetration is a standard practice for UV filters to determine whether systemic hazard endpoint assessments are needed. If systemic toxicity is needed, then effects can be evaluated using standardized testing, and MoE or MoS can be calculated. The resulting MoE/MoS value can be used to consider the human health risk from exposure to a given chemical, e.g., UV filter.

SYSTEMIC TOXICITY OF SUNSCREENS

The systemic toxicity of UV filters is done on a case-by-case basis. The chemical diversity of these materials makes sweeping generalizations unsuitable other than to reiterate that for the 16 UV filters approved for use by the Food and Drug Administration in the United States and the additional 20 or so used in Europe and elsewhere, systemic bioavailability is limited. UV filters are grouped into two categories: inorganic and organic UV filters. The systemic toxicity of each will be considered.

Inorganic UV Filters: Microfine (Nano-) Titanium Dioxide and Zinc Oxide

Inorganic UV filters are the metal oxides, titanium dioxide (TiO_2) and zinc oxide (ZnO), often referred to as physical sunscreens in the older sunscreen literature because of their ability to reflect and scatter UV. Technological advances in process manufacturing have led to the availability of microfine or nanoparticles, i.e., < 100 nm in at least two dimensions, of TiO_2 and ZnO. These TiO_2 and ZnO nanoparticles absorb as well as reflect/scatter UV and, below certain concentrations, are transparent on the skin thereby reducing any whiteness caused by reflectance of longer wavelengths of light on the skin.

Microfine (nano-) TiO_2 has an absorption profile, which is greater in shorter wavelengths, UVB (290–320 nm)/UVA II (320–340 nm), but extends into the long wavelength UVA I (340–400 nm). Microfine ZnO particles have a flat absorption profile, which spans UVB and UVA.

Until recently, TiO_2 and ZnO have been promoted as safe alternatives to organic UV filters based largely on their lack of chemical reactivity. However, concerns regarding potential skin penetration of microfine or "nano"-TiO_2/ZnO have led to a reconsideration of their toxicity. If these materials do not penetrate into or through the skin, then it would be reasonable to suggest that there is limited or no concern regarding systemic exposure to the material from topically applied products. There are multiple studies, which have examined the dermal penetration of pigmentary, i.e., particles > 100 nm, and nano-TiO_2/ZnO. These data support the view that these metal oxides, pigmentary or nano, do not penetrate through the skin but remain on the top layer, i.e., stratum corneum. As such, systemic toxicity of these inorganic UV filters is of limited concern.

Titanium Dioxide

A number of skin penetration studies have been conducted with microfine (nano-) TiO_2 and are summarized in Table 4. All these studies have found that TiO_2 does not penetrate beyond the stratum corneum. A detailed review of the dermal penetration of nano-TiO_2 is provided in the review by Nohynek et al. (25) and will be briefly discussed.

In one study, Tan et al. (26) suggest that the amount of titanium (Ti) in the dermis of the treatment group was higher compared with controls suggestive of penetration of microfine TiO_2. However, there was no statistically significant ($p = 0.14$) difference in the concentration of Ti in the epidermis and dermis of subjects who applied microfine TiO_2 compared with controls. The results of this study should be considered either inconclusive or demonstrating that microfine TiO_2 does not penetrate the skin. Dussert et al. (27) used scanning and transmission electron microscopy (TEM) to determine the distribution of TiO_2 in human skin. Neither intercellular nor intracellular penetration of TiO_2 was observed in this study using explants of human skin. The particles appeared to be confined to the stratum corneum. Similarly, in a carefully conducted in vitro pigskin penetration study, Pflucker et al. (28) found that there was no penetration of microfine TiO_2 beyond the outermost stratum corneum. Again, TEM was used to reveal no penetration of TiO_2 beyond the stratum corneum. Whereas traces of TiO_2 particles were seen at the hair follicle, there was no evidence of penetration into the skin. Lademann et al. (29) found no evidence of penetration of microfine TiO_2 into human skin based on tape strips and biopsy samples. Puccetti and Leblanc (30) used photoacoustic spectroscopy to measure the depth of penetration of TiO_2 particles (average diameter 80 nm) in human skin samples from cadavers. The three-dimensional depth profiles were unchanged up to 15 hours after application of TiO_2. Also, the UV light absorption profile seen ex vivo was unchanged compared with the absorption profile of an oil-based emulsion containing microfine TiO_2, which suggests no interaction between the TiO_2 particles and skin. Bennat and Muller-Goymann (31) determined the penetration of microfine TiO_2 particles into human skin using in vitro and in vivo experimental approaches. Although the authors reported a difference between oily and water dispersions of TiO_2 particles, neither preparation of TiO_2 showed penetration beyond the stratum corneum. Schulz et al. (32) examined the skin penetration of three "types" of micronized TiO_2 into the skin of human volunteers. The TiO_2 pigments were located exclusively on the outermost layer of the human stratum corneum regardless of the "type" of coating, formulation, or particle dimensions. In the study by Menzel et al. (33), particles of TiO_2 with a diameter of 15 nm

Table 4 Summary of Dermal Penetration Studies Conducted with Microfine (nano-) TiO₂ and/or ZnO

Type	Skin	Material	Methods	Results	References
In vitro	Human	SS; micronized TiO$_2$ and ZnO ~100 nm	TEM	No penetration beyond SC	Dussert et al., 1997
	Pig	SS; 4% TiO$_2$, 20 nm	SEM/TEM; tape strip	No penetration beyond SC	Pflucker et al., 1999
	Human	TiO$_2$ (80 nm) in mineral oil emulsion (concentration unknown)	Photoacoustical spectroscopy	No penetration beyond SC	Puccetti and LeBlanc, 2000
	Human	SS; 5% microfine TiO$_2$ (size not provided)	AAS; tape strip and receptor fluid	No penetration beyond SC	Bennat and Muller-Goymann, 2000
	Pig	SS; 4.5–40% micronized TiO$_2$; 45–150 nm long, 17–35 nm wide	Ion beam analysis for frozen sections	No penetration beyond SC/SG; no particles in follicles	Menzel et al., 2004
	Pig	SS; 10% microfine ZnO (<160 nm); TiO$_2$ (30–60 × 10 nm needlelike)	AS, AAS, ICP-AES, ICP-MS; tape strip and receptor fluid	No penetration beyond SC	Gamer et al., 2006
	Human	SS; 20% ZnO (ZinClear); 60% dispersion ZnO (ZinClear-S)	ICP-MS; TEM	No penetration beyond SC	Cross et al., 2007
In vivo	Human	SS; 8% microfine TiO$_2$ (size not provided)	ICP-MS; cyanoacrylate strips	No statistical difference; authors suggest trend	Tan et al., 1996
	Human	SS; TiO$_2$ microparticles (size not provided)	UV/VIS spectroscopy, X ray fluorescence	No penetration beyond SC; particles in follicles	Lademann et al., 1999
	Human	SS; 5% microfine TiO$_2$ (size not provided)	AAS; tape strips	No penetration beyond SC; particles in follicles	Bennat and Muller-Goymann, 2000
	Human	SS; micronized TiO$_2$ (10–100 nm)	Light and TEM punch biopsies	No penetration beyond SC	Schulz et al., 2002
	Human	SS; 15% 38 nm ZnO and 15% 398 nm ZnO	Tape stripping; ICP-AES	No difference between nano- and micro-ZnO. Recovery was lower for both at 2 hours after application	Casey et al., 2006

Abbreviations: AAS, flame atomic absorption spectroscopy; AS, atomic spectrometry; ICP-AES, inductively coupled plasma atomic emission spectroscopy; ICP-MS, inductively coupled plasma mass spectrometry; SC, stratum corneum; SG, stratum granulosum; SS, sunscreen; SEM, scanning electron microscopy; TEM, transmission electron microscopy; UV/VIS, ultraviolet/visible radiation.

penetrated through the stratum corneum into the stratum granulosum but no further (i.e., no particles in stratum spinosum). The hair follicle was not an important route for penetration. Finally, Gamer et al. (41) were the most recent group to show that TiO_2 particles do not penetrate beyond the stratum corneum. This study was done in accordance with OECD testing guidelines for skin penetration using pigskin explants.

On the basis of these data using in vitro pigskin, and in vivo human and pigskin, there is no evidence of penetration of TiO_2 beyond the stratum corneum regardless of the particle size or coating. The absence of dermal penetration of nano-TiO_2 corroborates earlier study results with uncharacterized test material and is supportive of the view that systemic toxicity is not a concern following topical exposure to TiO_2.

Zinc Oxide

The human safety profile of ZnO is based on an extraordinary volume of studies conducted during the past century. Much experience with topical treatments containing ZnO, e.g., calamine lotion, exists given that such therapies are some of the first recorded treatments of dermatological conditions. ZnO creams, ointments, salves, etc., have been applied to human skin with therapeutic benefits and very little in the way of adverse or toxicological consequences. This is even more remarkable when considering studies of wound-healing benefits of ZnO where it has been applied to damaged skin in some cases covering large portions of the body, i.e., burn victims or psoriasis. Suffice it to say that ZnO is nonirritating and without sensitization potential (34).

As is the case with microfine TiO_2, concerns related to the skin penetration of nano ZnO particles have been raised. The major difference between TiO_2 and ZnO is that the zinc salt is slightly soluble (pH dependent) forming zinc ions. Of course, zinc is an essential element with dietary requirements of 10 to 15 mg/day such that topical application may have some physiological benefits. Regardless, studies of ZnO skin penetration have demonstrated some penetration using pigmentary grade ZnO (35–38). These studies used suction blister to detect zinc, and this technique may have contributed to its detection. However, in one study, whole-body application of ZnO did not change serum concentrations of zinc, suggestive that systemic absorption was limited (39). The absence of any measurable change in serum or plasma zinc concentrations may be attributed to its controlled regulation in the human body (40).

Dermal penetration of microfine (nano-) ZnO has been investigated by Gamer et al (41), Casey et al. (42) and Cross et al. (43). In the studies by Gamer et al. and Cross et al., there was no evidence of penetration of ZnO beyond the stratum corneum, consistent with studies of microfine TiO_2. The study by Casey et al. was more difficult to interpret as the recovery of ZnO, nano or micron size, for up to 18 tape strips was reduced two hours after application. The authors raise several possibilities, none of which would explain the disappearance of the ZnO in such a rapid time, e.g., two hours. It is possible that the ZnO was dissolved, in which case, the zinc ions would in all probability be taken up by cellular machinery in tight control of intracellular zinc.

In summary, the studies conducted to date are supportive of the view that nanoparticles of TiO_2 or ZnO do not penetrate the skin. On the basis of the absence of penetration, systemic toxicity of such materials is of little concern.

Organic UV Filters

The major classes of organic filters are benzophenones, camphors, cinnamates, *p*-aminobenzoic acids, and salicylates with individual ones: butyl methoxydibenzoylmethane (avobenzone), octocrylene, and phenylbenzimidazole sulfonic acid (44). The most commonly used UV filters have relatively complete safety dossiers, although many of these are based on older toxicology studies, i.e., pre-guideline, conducted through 1970s to 1980s. More recent examples, such as Tinosorb M: Bisoctrizole; methylene bis-benzotriazolyl tetramethylbutylphenol, and Tinsorb S: Bemotrizinol; bis-ethylhexyloxyphenol methoxyphenyl triazine, have extensive human safety dossiers (45). Because some UV filters have been measured systemically, concerns related to toxicity have been raised. A comprehensive review of the systemic toxicity of all UV filters is beyond the scope of this paper, rather a limited number of examples will be discussed.

Benzophenone-3 (oxybenzone)

Benzophenone-3 (oxybenzone) has been measured in the blood and urine of humans (4,5,46,47) and rats (48), following topical application. Estimates of dermal penetration of benzophenone-3 using human skin explants have been up to 10% of the applied dose (2). Studies with rodents have found that benzophenone-3 is absorbed after dermal or oral exposure and metabolized (conjugated) and excreted in urine and feces (49–52). Thus, topical application of benzophenone-3 results in systemic exposure. Compared with other UV filters, benzophenone-3 is the most bioavailable following topical application. The bioavailability of benzophenone-3 is, in and of itself, not a toxicological concern but simply warrants some attention to systemic toxicological endpoints (53).

A systemic critical effect of concern for benzophenone-3 is endocrine disruption. This has been investigated using in vitro and in vivo methods. Janjua et al. (47) determined the concentration of benzophenone-3 in the plasma of 32 healthy volunteers exposed to daily whole-body topical application of 2 mg/cm^2 of sunscreen formulation for four days. The maximum median plasma concentration of benzopheneone-3 was 238 ng/mL detected in female subjects. On the basis of a 28-day repeat-dose study in rats, the NOAEL for benzophenone-3 is 100 mg/kg (52). The plasma concentration of benzophenone-3 in rats after topical application of 100 mg/kg in petrolatum to shaved back skin was 35.02 ug/mL or 35,020 ng/mL. Dividing the NOAEL by human dose yields $\frac{35,020}{238} = 147$. Thus, the plasma concentration of benzophenone-3 in the rat at a dose, which has no systemic toxicity, is 147 times higher than the human plasma concentration. Thus, the exposure to benzophenone-3 in humans would not be expected to have systemic toxicological effects.

Octyl Methoxycinnamate

Octyl methoxycinnamate or OMC is the most common UV filter used in the world (54). Like benzophenone-3, OMC has been measured in human plasma following topical application (6,47). Using in vivo and in vitro models, OMC has been reported to have endocrine-disrupting properties (55–58). Most of these studies are investigative research studies, which are not part of a systematic, toxicological evaluation of a test material. A two-generation reproduction toxicity study was conducted in accordance with OECD test guideline 416 (59). The NOAEL of OMC by continuous dietary administration in this study was 450 mg/kg/day for fertility and reproduction parameters and for systemic parental and developmental toxicity. Dividing the NOAEL by the estimated human systemic exposure dose (55) to OMC at 10% in a sunscreen product yields $\frac{450 \text{ mg/kg/day}}{0.96 \text{ mg/kg/day}} = 468$. This means the dose of OMC in rats that has no adverse effect on reproductive endpoints is 468 times higher than the estimated human exposure. Using experimental endpoints of reproductive toxicity as the critical effect, i.e., estrogen receptor β-gene expression, Klammer et al. (55) determined a NOAEL for OMC to be 100 mg/kg, which is 100 times higher than the estimated human dose. Interestingly, Klammer et al. made additional calculations using BMD and concluded that the concentration of OMC should be restricted. Regardless of this, using guideline study NOAEL and estimated human exposure, the systemic toxicological concern associated with topical application of OMC is minimal.

For other UV filters, similar concerns of endocrine disruption or more general systemic toxicity have been raised (53). In the paper by Greim (60), which discusses endocrine disruption, the following observation is offered: "Overall, the science-based knowledge on the robustness of the endocrine system, the well-understood principles of substrate-receptor interactions, and the generally low exposure of humans to potentially endocrine-disrupting chemicals make it unlikely that the latter play a causative role in diseases and abnormalities observed in children and in the human population in general." Whereas work continues in understanding the human impact of endocrine disruption, in the case of exposure to UV filters from sunscreens, the benefit of photoprotection from the use of such products would seem to outweigh the potential risk.

SUMMARY AND CONCLUSION

The human toxicological evaluation of UV filters applied topically is largely focused on site-of-contact safety studies, e.g., skin irritation, sensitization, together with functional toxicity, e.g., photoirritation, photoallergenicity. Determination of systemic toxicity for UV filters is predicated on their bioavailability. For topically applied products such as sunscreens, this means that UV filters must penetrate the skin, gaining access to the circulation for potential effects at sites beyond the skin. Demonstration of bioavailability may necessitate additional toxicological testing to assess systemic toxicity of UV filters. Such testing follows an organized set of guideline studies from which a critical effect is identified and NOAEL established. Together with estimates of human exposure, an MoE or MoS can be determined and used to quantitatively evaluate human risk.

For inorganic UV filters, there is no evidence of dermal penetration, even for the nanoparticles of TiO_2 or ZnO. The systemic toxicity of these materials is of limited or no concern. For organic UV filters, skin absorption has been reported in humans following topical application, although the extent is limited. Nonetheless, for the commonly used UV filters, there is an acceptable MoE supporting their safe use by humans.

As the field of biomonitoring expands and analytical methods become more sensitive and comprehensive, the list of UV filters detected in human samples will grow. Provided there is rational judgment applied to such discoveries, a calculated risk to human health can be evaluated most likely with available data or, if necessary, new studies. If, on the other hand, there is a rush to conclude that the detection of a chemical is equivalent to "toxicity," then we can anticipate unfavorable new reports implicating UV filters and potentially undermining consumer confidence in sunscreen products.

REFERENCES

1. Tanner PR. Sunscreen product formulation. Dermatol Clin 2006; 24(1):53–62.
2. Jiang R, Roberts MS, Collins DM, et al. Absorption of sunscreens across human skin: an evaluation of commercial products for children and adults. Br J Clin Pharmacol 1999; 48(4): 635–637.

3. Hayden CGJ, Cross SE, Anderson C, et al. Sunscreen penetration of human skin and related keratinocyte toxicity after topical application. Skin Pharmacol Physiol 2005; 18(4):170–174.

4. Hayden CG, Roberts MS, Benson HA. Systemic absorption of sunscreen after topical application. Lancet 1997; 350(9081):863–864.

5. Gustavsson Gonzalez H, Farbrot A, Larkö O. Percutaneous absorption of benzophenone-3, a common component of topical sunscreens. Clin Exp Dermatol 2002; 27(8):691–694.

6. Janjua NR, Mogensen B, Andersson AM, et al. Systemic absorption of the sunscreens benzophenone-3, octyl-methoxycinnamate, and 3-(4-methyl-benzylidene) camphor after whole-body topical application and reproductive hormone levels in humans. J Invest Dermatol 2004; 123(1):57–61.

7. Angerer J, Ewers U, Wilhelm M. Human biomonitoring: state of the art. Int J Hyg Environ Health 2007; 210(3–4):201–228.

8. Calafat AM, Ye X, Silva MJ, et al. Human exposure assessment to environmental chemicals using biomonitoring. Int J Androl 2006; 29(1):166–171.

9. Risk Assessment in the Federal Government: Managing the Process. Committee on the International Means for Assessment of Risks to Public Health, Commission Life Sciences, NRC 1983.

10. Cosmetic Ingredient Review, . Final report on the safety assessment of benzophenones-1, -3, -4, -5, -9 and -11. J Am Coll Toxicol 1983; 2(5):35–77.

11. Thune P. Contact and photocontact allergy to sunscreens. Photodermatol 1984; 1(1):5–9.

12. Menz J, Muller SA, Connolly SM. Photopatch testing: a six-year experience. J Am Acad Dermatol 1988; 18(5 pt 1):1044–1047.

13. Nohynek GJ, Schaefer H. Benefit and risk of organic ultraviolet filters. Regul Toxicol Pharmacol 2001; 33(3):285–299.

14. Chatelain E, Gabard B, Surber C. Skin penetration and sun protection factor of five UV filters: effect of the vehicle. Skin Pharmacol Appl Skin Physiol 2003; 16(1):28–35.

15. Geinoz S, Guy RH, Testa B, et al. Quantitative structure-permeation relationships (QSPeRs) to predict skin permeation: a critical evaluation. Pharm Res 2004; 21(1):83–92.

16. Walters KA, Brain KR, Howes D, et al. Percutaneous penetration of octyl salicylate from representative sunscreen formulations through human skin in vitro. Food Chem Toxicol 1997; 35(12):1219–1225.

17. Benech-Kieffer F, Wegrich P, Schwarzenbach R, et al. Percutaneous absorption of sunscreens in vitro: interspecies comparison, skin models and reproducibility aspects. Skin Pharmacol Appl Skin Physiol 2000; 13(6):324–335.

18. Nielsen JB, Nielsen F, Srensen JA. Defense against dermal exposures is only skin deep: significantly increased penetration through slightly damaged skin. Arch Dermatol Res 2007; 299(9):423–431.

19. Borm PJA, Robbins D, Haubold S, et al. The potential risks of nanomaterials: a review carried out for ECETOC. Particle Fibre Toxicol 2006; 3:11.

20. Stender IM, Andersen JL, Wulf HC. Sun exposure and sunscreen use among sunbathers in Denmark. Acta Derm Venereol 1996; 76(1):31–33.

21. Stenberg C, Larko O. Sunscreen application and its importance for the sun protection factor. Arch Dermatol 1985; 121(11):1400–1402.

22. Pruim B, Green A. Photobiological aspects of sunscreen re-application. Australas J Dermatol 1999; 40(1):14–18.

23. Gasparro FP, Mitchnick M, Nash JF. A review of sunscreen safety and efficacy. Photochem Photobiol 1998; 68(3):243–256.

24. Nash JF. Human safety and efficacy of ultraviolet filters and sunscreen products. Dermatol Clin 2006; 24(1):35–51.

25. Nohynek GJ, Lademann J, Ribaud C, et al. Grey goo on the skin? Nanotechnology, cosmetic and sunscreen safety. Crit Rev Toxicol 2007; 37(3):251–277.

26. Tan MH, Commens CA, Burnett L, et al. A pilot study on the percutaneous absorption of microfine titanium dioxide from sunscreens. Australas J Dermatol 1996; 37(4):185–187.

27. Dussert A-S, Gooris E, Hemmerle J. Characterization of the mineral content of a physical sunscreen emulsion and its distribution onto human stratum corneum. Int J Cosmet Sci 1997; 19:119–129.

28. Pflucker F, Hohenberg H, lzle E, et al. The outermost stratum corneum layer is an effective barrier against dermal uptake of topically applied micronized titanium dioxide. Int J Cosmet Sci 1999; 21(6):399–411.

29. Lademann J, Weigmann H, Rickmeyer C, et al. Penetration of titanium dioxide microparticles in a sunscreen formulation into the horny layer and the follicular orifice. Skin Pharmacol Appl Skin Physiol 1999; 12(5):247–256.

30. Puccetti G, Leblanc RM. A sunscreen-tanning compromise: 3D visualization of the actions of titanium dioxide particles and dihydroxyacetone on human epiderm. Photochem Photobiol 2000; 71(4):426–430.

31. Bennat C, Muller-Goymann CC. Skin penetration and stabilization of formulations containing microfine titanium dioxide as physical UV filter. Int J Cosmet Sci 2000; 22(4):271–283.

32. Schulz J, Hohenberg H, Pflucker F, et al. Distribution of sunscreens on skin. Adv Drug Deliv Rev 2002; 54(suppl 1):S157–S163.

33. Menzel F, Reinert T, Vogt J, et al. Investigations of percutaneous uptake of ultrafine TiO2 particles at the high energy ion nanoprobe LIPSION. Nucl Instrum Methods Phys Res B 2004; 219–220:82–86.

34. Lansdown AB. Interspecies variations in response to topical application of selected zinc compounds. Food Chem Toxicol 1991; 29(1):57–64.

35. Hallmans G, Lasek J. The effect of topical zinc absorption from wounds on growth and the wound healing process in zinc-deficient rats. Scand J Plast Reconstr Surg 1985; 19(2):119–125.

36. Agren MS. Percutaneous absorption of zinc from zinc oxide applied topically to intact skin in man. Dermatologica 1990; 180(1):36–39.

37. Agren MS, Krusell M, Franzen L. Release and absorption of zinc from zinc oxide and zinc sulfate in open wounds. Acta Derm Venereol 1991; 71(4):330–333.

38. Agren MS. Influence of two vehicles for zinc oxide on zinc absorption through intact skin and wounds. Acta Derm Venereol 1991; 71(2):153–156.

39. Derry JE, McLean WM, Freeman JB. A study of the percutaneous absorption from topically applied zinc oxide ointment. JPEN J Parenter Enteral Nutr 1983; 7(2):131–135.

40. Schwartz JR, Marsh RG, Draelos ZD. Zinc and skin health: overview of physiology and pharmacology. Dermatol Surg 2005; 31(7 pt 2):837–847.

41. Gamer AO, Leibold E, Van Ravenzwaay B. The in vitro absorption of microfine zinc oxide and titanium dioxide through porcine skin. Toxicol In Vitro 2006; 20(3):301–307.

42. Casey PS, Chau N, Finnin B. Issues relating to the use of Micro and nanoparticle zinc oxide in personal care products based on skin penetration studies. NSTI Nanotech Technical Proceedings, 2006, 1:541–544.

43. Cross SE, Innes B, Roberts MS, et al. Human skin penetration of sunscreen nanoparticles: in-vitro assessment of a novel micronized zinc oxide formulation. Skin Pharmacol Physiol 2007; 20(3):148–154.

44. Evolution of Sunscreen Chemicals. New York, United States: Felton Worldwide, 1990.

45. Tuchinda C, Lim HW, Osterwalder U, et al. Novel emerging sunscreen technologies. Dermatol Clin 2006; 24(1):105–117.

46. Gonzalez H, Farbrot A, Larkö O. Percutaneous absorption of the sunscreen benzophenone-3 after repeated whole-body applications, with and without ultraviolet irradiation. Br J Dermatol 2006; 154(2):337–340.

47. Janjua NR, Kongshoj B, Andersson AM, et al. Sunscreens in human plasma and urine after repeated whole-body topical application. J Euro Acad Dermatol Venereol 2008; 22(4):456–461.

48. Okereke CS, Abdel-Rhaman MS, Friedman MA. Disposition of benzophenone-3 after dermal administration in male rats. Toxicol Lett 1994; 73(2):113–122.

49. el Dareer SM, Kalin JR, Tillery KF, et al. Disposition of 2-hydroxy-4-methoxybenzophenone in rats dosed orally, intravenously, or topically. J Toxicol Environ Health 1986; 19(4):491–502.

50. Okereke CS, Kadry AM, Abdel-Rahman MS, et al. Metabolism of benzophenone-3 in rats. Drug Metab Dispos 1993; 21(5):788–791.

51. Kadry AM, Okereke CS, Abdel-Rahman MS, et al. Pharmacokinetics of benzophenone-3 after oral exposure in male rats. J Appl Toxicol 1995; 15(2):97–102.

52. Okereke CS, Barat SA, Abdel-Rahman MS. Safety evaluation of benzophenone-3 after dermal administration in rats. Toxicol Lett 1995; 80(1–3):61–67.

53. Benson HA. Assessment and clinical implications of absorption of sunscreens across skin. Am J Clin Dermatol 2000; 1(4):217–224.

54. Rastogi SC. UV filters in sunscreen products—a survey. Contact Dermatitis 2002; 46(6): 348–351.

55. Klammer H, Schlecht C, Wuttke W, et al. Multi-organic risk assessment of estrogenic properties of octyl-methoxycinnamate in vivo: a 5-day sub-acute pharmacodynamic study with ovariectomized rats. Toxicology 2005; 215(1–2):90–96.

56. Wuttke D, Christoffel J, Rimoldi G, et al. Comparison of effects of estradiol with those of octylmethoxycinnamate and 4-methylbenzylidene camphor on fat tissue, lipids and pituitary hormones. Toxicol Appl Pharmacol 2006; 214(1):1–7.

57. Wuttke D, Jarry H, Christoffel J, et al. Comparison of effects of estradiol (E2) with those of octylmethoxycinnamate (OMC) and 4-methylbenzylidene camphor (4MBC)—2 filters of UV light—on several uterine, vaginal and bone parameters. Toxicol Appl Pharmacol 2006; 210(3): 246–254.

58. Szwarcfarb B, Carbone S, Reynoso R, et al. Octyl-methoxycinnamate (OMC), an ultraviolet (UV) filter, alters LHRH and amino acid neurotransmitters release from hypothalamus of immature rats. Exp Clin Endocrinol Diabetes 2008; 116(2):94–98.

59. Schneider S, Deckardt K, Hellwig J, et al. Octyl methoxycinnamate: two generation reproduction toxicity in Wistar rats by dietary administration. Food Chem Toxicol 2005; 43(7): 1083–1092.

60. Greim H. Chemicals with endocrine-disrupting potential: a threat to human health? Angew Chem Int Ed Engl 2005; 44(35):5568–5574.

11

New and Emerging Sunscreen Technologies

Julian P. Hewitt

Croda Suncare & Biopolymers, Ditton, Cheshire, U.K.

SYNOPSIS

- Over the past 10 years, a number of UVB, UVA, and broad-spectrum UVB/UVA filters have been developed and are available in many parts of the world.
- Many developments in coating and dispersion technologies to improve ease of use, compatibility with other ingredients, and photostability of inorganic sunscreens have been achieved.
- Botanical extracts have been investigated for their property to protect the skin by mechanisms other than UV absorption (e.g., anti-inflammatory, antioxidative property).
- Developments in the delivery system include encapsulation of UV filters, submicron encapsulation, SLN, and NLC.
- Technology to enhance SPF includes emollient/solvent systems, rheological additives, film-forming polymers, and light-scattering particles.
- In the past few years, the issue of photolabile filters has been addressed by combining them with UV filters known to have photostabilizing effects, by the use of molecules that are not UV filters and that have been specifically designed to quench the excited states of photolabile UV filters, and by the use of Mn-doped TiO_2.

INTRODUCTION

The last 30 years have seen a rapid development of sun protection technology. As consumers have become more aware of the damage that UV radiation can cause to the skin, and clinicians have increased their understanding of the mechanisms of such damage, the demand for ever more effective UV protection products has stimulated many innovations. This process continues today, with the development of novel sunscreen actives and more effective ways to deliver these actives onto skin.

Therefore, in writing a chapter titled "New and Emerging Sunscreen Technologies," it might seem at first that there is plenty of material to use. But the first fundamental question which must be asked is: How exactly do we decide what is "new"? If one takes the cutting-edge approach, i.e., to discuss sunscreen actives that have only just been invented or are still being developed, then this chapter would contain little information of practical use, at least in the short-to-medium term. The long timescales involved in achieving regulatory approval for new sunscreens, especially in the United States, mean that technologies that are *that* new cannot actually be used yet.

Therefore, in the context of this chapter, the definition of "new" has been expanded somewhat to encompass technologies that have been around long enough to have achieved regulatory approval and hence are in commercial use in at least some parts of the world, but which are still recent enough to be generally considered as innovative and novel.

One must also remember that a new "sunscreen technology" might not necessarily involve a new UV-absorbing molecule or material. Because of the difficulties (not to mention expense) inherent in developing and commercializing new UV filters, much scientific effort in recent years has been focused on how to get more out of the existing UV filters; hence, this chapter also includes sections devoted to novel delivery systems such as encapsulation, "sun protection factor (SPF) booster" technologies, and novel finished product forms.

DEVELOPMENTS IN UV FILTER TECHNOLOGY

Novel Organic UV Filters

In addition to providing effective absorption of UV radiation in the wavelength range 290 to 400 nm, the ideal sunscreen molecule should also possess the following characteristics:

- Safe for use on skin, i.e., nontoxic, nonirritating, nonsensitizing, and non-comedogenic
- Does not penetrate into or through the skin.
- Good solubility in cosmetic emollients
- Photostable, i.e., does not decay on exposure to UV
- UV spectral profile not significantly affected by solvents
- Compatible with other cosmetic ingredients
- Does not produce an odor or color in the final formulation or on skin
- Chemically stable
- Compatible with most packaging materials

Most common UV filters are defective in at least one of these areas. For example, ethylhexyl methoxycinnamate (octinoxate) and butyl methoxydibenzoylmethane (avobenzone) are photolabile; avobenzone can also be difficult to solubilize, as can benzophenone-3 (oxybenzone). New developments in organic UV filters tend to be targeted at either addressing these shortcomings or improving the UV absorption efficacy. The latter could mean increasing the extinction coefficient or broadening the spectral coverage; in particular, the growing awareness of the skin damage caused by UVA radiation has prompted the development of a number of new UVA filters in recent years.

A common design feature of new UV absorber molecules is the presence of double, triple, or extended chromophores. This results in UV filters that are more effective (because of the presence of more than one chromophore in the same molecule), more photostable, and show very low skin penetration because of the size of the molecules. The guiding principle here is the "500 Dalton rule"; molecules with a molecular weight of 500 Dalton or more are too large to penetrate the skin. Another approach to minimizing the potential for skin penetration is to attach UV-absorbing chromophores onto a polymer backbone, thereby creating a very large molecule.

The following are some of the new UV filters introduced within the last 10 years and which are now approved (and used) in Europe and elsewhere. At the time of writing, however, none of these has been added to the list of approved UV filters on the Food and Drug Administration (FDA) Sunscreen Monograph in the United States (1). The chemistry and properties of these materials are covered in detail elsewhere in this book (chap. 2), so the following is only a brief review.

UVB Filters

Ethylhexyl triazone has a triple chromophore, giving it a molecular weight of 823 Dalton and a very high specific extinction coefficient [E(1%, 1cm)] of 1450. Its wavelength of maximum absorption (λ_{max}) is 314 nm.

Diethylhexyl butamido triazone has a similar structure to ethylhexyl triazone, and therefore similar properties: Molecular weight is 766 Dalton, E (1%, 1cm) is 1460, and λ_{max} is 312 nm. However, by changing one of the side groups, the molecule is no longer symmetrical, and this gives improved solubility in cosmetic emollients.

Polysilicone-15 was developed by taking the alternative molecular design approach mentioned above—that of attaching chromophores onto a polymer backbone. This results in a lower extinction coefficient [E(1%, 1cm) is 160–190], because the proportion of UV-absorbing chromophores in the overall molecule is quite low; λ_{max} is 312 nm. However, the polymer structure provides for improved film-forming properties (2).

UVA Filters

Diethylamino hydroxy benzoyl hexyl benzoate (DHHB) is essentially a benzophenone derivative with an extended chromophore, providing for a high extinction coefficient in the UVA region [E(1%, 1cm) = 900, λ_{max} = 354 nm].

Disodium phenyl dibenzimidazole tetrasulfonate (DPDT) is a water-soluble UVA filter. The molecular design in this case was once again derived from an existing filter—phenyl benzimidazole sulfonic acid. The latter is a UVB filter (λ_{max} = 302 nm), but by extending the chromophore, the λ_{max} is increased to 335 nm.

Terephthalylidene dicamphor sulfonic acid (TDSA; ecamsule) is also water soluble and is one of a group of UV filters that are proprietary to L'Oréal under the trade name Mexoryl®. It has a λ_{max} of 345 nm. Although not yet on the list of approved sunscreens in the FDA Sunscreen Monograph, a new drug application for a finished product containing this active (Anthelios SX) was approved in the United States in 2006.

UVA/B Filters

Bis-ethylhexyloxyphenol methoxyphenyl triazine (BEMT; bemotrizinol) is yet another example of an extended chromophore design, which in this case provides a molecule with two absorption maxima (310 and 343 nm), making it a true broad-spectrum filter.

Drometrizole trisiloxane (DTS) is another example of L'Oréal's captive Mexoryl filters. Like BEMT, this molecule has absorption maxima in both the UVB (303 nm) and UVA (341 nm).

Methylene bis-benzotriazolyl tetramethylbutylphenol (MBBT; bisoctrizole) once again has a double chromophore and once again has two absorption maxima (305 and 360 nm). This material is unique among organic UV filters in that it is not soluble in

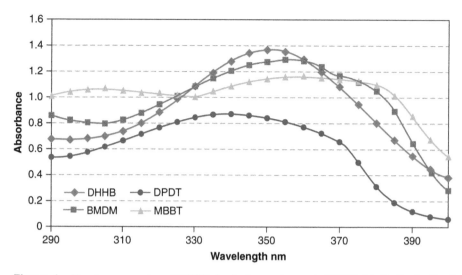

Figure 1 Absorbance spectra of DHHB (aminobenzophenone), DPDT (bisdisulizole disodium), and MBBT (bisoctrizole) compared to BMDM (avobenzone) (measured at 5% active in a sunscreen formulation).

either water or cosmetic oils; it is a particulate material, supplied as a 50% aqueous dispersion.

Figure 1 shows absorbance spectra measured in the Croda laboratories for DHHB, DPDT, and MBBT, compared to butyl methoxydibenzoylmethane (BMDM; avobenzone). Each filter was incorporated into a standard formulation at a level of 5% active. Formulations were applied onto Transpore™ tape at a dosage of 2 mg/cm^2, and absorbance spectra were measured on an Optometrics SPF-290 analyzer.

Novel Inorganic Sunscreens

The list of inorganic sunscreen actives is short: only titanium dioxide (TiO$_2$) and ZnO are of commercial importance, and these can no longer really be considered as new technologies. Sunscreen grades of these materials (variously described as "fine particle," "micronized," "microfine," "nanofine," or "nanoparticle" forms) have been used for around 20 years. TiO$_2$ is now used in over 60% of commercial sunscreen products in Europe (3) and elsewhere in the world; for example, in Japan, the proportion is even higher. There have been many developments in coating and dispersion technologies to improve ease of use, compatibility with other ingredients, and photostability of inorganic sunscreens; also, recent developments in optimization of particle size distribution have resulted in grades of TiO$_2$ and ZnO, which are transparent on skin and avoid whitening, which is traditionally associated with these products (4). However, the basic technology remains essentially the same. Other inorganic materials have been tried as sunscreens, for example, iron oxides, and boron nitride, but their efficacy is too low for them to be commercially useful.

However, one recent development in inorganic sunscreen technology can genuinely be described as new, and this development transforms TiO$_2$ from a simple UV filter into a multifunctional ingredient. This technology involves the doping of TiO$_2$ with a low level of manganese (Mn); the Mn ions are located both within the structural lattice of the TiO$_2$ and at the surface of the particles (Optisol™, Croda, Yorkshire, England). As reported in the literature (5), uncoated TiO$_2$ has the capacity to act as a photocatalyst, generating free

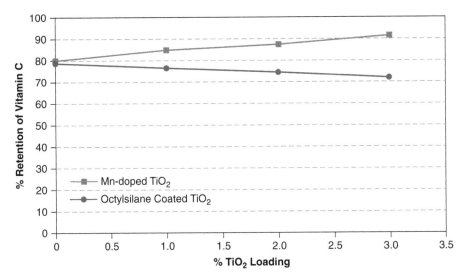

Figure 2 Retention of vitamin C in a water-oil-water (W/O/W) emulsion after two hours of UV exposure, in conjunction with conventional coated TiO_2 and manganese-doped TiO_2. *Source*: From Ref. 7.

radicals because of absorption of UV radiation. The conventional way to prevent this photocatalytic action is by coating the TiO_2 particles, and the coatings used nowadays on sunscreen grades of TiO_2 have been developed to be very effective in this regard. However, by doping the lattice with Mn ions, the generation of free radicals is prevented (6), so that coating is unnecessary. The resulting doped TiO_2 also provides increased UVA protection and has the ability to scavenge free radicals from the external environment. This means that it can photostabilize other ingredients such as photolabile organic UV filters or vitamins (6,7). For example, Figure 2 shows the percentage of vitamin C retained in a water-oil-water (W/O/W) emulsion after two hours of irradiation. With no TiO_2 present, the retention is about 80%, i.e., there has been a 20% decay in the level of vitamin C present. With increasing levels of a conventional TiO_2 in the formulation, there is a slight increase in the decay, whereas with the Mn-doped material, there is an increase in the percentage retention, showing that the photostability of the vitamin C has been improved. Since vitamins are themselves used as antiaging actives, the fact that Mn-doped TiO_2 stabilizes them means that it provides a functional benefit in antiaging skin care products as well as giving UV protection.

The one drawback of this material is that the Mn doping results in a colored material; typically, it is light brown or beige. However, this can in fact be advantageous, as in formulations the color shows as a natural-looking skin tone, masking the whitening usually seen with TiO_2.

Natural Sunscreens

The use of more "natural" ingredients is a growing marketing trend in all areas of personal care, and sun protection is no exception. However, to find a truly natural sunscreen active is problematic. All organic ("chemical") UV filters are synthetic materials. The inorganic sunscreens are perceived to be more "natural," as they are derived from natural mineral sources, and many commercial sun care products, which use only inorganic filters, have been marketed as "all natural," "contains natural mineral filters," "no chemical sunscreens," etc. Some nongovernmental organizations, which provide certification of "organic" consumer products, have, for the time being at least, chosen to exclude sunscreen grades of TiO_2 and ZnO, saying that they will not certify any products that contain nanoparticles. However, this exclusion is not because the TiO_2 and ZnO are not natural, but is rather based on ill-founded concerns over the safety of nanoparticulate forms of these materials. This is unfortunate, since the safety of TiO_2 and ZnO nanoparticles has been the subject of numerous studies (8–11), which have repeatedly demonstrated that they do not penetrate through the stratum corneum and they are completely safe for topical application. If a natural sunscreen claim is desired, TiO_2 and ZnO still represent the most natural and the safest option.

Various botanical extracts have been shown to have sun-protective effects, by virtue of containing antioxidants, or chemical species, which can act as UV filters. Bobin et al. measured the UV-filtering properties of about 100 natural extracts and found some that showed significant UV absorption (12), but the extinction coefficients were relatively low (compared with synthetic UV filters), and in many cases the absorption maxima lie in the UVC wavelengths at too short a wavelength to be of practical use to sunscreen products. Kapsner et al. (13) discussed the formulation of natural sun care products and mentioned significant UV absorption from the following natural extracts:

- Annatto
- Gamma oryzanol (extracted from rice bran oil)
- Liquorice (*Glycyrrhiza glabra*)
- Calophylum inophylum seed oil
- Pongamol (provides UVA protection)

Epstein (14) further reviewed botanicals with UVB absorbing or "SPF boosting" properties. To date, however, none of these botanical actives have been approved as UV filters, and their relatively weak UV-absorbing properties would indicate that none are likely to be pursued commercially for this function alone.

A more promising avenue may be the use of natural extracts, which can protect the skin by mechanisms other than UV absorption (chap. 16). For example, Yusuf and his group have studied the potential of green tea polyphenols as photoprotectants (15). They have found that these extracts can protect against sunburn (erythema), non–melanoma skin cancers, UV-induced immunosuppression, and photoaging. *Polypodium leucotomos,* a Central American fern plant extract, has been shown in oral and topical forms to be photoprotective against UVB- and PUVA-induced phototoxicity, to be photoprotective against the induction of polymorphous light eruption and solar urticaria, and to increase the doses needed for immediate pigment darkening, minimal erythema dose, minimal phototoxic dose, and minimal melanogenic dose. It has been shown to have antioxidantive and anti-inflammatory properties (16). Other possibilities are provided by marine biotechnology, for example Artemia extract, prepared from the plankton *Artemia salina* (17). The chief component of this extract was found to protect DNA and decrease DNA damage. Artemia extract also induces a heat shock protein, Hsp70, providing further protection for cells, as well as having an anti-inflammatory effect.

DELIVERY SYSTEMS AND FORMULATION EXCIPIENTS

As mentioned in the introduction, the difficulty and expense associated with developing new UV filters and gaining regulatory approval for them, means that much of the new technology in the sunscreen field is related to maximizing the efficacy of existing actives.

This section deals with some of the delivery systems and other ingredients that have been developed with this objective in mind.

Encapsulation

Encapsulation technologies have been, and continue to be, investigated for many applications in both the personal care and health care fields, as well as in a number of other industries. The thinking behind the use of encapsulation is usually based on one or more of the following rationales:

- Controlled release of actives over an extended period of time
- Enhancing delivery of actives to a particular site
- Protection of sensitive actives from interaction with other components of a formulation

In the case of sunscreen actives, the first of these rationales is not usually relevant; ideally, we want sunscreens to be distributed on the skin as quickly as possible. However, the other two rationales do apply, and there is also a further reason for encapsulation of organic sunscreen actives. Concern over the possible penetration of organic UV filters into or through the skin has led to the investigation of encapsulation methods as a means of preventing such penetration, thereby enhancing the safety of the UV filters.

Encapsulation usually involves surrounding a core of the active with a shell (typically composed of a polymer) or a fatty wall (in the case of liposomes). In many applications, the capsules are designed to rupture (e.g., under the application of shear by rubbing) when they have reached the site where the active is to be released, but in the case of sunscreens, such a release is not required or even desirable. This is because the site where we want the actives to be for optimum efficacy and safety is on the surface of the skin; with microencapsulated organic sunscreens, this is best achieved if the capsules remain intact. If the purpose of microencapsulation is to protect or stabilize the actives themselves, this too requires that the capsules remain intact.

The use of microencapsulation for sunscreens has been developed into a range of commercially available encapsulated UV filters (18). Production of these involves a sol-gel process, encapsulating the organic UV filter in a silica glass shell. The capsules are produced at room temperature and contain about 80% by weight of the UV filter. They are supplied as aqueous dispersions; the UV filter content in the dispersion is approximately 35%. In this way, hydrophobic UV filters can be incorporated into the aqueous phase of the emulsion. The microcapsules were shown to remain intact after application on skin, and an in vitro study showed almost no diffusion of the active [ethylhexyl methoxycinnamate, United States Adopted Name (USAN): octinoxate] through a lipophilic membrane. This was in contrast to a formulation containing free octinoxate, which showed significant diffusion. Further penetration studies using human epidermis indicated no significant penetration through the epidermis even with free octinoxate, although encapsulation did give a threefold decrease in the level of active taken up within the epidermis. It was also demonstrated that microencapsulation in this way improved photostability of photolabile organic UV filters; this topic is discussed in more detail in section "Photostabilizers."

Fairhurst and Mitchnick (19) described a different encapsulation technology, which they termed "submicron encapsulation," in which each particle consists of a homogeneous mixture of the active with a "matrix" material, typically a polymer or wax. The particles thus produced are an order of magnitude smaller than conventional microcapsules, with a typical diameter of 250 to 500 nm. As with the silica microcapsules described above, the capsules are dispersed in water for ease of formulation; the UV filter content of the dispersion is typically 20% but can be as high as 35%. Fairhurst and Mitchnick prepared such capsules containing not only single sunscreens but also mixtures of UV filters. They were able to demonstrate dramatically improved SPF values from the encapsulated materials, compared with using the "free" sunscreen actives.

Two similar technologies, which have been the subject of considerable research in recent years, are solid lipid nanoparticles (SLN) and nanostructured lipid carriers (NLC). Given the growing controversy about nanotechnology, this terminology is perhaps unfortunate, especially bearing in mind the fact that the particle sizes in SLN and NLC systems are typically greater than 200 nm, and hence they lie outside the most commonly accepted definitions of nanoparticles. As with the submicron encapsulation described by Fairhurst and Mitchnick, SLN and NLC systems involve the incorporation of an active into a lipid matrix. The difference between them is that SLN systems are based on pure solid lipid, whereas NLC systems use a blend of solid and liquid lipids. Once again the delivery form of the system is typically an aqueous dispersion. Although such systems have been claimed to give improved UV absorbance (20), they are not yet in use in commercial sunscreen systems. The most likely reasons for this are that the manufacturing processes involved are quite complex, involving high temperatures and high-pressure homogenization, and the resultant loadings of active UV filter in the final dispersions tend to be quite low. The use of TiO_2, rather than organic UV filters, in SLN systems has also been reported (21), but this does not appear to be an encapsulation of TiO_2. The UV absorbance profiles reported were characteristic of pigment grade TiO_2 rather than sunscreen grade. Since TiO_2 pigment has a mean primary particle size of 200 to 300 nm, and the particles sizes reported for the SLN in this case were in the same range, it seems unlikely that the TiO_2 is within the lipid nanoparticles. The authors suggested that TiO_2 "molecules" might be absorbed on the surface of the lipid nanoparticles, but given the insolubility of TiO_2 and the size of the TiO_2 particles, this too seems unlikely. The authors reported that their SLN systems containing TiO_2 showed enhanced UV absorption, but this is more likely to be due to light scattering from the lipid nanoparticles themselves. Dahms (22) referred to this as a "pigment effect" of SLN systems; however, since no actual encapsulation of the UV active is involved, discussion of this phenomenon falls more correctly under the heading of "SPF Boosters" and is discussed in the next section of this chapter.

Efficacy Enhancers

As the "horsepower race" to achieve higher and higher SPFs in sun protection products has developed, so a number of different ingredients and technologies have been claimed to boost or enhance SPF, allowing the formulator to achieve their targets with lower levels of active ingredients. Such SPF boosters include the following:

- Emollient/solvent systems
- Rheological additives
- Film-forming polymers
- Light-scattering particles

In view of the now well-recognized need for sunscreen products to provide effective UVA protection as well as high SPF, such SPF boosters are more correctly described as "efficacy enhancers," since most, if not all, of these technologies are capable of boosting efficacy across the UV spectrum and hence will increase UVA protection factors as well as SPF.

A recent paper (23) described studies to assess the efficacy of some of these ingredients. It was found that each of the technologies is capable of boosting SPF in specific types of systems, but there is no "magic bullet" that works in all formulations. However, by matching the right technology for a given system, some spectacular boosts in SPF can be achieved, in some cases increasing SPF efficacy by over 50%.

Emollients

The selection of specific emollients or solvents to improve the efficacy of UV filters can hardly be described as new technology. It is well known that the vehicle in which a sunscreen active is dissolved or dispersed can influence the efficacy of that active (24,25). Most organic sunscreens are oil soluble, so the emollients used in a formulation act as solvents for the actives. Depending on the relative polarity of the solvent and the sunscreen, the solvent can shift the wavelength of maximum absorption (λ_{max}) to either a shorter wavelength (hypsochromic shift) or longer wavelength (bathochromic shift). If the shift is such that the absorption spectrum of the active more closely matches the erythemal effectiveness spectrum, then (theoretically at least) an improved SPF can be achieved. Also, the solubility of the active in the solvent can be of critical importance. Solid UV filters need to be adequately solvated to remain in solution. What is new is the use of knowledge of these factors to aid development of new emollients, which are claimed to boost SPF (26). In the study reported by Hine (23), it was concluded that any SPF-boosting effect from an emollient is specific to certain filters and/or certain formulation systems.

In the case of inorganic sunscreens, solubility is not relevant, since the active is insoluble. Also, there are no solvent shifts in λ_{max}. However, it has been shown that the emollients used can influence the degree of dispersion of the particles of inorganic sunscreen (27), and hence can influence SPF.

Rheological Additives and Film Formers

Previous work has shown that SPF can be significantly improved by optimizing the rheological behavior of a sunscreen formulation (27–30). For example, the use of waxes in water-in-oil (W/O) systems increases SPF by shortening the "recovery time" of the emulsion after spreading. Recovery time is the time taken to rebuild structure and viscosity in a thixotropic material after it has been subjected to high shear, for example, spreading on skin. A short recovery time means that the product maintains an even film over the skin, rather than flowing into the skin wrinkles.

Another way to achieve and maintain a more even film is to incorporate a film former into the formulation. Such ingredients, usually polymers, have also been shown to boost SPF (2,31,32).

Hine (23) studied SPF-boosting effects of a group of experimental polyol polyesters, which act as film formers, and some of which also modify the rheology of formulations. The results indicated that both mechanisms—rheology modification and film forming—play a role in enhancing the efficacy of sunscreen formulations.

Light-Scattering Additives

Jones (33) described a hollow sphere technology for boosting SPF. This involves synthesis of spheres composed of a styrene/acrylates copolymer, which on production and in the formulation, contain water. It is claimed that on application of the formulation onto the skin, the water migrates out of the polymer spheres, which can then scatter light because of the different refractive indices of the carrier medium, the polymer itself, and air inside the polymer shell. This scattering increases the path length for UV radiation to

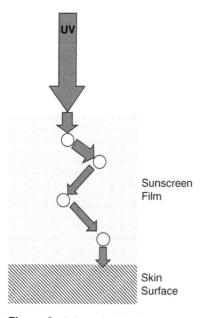

Figure 3 Schematic showing scattering of UV light by particles or hollow spheres in a sunscreen film, thereby increasing path length and hence UV absorbance.

traverse the sunscreen film (Fig. 3); from the Beer–Lambert law, the absorbance given by a UV filter depends on the path length that the light must travel, so by increasing this, the absorbance is increased. In vivo data showed that the polymer spheres themselves exhibit no UV-filtering effect, but when they were added to formulations containing organic UV filters, SPF was increased by 60% to 70%. In a system containing the UVA filter BMDM (avobenzone), the UVA absorbance was increased, showing that the effect operates across both UVB and UVA.

Dahms (22) described a similar SPF-boosting effect from the use of membrane-structured solid nanoparticles (MSSN). These are similar in concept to the SLN described earlier, and their main purpose, as with SLN, is encapsulation of actives. The claimed advantage of MSSN is that each particle consists of a continuous liquid crystalline membrane, which facilitates the homogeneous incorporation of amphiphilic molecules such as retinol or tocopherol. Dahms reported an SPF-boosting effect when unloaded MSSN were incorporated into a sunscreen formulation containing ethylhexyl salicylate. This improvement in UV efficacy, however, was attributed not to encapsulation of the UV filter but rather to scattering of light, thus increasing the path length through the sunscreen film as discussed above. As mentioned earlier, this is also the most likely explanation for the improved absorption from TiO_2 systems with SLN, as reported by Cengiz et al. (21).

Photostabilizers

As mentioned earlier, a weakness of some of the most commonly used organic UV filters is that they photo-decay, i.e., they undergo chemical changes because of absorption of UV, converting to isomers, tautomers, or dimers, which are less-effective sunscreens. Therefore, their efficacy decreases over time when in use (1,34). This decay is automatically accounted for during in vivo SPF testing, as this is a time-resolved experiment, so the measured SPF value is still a valid representation of the level of sunburn protection offered by the product. However, if the decay can be prevented, the efficacy of the actives can be increased. Also, most modern in vitro techniques for measuring UVA protection efficacy, including the recently released FDA proposal, involve a pre-irradiation step (35–37), so the filter system needs to be photostable to perform well on these tests. As discussed in the section "Novel Organic UV Filters," most new UV filters have been developed with photostability as a key requirement; however, these filters are expensive and are not yet globally approved, so, many formulations still make use of standard UV filters such as EHMC (octinoxate) and BMDM (avobenzone). These are the two most notoriously photounstable UV filters, and when they are used together, the degree of photo-decay increases even further because of a 2+2 cycloaddition reaction (1,38). Therefore, the development of excipients, which can photostabilize these materials, has been the subject of much research in recent years.

Several other UV filters are known to have photostabilizing effects on the photolabile filters. The best known is the use of octocrylene to stabilize avobenzone, but this strategy is covered by patents (34), and in any case, it is much less effective when avobenzone is combined with octinoxate (38). Methylbenzylidene camphor (MBC) is another filter which has been shown to photostabilize avobenzone, but this filter is not yet approved in the United States and has fallen out of favor in Europe. Two of the newer UV filters, MBBT (bisoctrizole) and BEMT (bemotrizinol), have also been reported to boost photostability; the latter has been reported to increase photostability of the avobenzone/octinoxate combination (39).These UV filters stabilize avobenzone by "quenching" the triplet-excited state of the molecule before it can undergo the photochemical reactions that lead to loss of UV efficacy.

Other molecules, which are not UV filters, have been specifically designed to quench the excited states of photolabile UV filters in a similar way. The first of these was diethylhexyl-2,6-naphthalate, reported by Bonda and Steinberg (40). This was found to be extremely effective in photostabilizing avobenzone, but even this could not completely photostabilize the avobenzone/octinoxate combination. More recently, Bonda has reported the development of new materials that are effective in stabilizing this combination (38).

There are other strategies for improving photostability of these photolabile materials. As mentioned in the section "Encapsulation," encapsulation of the filters can render them more photostable. Pflucker et al. were able to demonstrate that in octinoxate/avobenzone combinations, when the octinoxate is encapsulated, the rate of decay of avobenzone is reduced compared with the rate measured when free octinoxate is used (18). Citernesi (41) studied the photostability of UV filters complexed in either phospholipids or cyclodextrin; he found that while complexing in phospholipid systems shows no improvement in photostability, the cyclodextrin complexes were effective in preventing photo-decay.

Still another approach is to make use of the Mn-doped TiO_2 discussed in section "Novel Inorganic Sunscreens." This was shown to have a substantial photostabilizing effect on avobenzone and octinoxate (7), due partly to the absorption of UV by the TiO_2, but also from scavenging of reactive oxygen species (ROS) by Mn ions at the surface of the particles, as shown in the following reaction scheme:

$$Mn^{2+} \Leftrightarrow Mn^{3+} + e^-$$
$$Mn^{2+} + OH\cdot \Rightarrow Mn^{3+} + OH^-$$
$$Mn^{3+} + \cdot O_2 \Rightarrow Mn^{2+} + O_2$$

A more recent study (42) further showed that the Mn-doped TiO_2 is even more effective in stabilizing avobenzone and octinoxate when it is used in a predispersed form, because the improved dispersion of the particles means that more particle surface is exposed, enhancing the free-radical scavenging effect.

NOVEL PRODUCT FORMS

Another aspect of sun protection, which has been the subject of considerable recent innovation, is the physical form of the final consumer product. The driving force for these developments has been greater convenience, leading hopefully to improved consumer compliance. Historically, the vast majority of sunscreen products have been formulated as creams or lotions; application of such products is messy and time consuming. This can be particularly problematic with the most important target group for sun protection, namely children and teenagers.

The need for products that are easier to apply has led to a rapid growth in the use of spray formulations as a vehicle for sunscreens. Single-phase oil spray sunscreen products have been around for many years, but the rheology of such products means they tend to be limited to low SPF values. Recent years have seen the development of sprayable emulsion systems (especially prevalent in the European market) and aerosol sprays (now commanding a large share of the U.S. market).

The development in emulsion sprays has been made possible by advances in emulsification technology (43), facilitating the development of stable low-viscosity systems. Initially, sunscreen products based on emulsion sprays were limited to low SPF values (5 or 10), but now such products are available with SPFs of 30 or even 50.

The aerosol sprays are often promoted as "continuous spray sunscreen" or "no-rub sunscreen," and mostly consist of a simple one-phase alcohol-based formulation with a film-forming polymer. The concept is that with a very fine spray and the polymer to aid film formation on skin, the product distributes evenly over the skin with no need for rubbing in and gives a dry, nongreasy, and nonoily skin feel.

Another novel vehicle is the sunscreen wipe. In this case, a thin liquid emulsion containing the sunscreen actives is impregnated into a wipe. Again the objective is convenience, particularly for applying sunscreen onto small children. However, this type of product has remained something of a niche application and has not achieved the same popularity as sprays.

Sunscreen sticks have been around for many years but have been mainly for protection of the lips. Now this format is also finding wider usage in products for the face; for example, one target group of users is golfers, who need sun protection but, for obvious reasons, do not want greasy sun lotion on their hands.

CONCLUSIONS

The last 20 years have seen rapid advancement in sun protection technology. Increasing awareness of the dangers of the sun has driven the demand for ever-increasing SPF values and broad-spectrum protection products, which in turn has provided the impetus for development of new sunscreen actives and more efficient vehicles for those actives. Many of the new actives have yet to achieve global regulatory approval and therefore can still be viewed as emerging technologies, even though they have actually been around for a few years. Much of the newest technology in the sunscreen field is concerned with delivery of the actives in such a way that they are more efficient, safer, and more stable, thereby providing high protection factors without the use of excessively high concentrations of UV filters. Meanwhile, development of novel formats for final products is aimed at making topical sun protection products more convenient to use.

REFERENCES

1. Shaath NA. The Encyclopedia of Ultraviolet Filters. Carol Stream, IL: Allured Publishing Corporation, 2007.
2. Schwarzenbach R, Huber U. Optimization of sunscreen efficacy. In: Sun Protection. Augsburg, Germany: Verlag für chemische Industrie, H. Ziolkowsky GmbH, 2003:131–137.
3. Johncock W. Market situation of sun products—a review of latest innovations. In: Sun Protection. Augsburg, Germany: Verlag für chemische Industrie, H. Ziolkowsky GmbH, 2003:281–286.
4. Hewitt JP. UV Protection in "Prestige" Products. Presented at: the eighth Florida Sunscreen Symposium; April 2002, Orlando, FL.
5. Schlossman D, Shao Y. Inorganic ultraviolet filters. In: Shaath NA, ed. Sunscreens: Regulations and Commercial Development. 3rd ed. Boca Raton, FL: Taylor & Francis, 2005:239–279.
6. Wakefield G, Lipscomb S, Holland E, et al. The effects of manganese doping on UVA absorption and free radical generation of micronised TiO_2 and its consequences for the photostability of UVA absorbing organic sunscreen components. Photochem Photobiol Sci 2004; 3:648–652.
7. Wakefield G, Stott J. Photostabilisation of organic UV-absorbing and anti-oxidant cosmetic components in formulations containing micronized manganese doped titanium dioxide. J Cosmet Sci 2006; 57:385–395.
8. Nohynek GJ, Lademann J, Ribaud C, et al. Grey goo on the skin? Nanotechnology, cosmetic and sunscreen safety. Crit Rev Toxicol 2007; 37:251–277.
9. Pflücker F, Wendel V, Hohenberg H, et al. The human stratum corneum layer: an effective barrier against dermal uptake of different forms of topically applied micronised titanium dioxide. Skin Pharmacol Appl Skin Physiol 2001; 14(suppl 1):92–97.
10. Schulz J, Hohenberg H, Pflücker F, et al. Distribution of sunscreens on skin. Adv Drug Deliv Rev 2002; 54(suppl 1):S157–S163.
11. Gelis C, Miquel C, Mavon A. In vivo and ex vivo study of the skin penetration of mineral and organic sunscreens and assessment of the efficiency of this photoprotection on a reconstituted human epidermis. Presented at: 23rd IFSCC International Congress; Oct 24–27 2004; Orlando, Florida, poster 111.
12. Bobin MF, Raymond M, Martini MC. Natural UVA/UVB absorbers. Cosmet Toilet 1994; 109(11): 63–70.
13. Kapsner T, Matravers P, Shiozawa K, et al. Formulating natural sun care products . In: Shaath NA, ed. Sunscreens: Regulations and Commercial Development. 3rd ed. Boca Raton, FL: Taylor & Francis, 2005:507–521.
14. Epstein H. Botanicals in sun care products. In: Shaath NA, ed. Sunscreens: Regulations and Commercial Development. 3rd ed. Boca Raton, FL: Taylor & Francis, 2005:657–671.
15. Yusuf N, Irby C, Katiyar SK, et al. Photoprotective effects of green tea polyphenols. Photodermatol Photoimmunol Photomed 2007; 23(1):48–56.
16. Caccialanza M, Percivalle S, Piccinno R, et al. Photoprotective activity of oral polypodium leucotomos extract in 25 patients with idiopathic photodermatoses. Photodermatol Photoimmunol Photomed 2007; 23(1):46–47.
17. Domloge N, Bauza E, Cucumel K, et al. Artemis extract: toward more extensive sun protection. Cosmet Toilet 2002; 117(2):69–78.
18. Pflucker F, Guinard H, Lapidot N et al. Sunglasses for the skin: reduction of dermal UV filter uptake by encapsulation. In: Sun Protection. Augsburg, Germany: Verlag für chemische Industrie, H. Ziolkowsky GmbH, 2003:97–105.
19. Fairhurst D, Mitchnick M. Submicron encapsulation of organic sunscreens. Cosmet Toilet 1995; 110(9):47–50.
20. Xia Q, Saupe A, Müller RH, et al. Nanostructured lipid carriers as novel carrier for sunscreen formulations. Int J Cosmet Sci 2007; 29(6):473–482.
21. Cengiz E, Wissing SA, Müller RH, et al. Sunblocking efficiency of various TiO_2-loaded solids lipid nanoparticle formulations. Int J Cosmet Sci 2006; 25(5):371–378.

22. Dahms GH. Membrane structured solid nanoparticles—a novel nanotechnology for delivery of cosmetic active ingredients. IFSCC Magazine 2008; 8(3):193–198.

23. Hine HA, Hewitt JP. Magic bullets? As assessment of SPF boosting technology. In: Proceedings of the 42nd Annual Conference of the Australian Society of Cosmetic Chemists; 2008 Mar 6–9; Gold Coast, Australia.

24. Shaath NA. On the theory of ultraviolet absorption by sunscreen chemicals. J Soc Cosmet Chem 1987; 82:193–207.

25. Agrapidis-Paloympis LE, Nash RA, Shaath NA. The effects of solvents on the ultraviolet absorbance of sunscreens. J Soc Cosmet Chem 1987; 38:209–221.

26. Cernasov D, Macchio R, Mesiha M, et al. Octyldodecyl neopentanoate: its effect on the performance of sunscreen formulations. Cosmet Toilet 1997; 112(6):75–82.

27. Hewitt JP, Woodruff J. factors influencing efficacy of oil-dispersed physical sunscreens. IFSCC Magazine 2000; 3(1):18–23.

28. Dahms GH. Influence of thixotropy on the UV absorption of sun protection emulsions. Parf Kosmet 1994; 75:675–679.

29. Hewitt JP, Dahms GH. The influence of rheology on efficacy of physical sunscreens. In: Proceedings of the IFSCC Between-Congress Conference; 1995; Switzerland:Montreux, 313–323.

30. Floyd DT, Macpherson BA, Bungard A, et al. Formulation of sun protection emulsions with enhanced SPF response. Cosmet Toilet 1997; 112(6):55–64.

31. Angelinetta C, Barzaghi G. Influence of oil polarity on SPF in liquid crystal emulsions with ultrafine TiO_2 pre-dispersed in oil, and cross-linking polymers. Cosmet News (Italy) 1995; 100:20–24.

32. Hunter A, Trevino M. Film formers enhance water resistance and SPF in sun care products. Cosmet Toilet 2004; 119(7):51–56.

33. Jones CE. Hollow sphere technology for sunscreen formulation. In: Sun Protection. Augsburg, Germany: Verlag für chemische Industrie, H. Ziolkowsky GmbH, 2003: 106–113.

34. Bonda CA. The Photostability of organic sunscreen actives: a review. In: Shaath NA, ed. Sunscreens: Regulations and Commercial Development. 3rd ed. Boca Raton, FL: Taylor & Francis, 2005:321–349.

35. COLIPA Guideline: Method for the in-vitro determination of UVA protection provided by sunscreen products, 2007a. Available at: http://www.colipa.com/site/index.cfm?SID=15588&OBJ=28546&back=1.

36. Food and Drug Administration. Sunscreen Drug Products for Over-The-Counter Human Use: Proposed Amendment of Final Monograph. 21 CFR Part 352, §352.71 paragraph (h) (72 FR 49119 – 49120), Aug. 27, 2007.

37. Boots UK Ltd. Measurement of UVA: UVB Ratios According to the Boots Star Rating System (2008 Revision). January 2008; Nottingham, UK.

38. Bonda CA. Research Pathways to New Performance Additives for Broad Spectrum Sunscreens. In: Proceedings of the 11th Florida Sunscreen Symposium; Sep 6–9 2007; Orlando, FL.

39. Chatelain E, Gabard B. Photostabilization of butyl methoxy dibenzoylmethane (avobenzone) and ethylhexyl methoxycinnamate by bis-ethylhexyloxyphenol methoxyphenyl triazine (Tinosorb S), a new UV broadband filter. Photochem Photobiol 2001; 74:401.

40. Bonda CA, Steinberg DC. A new photostabilizer for full spectrum sunscreens. Cosmet Toilet 2000; 115(6):37–45.

41. Citernesi U. Photostability of sun filters complexed in phospholipids or β-Cyclodextrin. Cosmet Toilet 2001; 116(9):77–86.

42. Hewitt JP, Stott J, Duggan A. Using inorganic sunscreens to enhance the photostability of organic sunscreens: dispersion effects. In: Proceedings of the 42nd Annual Conference of the Australian Society of Cosmetic Chemists; 2008 Mar 6–9; Gold Coast, Australia.

43. Tadros T, Taelman M-C, Leonard S. Principles of formulation of sprayable emulsions. International Conference on Sun Protection: A Time of Change. London: Summit Events Ltd, 2003.

12
DNA Repair and Photoprotection

Daniel B. Yarosh and Kenneth A. Smiles
AGI Dermatics, Freeport, New York, U.S.A.

SYNOPSIS

- UV produces DNA damage. UVB is the predominant wavelength that results in the formation of CPDs and <6-4>PPs; 8oGua is formed secondary to exposure to UVA.
- CPDs and <6-47>PPs are repaired by NER pathway. It takes about 24 hours to remove 50% of the CPDs formed, while 50% of <6-4>PPs are removed in 30 minutes.
- Damage to single bases such as 8oGua is repaired by BER pathway.
- Liposomes carrying DNA repair enzymes (T4 endonuclease V, photolyase) have been shown to enhance CPD repair in mammalian cells and in human skin. T4 endonuclease V containing lipososmes have been demonstrated to decrease the formation of actinic keratosis and basal cell carcinoma in patients with xeroderma pigmentosum.
- Liposomes carrying OGG1 have been shown to enhance removal of 8oGua in an animal model.
- Enhancing DNA repair may be essential to extend our strategy for photoprotection.

INTRODUCTION TO DNA REPAIR AND PHOTOPROTECTION

The development of materials that substantially diminish the amount of UV radiation delivered to skin has been to date the primary strategy for sun protection. Thus the use of clothing, shade, and topical sunscreen products containing both organic/chemical and inorganic/physical UV filters are principal strategies for avoiding both the short- and long-terms effects of UV damage. No matter how effective a UV filter is, however, some radiation is still going to damage targets in the skin either directly, such as DNA damage, or indirectly, such as oxidative damage to vital cellular components. Recent work has pointed out two new strategies for overcoming the practical limitations of UV filter–based sunscreens (1). One involves the use of potent antioxidants to limit the amount of cellular damage induced primarily by reactive oxygen species and the other involves helping the skin to more effectively and quickly repair the UV damage to DNA. This chapter will review the progress made recently in incorporating active ingredients into topical products that effectively boost overall protection against UV radiation and help repair the primary DNA damage.

SUN DAMAGE TO DNA

Wavelengths of Sunlight that Damage DNA

In large part, because of the aromatic rings in the DNA purine and pyrimidine bases, DNA absorbs readily in the UV portion of the solar spectrum. Although the shorter UVC wavelengths (200–280 nm) do not actually reach the earth's surface because of their absorption by the ozone layer, the longer wavelength UVB (280–315 nm) is still relatively efficient in causing direct damage to the DNA bases and penetrates largely only into the epidermis (2). The even longer wavelength UVA (315–400 nm) penetrates into the dermis; however, since these photons carry less energy, they are relatively less efficient in producing direct damage to DNA than UVB but still create reactive oxygen species in the skin cells that indirectly damage DNA (3). Recent evidence suggests that very high doses of visible light can produce indirect DNA damage through the formation of reactive oxygen species (4).

Photoproducts

Solar UV directly causes an instantaneous photochemical reaction in DNA that links together adjacent pyrimidine bases (cytosine or thymine) (5). This cyclobutane pyrimidine dimer (CPD) is the most common form of DNA damage and is formed by all UV wavelengths, including UVA, UVB, and UVC (6) (Table 1). After a sunburn dose, on the order of 100,000 CPDs are formed in the DNA of every sun-exposed cell. In a much less common reaction, solar UV can directly link together these bases by a single twisted bond, resulting in a 6-4 photoproduct (<6-4>PP) (6).

Solar UV can also cause DNA damage by an indirect method, through the formation of reactive oxygen species that attack DNA, particularly the guanine base. This oxidation

Table 1 DNA Photoproducts, Their Cause and Course of Repair

DNA photoproduct	Peak UV region	Direct (UV absorption) or indirect (oxidation)	Percent of all DNA damage from sunlight	Repair mechanism	Speed of repair (time to remove 50% of damage)
Cyclobutane pyrimidine dimer	UVB	Direct	75%	Nucleotide excision repair (NER)	24 h
6-4 Photoproduct	UVB	Direct	15%	Nucleotide excision repair (NER)	30 min
8-oxo-guanosine	UVA	Indirect	10%	Base excision repair (BER)	2 h

reaction most often results in 8-oxo-guanosine (8oGua), but even after UVA exposure, CPDs are much more common than 8oGua (7). Oxidation of DNA can also result in single-stranded breaks, but under physiological conditions, these are very difficult to detect. When single-stranded breaks are found after UV irradiation, they are almost all caused by DNA repair enzymes cutting the DNA in an intermediate step in repair.

MECHANISMS OF DNA REPAIR

Despite the many types of potential DNA photoproducts, human cells funnel the lesions into one of two basic pathways for removing and repairing the damaged strands.

Nucleotide Excision Repair

Major damage to DNA, such as CPDs or <6-4>PPs, interferes with its coding ability and must be repaired for that stretch of DNA to function. Each of these is removed in a patch of about 30 DNA nucleotides by a process termed "nucleotide excision repair" (NER) (8). A dozen or more proteins may cooperate to complete NER. One subset of these proteins recognizes CPDs throughout the genome because they distort the regular turns of the DNA helix, and they initiate global genomic repair (GGR). However, an additional set of proteins are especially tuned to CPDs in regions of DNA actively transcribing RNA, and they are able to more quickly mobilize the NER machinery to these regions of DNA vital to cell function to initiate transcription-coupled repair (TCR).

Once these recognition proteins bind to the site of DNA damage, they recruit additional enzymes that pry open the DNA, make a single-stranded break on either side of the CPD, and release the 30-nucleotide piece of DNA. The strand is then patched by DNA polymerases that use the opposite strand of the DNA as a template. Each cell has several varieties of DNA polymerases, and most of them copy DNA very accurately. However, a few types are much more error prone, and when they are called into service, they introduce mutations where incorrect bases are incorporated into the patch (9).

NER of CPDs is not a very efficient process. After UV exposure that produces a sunburn in human skin, it takes about 24 hours to remove 50% of the damage. NER repair of <6-4>PPs is much quicker: about 50% are removed in 30 minutes. This is because <6-4>PPs are less frequent, and they so greatly distort DNA that they are easier for the NER proteins to locate and excise.

Base Excision Repair

Damage to single bases such as 8oGua is much less distorting to DNA, and is repaired by a second pathway termed "base excision repair" (BER) (8). Here a DNA repair enzyme termed an "oxo-guanine glycosylase-1" (OGG1) specifically recognizes 8oGua and clips it from the DNA. A second enzyme recognizes this site and makes a single stranded break. A few bases on either side of the break are removed, and the short patch is again resynthesized using the opposite strand as a template. This is a speedy process, and half of the 8oGua introduced by solar UV are repaired in about two hours (10).

In human cells, CPDs are not repaired by BER because there is no glycosylase to recognize them. However, the bacteriophage enzyme T4 endonuclease V recognizes CPDs and clips one side of the dimer from the DNA, initiating BER. Amazingly, when delivered into human cells, this enzyme functions quite well to initiate repair of CPDs by BER.

Photoreactivation

An additional pathway of DNA repair is used by plants, fish, reptiles, and amphibians, but it is not present in humans or other mammals. This repair is accomplished by the enzyme photolyase, which directly reverses CPD by capturing long-wavelength UV and visible light and using the energy to split the bonds that bind together the pyrimidine bases in a CPD (11). This restores the DNA to normal without producing a single strand break or removing any DNA. Once again, while human cells have no photolyase enzymes, when these enzymes are introduced into human cells, they function quite well in repairing CPDs.

Diseases of DNA Repair

Much has been learned by studying rare genetic diseases with defects in DNA repair. This has revealed not only each of the proteins and their functions, but also the fact that many DNA repair proteins have multiple functions in the cell.

Xeroderma Pigmentosum, Trichothiodystrophy, Cockayne Syndrome

Xeroderma pigmentosum (XP) is characterized by mild to extreme photosensitivity, often with areas of hypo- and hyperpigmentation, an increased risk of skin cancer, and a shortened life expectancy (12). There are seven complementation groups of XP (A–G), corresponding to defects in one of seven genes that code for proteins involved in NER and a variant group with a defect in repair synthesis. Stringent photoprotection from an early age can greatly reduce actinic damage but does not prevent neurological defects that are a hallmark of some of the complementation groups. This may be because some of these genes are also involved in non-DNA repair gene transcription.

Trichothiodystrophy (TTD) patients have a defect in the same gene as XP-D patients, but at different locations within the gene, so they manifest photosensitivity, stunted growth, and brittle hair, but not an increase in skin cancer (12). This highlights that subtle differences in a DNA repair protein can produce drastic differences in human development and morphology. Patients with Cockayne Syndrome (CS) have mutations in one of two genes that code for proteins controlling TCR, and they also have growth and developmental abnormalities, but surprisingly little increased risk of skin cancer (12).

DNA Repair Gene Polymorphisms

The genes implicated in these genetic diseases code for proteins that participate not only in DNA repair but also in other routine developmental programs and cell functions. The general population carries many forms of these genes with other, less serious mutations, and these forms are called genetic polymorphisms. While some of these polymorphisms are innocuous, groundbreaking research shows that some gene forms increase the risk of cancer, including skin cancer (13).

CELLULAR EFFECTS OF DNA DAMAGE

Cellular Effects of DNA Damage

A complex system regulates the cell's progression through division to ensure that only undamaged ones replicate, in order to avoid genetic instability and cancer (14,15). As cells approach commitment to DNA synthesis (S phase), proteins encoded by checkpoint genes delay entry if DNA damage is present. DNA proteins kinases, such as ATM (ataxia-telangiectasia mutated) and ATR (ataxia-telangiectasia mutated and Rad3 related), then initiate signaling cascades resulting in DNA damage responses that include activation of the p53 protein. This tumor suppressor plays a central role in whether a cell repairs the damage (16) or is diverted into programmed cell death (apoptosis), cell cycle arrest, or senescence (14).

Mitochondrial DNA is damaged largely as a result of oxidative damage secondary to the production of excess ROS by UV or normal metabolism. Sufficient levels of this damage cause release of mitochondrial factors, such as cytochrome C, which binds to the apoptotic protease–activating factor 1 (Apaf-1), resulting in the formation of the apoptosome. This critical event leads to the activation of caspase-9 and the initiation of the mitochondrial apoptotic pathway through caspase-3 activation (17). Apoptosis is a critical event preventing damaged cells from progressing to malignancy.

One new photoprotection strategy is to selectively target DNA-damaged cells for apoptosis, while leaving normal cells unaffected. Oral administration of caffeine or green tea (which often contains high levels of caffeine) in amounts equivalent to three to five cups of coffee per day to UVB-exposed mice increased levels of p53, slowed cell cycling, and increase apoptotic sunburn cells in the epidermis (18). It should be noted that the antioxidant property of polyphenols in green tea also contributes to its ability to downregulate UV-induced cutaneous inflammation (see chap. 16).

Mutations and Skin Cancer

Most of the solar UV–induced DNA damage distorts the double helix. In attempting to replicate past CPD lesions, the cell often makes the same mistake of misincorporating two consecutive bases, resulting in mutations characteristic of UV damage (19). In many cases these mutations have no effect on the cell, but if they occur at critical locations in tumor suppressor genes, they abrogate apoptosis and initiate the process of carcinogenesis. These UV "signature" mutations are often found in mutated p53 genes, a key tumor suppressor gene, in human squamous cell carcinoma, and basal cell carcinoma (19). This is the key link between UV exposure and skin cancer and directly implicates CPDs in carcinogenesis. These p53 signature mutations are also frequently found in precancerous actinic keratosis, suggesting that these mutations are an early step in the process of forming squamous cell carcinomas, and that later steps, such as additional gene mutations and immune suppression, determine if a cell goes on to malignancy.

The situation is less clear in melanoma. There appears to be many different tumor suppressor genes that can be mutated in melanoma, and the frequency of signature mutations is not as common as in squamous cell carcinoma (20).

Mitochondria generate energy for the cell, and they contain DNA that encodes many of the crucial proteins in the energy production machinery. This DNA is also subject to mutations, and mitochondria develop a peculiar type of mutation called the *common deletion,* in which a particular 477 base pair section of the DNA is deleted. The frequency of the common deletion in the mitochondria of human skin cells does not correlate with chronological age, but rather with sun exposure and photoaging (21). This implies that solar UV is responsible for the formation of the common deletion, and its contribution to the signs of photoaging is an active area of research.

SYSTEMIC EFFECTS OF DNA DAMAGE

Cytokines

DNA in skin acts like a sensor for UV damage on behalf of both exposed and unexposed cells in distal parts. DNA damage, particularly in keratinocytes, triggers the production and release of cytokines that act on the cell itself, as well as other cells with such cytokine receptors, to activate characteristic UV responses, such as wound healing and immune suppression (22). Triggers for such responses are stalled RNA transcription complexes or DNA replication forks, which activate DNA protein kinases to phosphorylate transcription factors that activate cytokine genes. Cytokines such as IL-1 and TNFα then induce a cascade of other cytokines that can activate collagen-degrading enzymes, suppress the immune system, dilate blood vessels, and attract inflammatory T cells. In this way, cells with DNA photodamage, even if they are destined to die, have profound effects on cells in the skin and elsewhere that may not have been UV exposed.

IL-12 plays a curious role in photoprotection. It is an immunostimulatory cytokine that is released by keratinocytes at late times after UV in order to counteract the suppressive effects of IL-10 (23). Recently, it has also been reported to stimulate the repair of CPDs in the DNA of keratinocytes in a manner yet to be understood (24).

Immune Suppression

UV-induced immune suppression is an essential event for skin cancer formation (25). It is important to note that this is not generalized immune suppression, but a reduced ability to respond to antigens presented just after exposure. There may be a genetic susceptibility to suppression, because skin cancer patients are more easily UV suppressed than cancer-free controls (26). At lower UV doses, the primary target is the Langerhans cell, which flees the epidermis, and those with DNA damage have impaired antigen-presenting ability (27). Higher doses produce systemic immune suppression, mediated by the generation of suppressor T cells, in which nonexposed skin becomes hampered in responding to antigens (25). In several experimental models, including humans, reducing DNA damage decreases the degree of immune suppression (28).

Photoaging

Photoaging is associated with particular signs of skin damage not apparent in areas protected from the sun. The major changes are found in the dermis and include a loss of collagen, brought about mainly by an increase in the secretion of degrading enzymes such as matrix metalloproteinase -1, or MMP-1 (29), a degradation of the dermal elastic fiber network and fragmentation of collagen matrix (30), and a corresponding decrease in the biophysical properties of the skin (31) reflected in a loss of skin strength and elasticity, flattening of the rete ridges, and the appearance of wrinkles and skin folds. Additionally, there are degradative vascular changes in the dermis resulting in telangiectasia, decreases in the capillary network and in skin blood flow (32).

A perhaps surprising finding is that many of the changes in the dermis may be due to signals initiated from the epidermis rather than as a direct effect of UV on either the fibroblasts or extracellular structural components of the dermis. This is illustrated in a series of experiments in which media collected from keratinocytes exposed to either increasing solar-simulating UV or a single UVB dose was transferred to unirradiated fibroblasts, which substantially increases MMP-1 production from fibroblasts and decreases the fibroblasts production of collagen (33). These experiments implicate soluble factors released by keratinocytes, including IL-1, IL-6, and TNF-α, in this paracrine effect (33,34). DNA damage is directly related to the release of soluble mediators since enhanced repair of keratinocyte DNA reduced the release of the mediators and lowered the effect of media transfer on unirradiated fibroblasts (35).

PHOTOPROTECTION

Sunscreens and DNA Damage

Sunscreens effective in blocking UVB radiation are effective in limiting the number of CPDs formed (36–38). A SPF 15 sunscreen might typically prevent better than 90% of the CPDs expected from a 15 minimal erythemal dose (MED) of UVB, leaving CPD numbers similar to a 0.5 to 1 MED dose. As noted earlier, however, some increase in CPDs is inevitable since some UVB still does get through the sunscreen layer, and more importantly in actual use, the sunscreen is likely not be applied at a high-enough dose per unit area (39), nor is it likely to be applied often enough (40) to give optimal protection (41). In addition, it is known that suberythemogenic doses of UV are sufficient to initiate photoaging and photoimmunosuppression. Thus additional ingredients to prevent or help repair UVB-induced DNA damage and other UV-induced changes would be useful.

Of perhaps more importance, however, are the DNA lesions caused directly and indirectly (42) by UVA wavelengths, since it is much more difficult to filter these much more prevalent photons. Up to 98.7% of the UV radiation reaching the earth's surface is UVA. UVA exposure is higher through most of the day and for a longer season than UVB (43). In addition to the issues mentioned for UVB, until recently, UVA protection in many sunscreen products hasn't been reliably photostable. Thus UVA protection can erode over time once the sunscreens have been applied, likely leading to more-than-anticipated UVA-associated skin damage. Marrot has shown directly (44,45) that a photostable sunscreen is more effective in preventing DNA damage and p53 accumulation in keratinocytes in culture as well as MMP-1 release in a three-dimensional in vitro skin model system.

Antioxidants

DNA is a target for oxygen radicals, and it has been estimated that every day as many as 10,000 oxidation reactions cause DNA damage in each human cell (46). The most common modifications are 8oGua and thymine glycol, which can be repaired by either base excision repair (BER) or nucleotide excision repair (NER) (47). Antioxidants that absorb oxygen radicals or stop radical propagation reduce the incidence of DNA damage, and they may also trigger cell death by apoptosis by breaking DNA at the site of oxidative damage (48).

One type of DNA damage that antioxidants cannot stop or repair is the CPD. CPDs are initiated when a pyrimidine absorbs a photon and becomes excited to a triplet-state and then forms a bond with an adjacent pyrimidine in a total of about 1 picosecond (10^{-9} seconds) – too fast for an antioxidant to intervene (49).

Antioxidants containing sulfur, such as *N*-acetyl cysteine, may have photoprotective effects independent of their DNA protection activity. These antioxidants increase p53 levels in cells, and in precarcinogenic cells (but not normal cells) they induce apoptosis (50). In this way they may clear the skin of transformed cells before they can become skin cancers.

DNA Repair Enzymes

Sunscreens and antioxidants are active before sun exposure, but it may be possible to stimulate mechanisms that act after the damage has been done in DNA, but before it takes effect. One approach to enhancing DNA repair is to accelerate the first, rate-limiting step of NER and BER—the recognition and incision at the site of lesions. DNA repair enzymes have been encapsulated in pH-sensitive liposomes in order to be internalized by cells into endosomes, where the lower pH triggers release. Within an hour, topically applied enzymes are delivered to the nuclei and mitochondria of the cells for the repair of DNA, where they supplement the endogenous processes that would excise only about half of daily damage by themselves (51). The repair enzymes localize within the epidermis with little delivery beyond the dermis or into circulation.

One advantage of this approach is that different enzymes can be used to target different DNA lesions. Liposomes carrying T4 endonuclease V, a CPD glycosylase derived from the bacteriophage T4, accelerate CPD repair in mammalian cells (52,53). Photolyase from the cyanobacterial plankton *Anacystis nidulans* has been encapsulated in liposomes and it accelerates CPD repair in human skin in a light-dependent reaction (54). The OGG1 enzyme from the mustard plant *Arabidopsis thalania* incorporated in liposomes targets 8oGua oxidative damage in both nuclear and mitochondrial DNA because it has functional nuclear and mitochondrial localization signals. Treatment of mice over 28 weeks with UVB followed by liposomal OGG1 reduces the level of 8oGua in their epidermis compared to placebo controls (55).

Enhanced repair of CPDs, using these DNA repair liposomes, reduced UV-induced immune suppression in humans in vivo (28,54). Accelerating repair of both CPD and 8oGua reduced the expression of MMP-1 following UV in cells in culture and in human skin in vivo (35), suggesting that these DNA repair liposomes may be tool in the prevention and treatment of photoaging. Most importantly, in a clinical study, XP patients who used a lotion with T4 endonuclease V liposomes daily over one year had lower rates of actinic keratosis and basal cell carcinoma than the placebo group (56).

These examples emphasize that DNA repair enzymes from other species and even other kingdoms can function efficiently in human cells. Enzymes delivered by liposomes are degraded by the host cells within a day, and therefore require repeated application to maintain increased repair capacity (57). Safety studies have shown no risk of irritation or sensitization with these DNA repair liposomes (58), in part due to the localization in the epidermis and minimal or no systemic delivery (52).

These results suggest that our efforts for photoprotection can extend beyond the prevention of the initial insult with sunscreens or antioxidants and include repair of DNA damage.

CONCLUSION

DNA damage to cells of the skin, particularly the keratinocytes, serves as a sensor for environmental insult and metabolic stress for the rest of the skin, and indeed the rest of the body. Lesions in cellular DNA disrupt cell cycling and invoke repair process; or if they fail, they initiate an apoptotic response to rid the skin of irreparable cells. Damaged cells also release soluble mediates, such as the cytokines IL-1, IL-10, and TNFα, that invoke responses that are both immune suppressive and wound healing from surrounding cells and cells that may not have suffered any damage. Over the long term, these repeated rounds of damage and response contribute to photoaging. If the lesions are not repaired,

DNA replication may insert erroneous basis, which can lead to mutations in key, tumor suppressor genes and initiate malignant transformation.

Photoprotection strategy should include seeking shade and the use of photo-protective clothing. In addition, use of both sunscreens, to attenuate the UV dose, and antioxidants, to minimize exposure to free radicals, are integral parts of the first lines of defense. Despite these protections, skin DNA suffers substantial damage from intentional and unintentional sun exposure.

Fortunately, we have an enzymatic system for repairing many forms of DNA damage, which is quite efficient when we consider the severity of the genetic diseases in which it malfunctions. Nevertheless, it can be improved at the first step, namely, the recognition of the DNA damage and initiation of repair. This has been accomplished experimentally and in vivo by delivery of exogenous DNA repair enzymes that accelerate these first steps of repair. This results in more rapid removal of DNA damage, a reduction in the release of the soluble mediators and the wounding responses, a lessening of the appearance of photoaging, and a reduction in the risk of skin cancer.

Enhancing DNA repair may be essential to extend our strategy beyond sunscreens and antioxidants for photoprotection.

REFERENCES

1. Vershooten L, Claerhout S, Laethem AV, et al. New strategies in photoprotection. Photochem Photobiol 2006; 82:1016–1023.
2. Yarr M, Gilchrest BA. Photoaging: mechanism, prevention and therapy. Br J Dermatol 2007; 157:874–887.
3. Cadet J, Sage E, Douki T. Ultraviolet radiation –mediated damage to cellular DNA. Mutat Res 2005; 571:3–7.
4. Mahmoud BH, Hexsel CL, Hamzavi IH, et al. Effects of visible light on the skin. Photochem Photobiol 2008; 84:450–462.
5. Schreier W, Schrader T, Koller, et. al. Thymine dimerization in DNA is an ultrafast photoreaction. Science 2007; 315:625–629.
6. Yoon J-H, Lee C-S, O'Connor T, et al. The DNA damage spectrum produced by simulated sunlight. J Mol Biol 2000; 299:681–693.
7. Courdavault S, Baudoin C, Charveron M, et al. Larger yield of cyclobutane dimers than 8-oxo-7, 8-dihydroguanine in the DNA of UVA-irradiated human skin cells. Mutat Res 2004; 556: 135–142.
8. Sancar A, Lindsey-Boltz L, Unsal-Kacmaz K, et al. Molecular mechanisms of mammalian DNA repair and the DNA damage checkpoints. Annu Rev Biochem 2004; 73:39–85.
9. Christmann M, Tomicic M, Roos, W, et al. Mechanisms of human DNA repair: an update. Toxicol 2003; 193:3–34.
10. Yarosh D, Canning M, Teicher D, et al. After sun reversal of DNA damage: enhancing skin repair. Mutat Res 2005; 571:57–64.
11. Carell T, Burgdorf L, Kundu L, et al. The mechanism of action of DNA photolyases. Curr Opin Chem Biol 2001; 5:491–498.
12. Cleaver J. Cancer in xeroderma pigmentosum and related disorders of DNA repair. Nat Rev 2005; 5:564–573.
13. Au W, Navasumrit P, Ruchirawat M. Use of biomarkers to characterize functions of polymorphic DNA repair genotypes. Int J Hyg Environ Health 2004; 207:301–304.
14. Funk JO. Cell cycle checkpoint genes and cancer. In: Encyclopedia of Life Sciences. Chichester, UK: John Wiley, 2005:1–5.
15. Harper JW, Elledge SJ. The DNA damage response: ten years after. Mol Cell 2007; 28: 739–745.

16. Sancar A, Lindsey-Boltz LA, Ünsal-Kamaz K, et al. Molecular mechanisms of mammalian DNA repair and the DNA damage checkpoints. Annu Rev Biochem 2004; 73:39–85.

17. Guzman E, Langowski JL, Owen-Schaub L. Mad dogs, Englishmen and apoptosis: the role of cell death in UV-induced skin cancer. Apoptosis 2003; 8:315–325.

18. Lu Y-P, Lou Y-R, Peng Q-Y, et al. Effect of caffeine on the ATR/Chk1 pathway in the epidermis of UVB-irradiated mice. Cancer Res 2008; 68:2523–2529.

19. Brash D. Sunlight and the onset of skin cancer. Trends Genet 1997; 13:410–414.

20. High W, Robinson W. Genetic mutations involved in melanoma: a summary of our current understanding. Adv Dermatol 2007; 23:61–79.

21. Berneburg M, Plettenberg H, Medve-Konig K. Induction of the photoaging-associated mitochondrial common deletion in vivo in normal human skin. J Invest Dermatol 2004; 122:1277–1283.

22. Kondo S. The roles of keratinocyte-derived cytokines in the epidermis and their possible responses to UVA-irradiation. J Investig Dermatol Symp Proc 1999; 4:177–183.

23. Barr R, Walker S, Tsang W, et al. Suppressed alloantigen presentation, increased TNF-α, IL-1, IL-1RA, IL-10, and modulation of TNF-R in UV-irradiated human skin. J Invest Dermatol 1999; 112:692–698.

24. Schwarz A, Ständer S, Berneburg M, et al. Interleukin-12 suppresses ultraviolet radiation-induced apoptosis by inducing DNA repair. Nat Cell Biol 2002; 4:26–31.

25. Kripke M. Immunologic unresponsiveness induced by UV radiation. Immunol Rev 1984; 80: 87–102.

26. Streilein J. Immunogenetic factors in skin cancer. N Engl J Med 1991; 325:884–887.

27. Vink A, Moodycliffe A, Shreedhar V, et al. The inhibition of antigen-presenting activity of dendritic cells resulting from UV irradiation of murine skin is restored by in vitro photorepair of cyclobutane pyrimidine dimers. Proc Natl Acad Sci U S A 1997; 94:5255–5260.

28. Kuchel J, Barnetson R, Halliday G. Cyclobutane pyrimidine dimer formation is a molecular trigger for solar-simulated ultraviolet radiation-induced suppression of memory immunity in humans. Photochem Photobiol Sci 2005; 4:577–582.

29. Yaar M, Gilchrest BA. Photoageing: mechanism, prevention and therapy. Br J Dermatol 2007; 157(5):874–887.

30. Fisher GJ, Varani, J, Voorhees, JJ. Looking older. Fibroblast collapse and therapeutic implications. Arch Dermatol 2008; 144:666–672.

31. Leveque J-C, Agache P, eds. Aging Skin: Properties and Functional Changes. Aulnoy-sous Bois, France: Informa Health Care, 1993.

32. Ryan T. The ageing of the blood supply and the lymphatic drainage of the skin. Micron 2004; 35: 161–171.

33. Fagot D, Asselineau D, Bernerd F. Direct role of dermal fibroblasts and indirect participation of epidermal keratinocytes in MMP-1 production after UV-B irradiation. Arch Dermatol Res 2002; 293:576–583.

34. Wlaschek M, Heinen G, Poswig A, et al. UVA-induced autocrine stimulation of fibroblast-derived collagenase/MMP-1 by interrelated loops of interleukin-1 and interleukin-6. Photochem Photobiol 1994; 59:550–556.

35. Dong K, Damaghi N, Picart S, et al. UV-Induced DNA damage initiates release of MMP-1 in human skin. Exp Dermatol (in press).

36. Liader S, Scaletta C, Panizzon R, et al. Protection against pyrimidine dimers, p53, and 8-hydroxy-2′-deoxyguanosine expression in ultraviolet-irradiated human skin by sunscreens: differences between UVB + UVA and UVB alone sunscreens. J Invest Dermatol 2001; 117: 1437–1441.

37. Mahroos MA, Yaar M, Phillips TJ, et al. Effect of sunscreen application on UV-induced thymine dimers. Arch Dermatol 2002; 138:1480–1485.

38. Wolf P, Yarosh DB, Kripke ML. Effects of sunscreens and DNA excision repair enzyme on ultraviolet radiation-induced inflammation, immune suppression and cyclobutane pyrimidine dimer formation in mice. J Invest Dermatol 1993; 101:523–527.

39. Autier P, Boniol M, Severi G. Quantity of sunscreen used by European students. Br J Dermatol 2001; 144:288–291.

40. Pincus MW, Rollings PK, Craft AB, et al. Sunscreen use on Queensland beaches. Australas J Dermatol 1991; 32:21–25.

41. Theiden E, Philipsen PA, Sandby-Møller J, et al. Sunscreen use related to UV exposure, age, sex and occupation based on personal dosimeter readings and sun exposure behavior diaries. Arch Dermatol 2005; 141:967–973.

42. Haywood R, Wardman P, Sanders R. Sunscreen inadequately protect against ultraviolet-A-induced free radicals in the skin: implications for skin aging and melanoma? J Invest Dermatol 2003; 121:862–868.

43. International Commission in Illumination. Solar spectral irradiance. CIE Technical Report 85, Vienna, Commission international de l'eclairage, 1985.

44. Marrot L, Belaïdi J-P, Meunier J-R. Importance of UVA photoprotection as shown by genotoxic related endpoints: DNA damage and p53 status. Mutat Res 2005; 571:175–184.

45. Marrot L, Belaïdi J-P, Lejeune F, et al. Photostability of sunscreen products influences the efficacy of protection with regard to UV-induced genotoxic or photoageing-related endpoints. Br J Dermatol 2004; 151:1234–1244.

46. Ames B. Endogenous oxidative DNA damage, aging and cancer. Free Radic Res Commun 1989; 7:121–128.

47. Moller P, Wallin H. Adduct formation and nucleotide excision repair of DNA damage produced by reactive oxygen species and lipid peroxidation product. Mutat Res 1998; 410:271–290.

48. Hadi S, Bhat S, Azmi A, et al. Oxidative breakage of cellular DNA by plant polyphenols: a putative mechanism for anticancer properties. Semin Cancer Biol 2007; 17:370–376.

49. Schreier W, Schrader T, Koller F, et al. Thymine dimerization in DNA is an ultrafast photoreaction. Science 2007; 315:625–629.

50. Harve P, O'Reilly S, McCormick J, et al. Transformed and tumor-derived human cells exhibit preferential sensitivity to the thiol antioxidants, N-acetyl cysteine and penicillamine. Cancer Res 2002; 62:1443–1449.

51. Yarosh DB. Liposomes in investigative dermatology. Photodermatol Photoimmunol Photomed 2001; 17:203–212.

52. Yarosh D, Bucana C, Cox P, et al. Localization of liposomes containing a DNA repair enzyme in murine skin. J Invest Dermatol 1994; 103:461–468.

53. Yarosh D, Kibitel J, Green L, et al. Enhanced unscheduled DNA synthesis in UV-irradiated human skin explants treated with T4N5 liposomes. J Invest Dermatol 1991; 97:147–150.

54. Stege S, Roza L, Vink A, et al. Enzyme plus light therapy to repair DNA damage in ultraviolet-B-irradiated human skin. Proc Natl Acad Sci U S A 2000; 97:1790–1795.

55. Wulff B, Schick J, Thomas-Ahner J, et al. Topical treatment with OGG1 enzyme affects UVB-induced skin carcinogenesis. Photochem Photobiol 2008; 84:317–321.

56. Yarosh D, Klein J, O'Connor A, et al. Effect of topically applied T4 endonuclease V in liposomes on skin cancer in xeroderma pigmentosum: a randomized study. Xeroderma Pigmentosum Study Group. Lancet 2001; 357:926–929.

57. Kripke M, Cox P, Bucana C, et al. Role of DNA damage in local suppression of contact hypersensitivity in mice by UV radiation. Exp Dermatol 1996; 5:173–180.

58. Yarosh D, Klein J, Kibitel J, et al. Enzyme therapy of xeroderma pigmentosum: safety and efficacy testing of T4N5 liposome lotion containing a prokaryotic DNA repair enzyme. Photoderm Photoimm Photomed 1996; 12:122–130.

13
Photoprotection in Moisturizers and Day Care Products

André Rougier and Sophie Seité
La Roche-Posay Pharmaceutical Laboratories, Asnières, France

Anny Fourtanier
L'Oréal Research, Clichy, France

SYNOPSIS

- Products designed for daily use containing broad-spectrum photostable UV filters can
  - prevent free radicals production induced by suberythemal UVA exposure,
  - prevent UVA induction of matrix metalloproteinase-1 (MMP-1) gene,
  - decrease pigmentation induced by suberythemal doses of UVA, and
  - prevent changes induced by solar-simulated radiation that are associated with photoaging.

INTRODUCTION

During usual daily activities, an appropriate protection against solar UV exposure should prevent clinical, cellular, and molecular changes potentially leading to photoaging. In skin areas regularly exposed to sun, UV damage is superimposed to tissue degeneration resulting from chronological aging (1–5).

Solar radiation reaching the surface of the earth, and thereby the surface of our skin, contains infrared, visible, and UV radiation (UVR). Dermatologists are particularly interested in the UV segment of radiation, as it is almost exclusively the cause of sun exposure–related skin disorders (6). The UVR component of sunlight reaching the earth's surface has radiation with wavelengths of 290 to 400 nm and accounts for almost 10% of the total energy emitted by the sun (Fig. 1).

There are three types of UVR: UVA (320–400 nm), UVB (290–320 nm), and UVC (200–290 nm). Shorter UV wavelengths are more energetic and potentially more

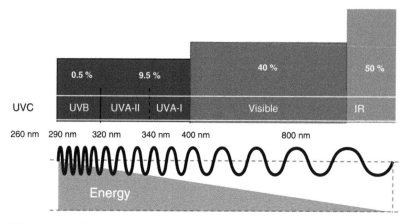

Figure 1 Light energy on the surface of the earth.

destructive than longer wavelengths. Fortunately, UVC, the shortest of wavelengths in the UV spectrum, is completely absorbed by the ozone layer. Therefore, UVR reaching the skin consists only of UVB and UVA. UVB reaches the earth in relatively small amounts (about 0.5% of the solar energy), but it is very efficient in producing biologic response. UVA photons carry less energy than UVB photons; nevertheless, UVA radiation is more abundant than in UVB radiation (about 9.5%). UVA can be further subdivided into UVA-I (400–340 nm) and UVA-II (340–320 nm) (Fig. 1).

The extent of an individual's exposure to UVR varies widely depending on a multiplicity of factors, such as weather, hour of the day, season, pollution, humidity, temperature, and also geographic factors such as altitude and latitude. These can be summarized below:

- In temperate climate, the quantity of UV reaching the skin is seasonal. UVB exposure is much greater in summer than in winter.
- There is greater amount of both UVA and UVB with decreasing latitude.
- The quantity of UVR transmission increases by 4% every 1000 ft above sea level. Indeed, as the atmospheric layer traveled by the UVR is thinner, the filtration effect is reduced.
- Time of day also plays an important part. UVB is strongest between 10 a.m. and 4 p.m., especially around midday, whereas UVA follows the variation of visible light.
- Finally, several environmental factors contribute to influence UV exposure. UV can be modified according to the nature of terrain, which induces different reflections of radiation. Furthermore, glass filters at least UVB (7).

UVB is far more sensitive to the above factors than UVA. Consequently, compared with that to UVB, there is more consistent exposure of the skin to UVA throughout the day (8,9). As the wavelength increases, there is a corresponding percentage increase in the depth of skin penetration of UVR (Fig. 2). UVB penetrates the epidermis and is almost fully absorbed in the upper dermis, while one quarter of the UVA reaches as far as the mid-dermis.

It has long been thought that the majority of sun exposure–induced lesions in humans were due to UVB rays (1). Unlike UVB rays, UVA rays do not trigger the well-known alarm signal of sunburn. Therefore, large amounts of UVA can accumulate without any immediate visible signs but, in the long term, can cause cumulative changes

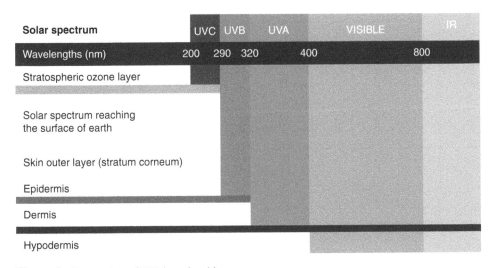

Figure 2 Penetration of UV into the skin.

(2) similar to those caused by long-term exposure to solar radiation (10), including epidermal hyperplasia with the presence of photodyskeratosic cells (a sign of damage to the DNA) (3,4,11), a reduction in Langerhans cells number (5,12,13), latent inflammation of the dermis with vascular and collagen damage (10,14,15), splitting of the lamina densa (4), disorganization of the elastic fibre network, and expression of lysozyme (16), leading to changes in the biomechanical properties of the skin (17). It has been shown that a dose of around 20 J/cm^2 of UVA for five weeks (11), which corresponds to a daily UVA dose received in temperate climate regions, or a dose of only 0.5 MED (minimal erythematous dose) of UVA for eight days (18), can produce all the effects referred above.

It is therefore important to know if moisturizers and day care products containing UVA absorbers combined with UVB ones are able to prevent these skin damages. This chapter summarizes clinical studies evaluating this topic.

REACTIVE OXYGEN SPECIES PREVENTION BY A DAY CARE PRODUCT

The involvement of activated states of oxygen generated after UVA irradiation in the photoaging process has been given particular attention (19).

During UVA-induced oxidative process and free radicals generation, part of the energy is released in the form of photons, a process termed "chemiluminescence." These photons can be detected and amplified by a photo-multiplier. This allows measurement of oxidative stress and protection afforded by topically applied formulations. As an example, the skin protection against oxidative stress of a day cream with photoprotection SPF 15, UVA-PF 12 [measured by the persistent pigment darkening method, PPD (Hydraphase XL, La Roche-Posay, France)] containing octocrylene (Uvinul® N539, BASF, Ludwigshafen, Germany), terephtalilydene dicamphor sulfonic acid (Mexoryl® SX, Chimex SA, le Thillay, France), drometrizole trisiloxane (Mexoryl® XL, Chimex SA) and butyl methoxy dibenzoylmethane (avobenzone®, Roche SA, Bale, Switzerland) applied at 2 mg/cm2, 20 minutes prior to a single exposure to a suberythemal dose of UVA (320–400 nm, 1 J/cm^2), has been assessed by means of induced chemiluminescence (20). Results obtained on 20 volunteers showed that the day cream leads to a decrease of

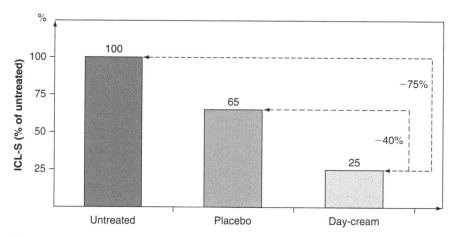

Figure 3 Induced chemiluminescence after UVA exposure and protection afforded by single application of a day cream (SPF 15, UVA-PF 12).

about 75% and 40% of chemiluminescence compared with untreated or placebo-treated skin respectively (Fig. 3). These results suggest that the use of a day cream with both UVB and UVA absorbers can possibly prevent free radicals production induced by suberythemal UVA exposure.

PREVENTION OF UVA INDUCTION OF MATRIX METALLOPROTEINASE-1 GENE EXPRESSION BY A DAY CARE PRODUCT

Induction of matrix metalloproteinases (MMPs) following UVR exposure is known to play an important role in photoaging (21). A study was done to evaluate the protective effect of a day cream SPF 15, UVA-PF 15 (measured by the PPD method) (Seité S, Rougier A, and Krutmann J, unpublished data). Buttock skin of 10 healthy subjects was exposed to 40 or 80 J/cm^2 of UVA (320–400 nm). These doses were previously shown to increase significantly MMP-1 mRNA expression 24 hours after exposure. Application at 2 mg/cm^2 of the day cream (Anthelios SX, La Roche-Posay, USA) composed of butyl methoxy dibenzoylmethane, terephthalilylidene dicamphor sulfonic acid, and octocrylene, 20 minutes before exposure resulted in significant inhibition of UVA-induced gene expression of MMP-1 (Fig. 4). This result demonstrated the effective protection offered by a broad-spectrum day cream in the prevention of UVA radiation-induced MMP-1 gene expression.

PIGMENTATION PREVENTION BY A DAY CARE PRODUCT

UVA is known to be involved in the development of pigmented skin lesions associated with skin aging. The effect of a day cream with broad-spectrum photoprotection (SPF 15, UVA-PF 12; Hydraphase XL) was evaluated in a bilateral comparison study using vehicle as control (22). Twenty healthy women were exposed on the neckline three times a week for three months to suberythemal doses of UVA (20, 25, 30 J/cm^2 respectively for the first, second, and third month). Evaluation of skin pigmentation was performed monthly by visual examination and by chromametry. Clinically and with Wood's lamp examination, pigmentation was found to be more intense on the vehicle-treated side.

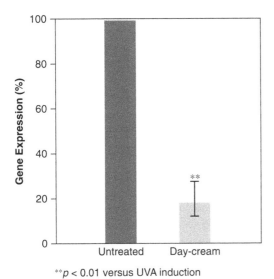

**p < 0.01 versus UVA induction

Figure 4 Relative expression of MMP-1 mRNA after UVA exposure and protection afforded by single application of a day cream (SPF 15, UVA-PF 15).

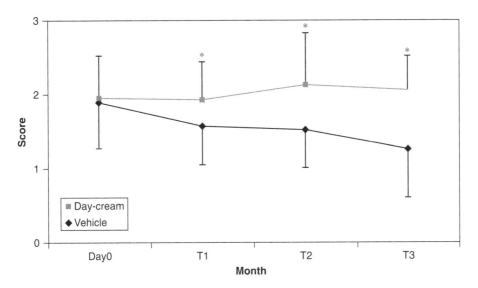

Figure 5 Evolution of pigmented skin lesion by clinical assessment after application of a day cream (SPF 15, UVA-PF 12) or vehicle. Data are mean $\pm$ SD. $^{*}p \leq 0.05$ compared with vehicle-treated site.

Moreover, clinical examination of actinic lentigines indicated that the pigmentation of these lesions was not changed on the vehicle-treated side, whereas it was significantly decreased on the daily cream–protected side (Fig. 5) (23). It thus appears that the use of a day cream containing broad-spectrum filtration in chronic UVA exposure conditions not only offers an efficient protection on the induction of pigmentation but also allows a lightening of pre-existing pigmented lesions.

PHOTOAGING PREVENTION

Clinically photoaged skin is characterized by roughness, fine and coarse wrinkling, sagging, mottled hyperpigmentation evidenced by lentigines and freckles, poor color quality, and telangectasias. There is compelling evidence to support an important role of UVB in this photodamage. It is only more recently that, in humans, the role of UVA was demonstrated (10).

Effects of Repeated SSR Exposure, and Protection by a Day Care Product

In order to evaluate the photoprotective efficacy of a cream for daily use containing a photostable combination of UV absorbers (butyl methoxy dibenzoylmethane, terephta-lilydene dicamphor sulfonic acid, and octocrylene) and providing a continuous absorption through the entire UV spectrum, an evaluation of molecular, morphological, functional, and structural cutaneous changes induced by a six-week exposure to 1 MED of solar-simulated radiation (SSR) (which average 0.86 J/cm^2 UVB and 11 J/cm^2 UVA) in young volunteers was performed (24). The SPF of this day cream was 8.39 $\pm$ 1.22 and the UVA-PF value, determined using the PPD method, was 7.4 $\pm$ 2.4.

SSR exposed, unprotected skin sites showed increased pigmentation, dryness and a significant alteration of the microtopography (Table 1). Histological examination revealed increased thickness of both the stratum corneum and the stratum granulosum (Table 1). The dermis showed an increased tenascin expression just below the dermal epidermal junction, as well as an enhanced lysozyme and α-1 antitrypsin deposition on elastin fibers associated with a reduced expression of type 1 pro-collagen (Table 1). These latest modifications are considered as early events of solar elastosis (25,26). The assessment of molecular changes by RT-PCR revealed a significant enhancement of collagenase-2 (MMP-2) mRNA induced by this regimen of SSR exposure. All these changes are observed in long-term sun exposed skin (24).

The day cream applied at 2 mg/cm^2, 30 minutes before each exposure on the same volunteers prevented all the SSR-induced damage (Table 1).

In conclusion, using repeated low doses of SSR for six weeks resulted in major alterations observed in long-term photoaging processes (deepening of skin furrows, reduced level of type I collagen precursor, increased lysozyme deposit on elastic fibers, etc.); these changes occurred even in subjects who developed brisk SSR-induced pigmentation, offering progressive skin auto-protection. This demonstrates the beneficial effect of a photostable combination of UV absorbers, providing a continuous absorption through the entire UV spectrum in the prevention of premature skin aging.

Effects of Repeated Simulated Daily UV Radiation Exposure, and Protection by a Day Care Product

In another clinical experiment (27), the protection afforded by the same day cream (SPF 8.4 and UVA-PF 7.4) against clinical, histological, and immunohistochemical damage induced by repeated simulated daily UV radiation (DUVR) exposure was evaluated. Simulated DUVR (28) is more typical of commonly encountered UVR exposure conditions because it has a UVA to UVB irradiance ratio of about 25, instead of about 10 for SSR, which has been used in the study above. We assessed protection against clinical, histological, and immunohistochemical damage induced by repeated DUVR exposure in 10 healthy volunteers. We compared unprotected and protected buttock skin after 19 exposures to 0.5 MED.

Table 1 Biological Effects Induced by 30 Repeated Exposures to 1 MED SSR and Protection Afforded by a Broad-Spectrum Day Cream Vs. Vehicle

Parameters (n = 12)	Control	+SSR	+SSR/+Veh	+SSR/+DC
ΔITA°	−1.90 ± 2.34	−39.02 ± 7.65[a]	−39.29 ± 7.85[a]	−6.30 ± 3.00[b,c]
Melanization (visual score)	1.3 ± 0.5	3.5 ± 1.0[a]	3.2 ± 0.7[a]	1.4 ± 0.7[b,c]
Microtopography (visual grade)	0.04 ± 0.14	3.71 ± 1.51[a,b]	1.92 ± 1.58[a,c]	0.08 ± 0.29[b,c]
Number of stratum corneum layers	14.5 ± 2.3	20.6 ± 4.2[a]	19.8 ± 3.6[a]	15.0 ± 1.4[b,c]
Number of stratum granulosum layers	1.0 ± 0.0	2.1 ± 0.6[a]	1.8 ± 0.7[a]	1.1 ± 0.2[b,c]
Viable epidermis thickness (μm)	79.7 ± 12.1	88.8 ± 5.8[a]	85.2 ± 8.8	90.0 ± 12.0[a]
Melanization (visual score)	1.3 ± 0.5	3.5 ± 1.0[a]	3.2 ± 0.7[a]	1.4 ± 0.7[b,c]
Tenascin (AU)	4.9 ± 3.4	8.2 ± 4.9[a]	8.9 ± 3.4[a]	4.8 ± 2.8[b,c]
Type I pro-collagen (AU)	7.7 ± 3.4	5.3 ± 3.9[a]	6.8 ± 4.2	8.7 ± 4.5[c]
Type III pro-collagen (AU)	3.0 ± 1.0	3.4 ± 1.7	3.6 ± 1.0	3.4 ± 0.8
Elastin (AU)	22.5 ± 5.7	21.6 ± 3.0	20.6 ± 5.3	20.8 ± 4.5
Lysozyme deposit (visual assessment)	0.1 ± 0.2	0.8 ± 0.5[a]	0.8 ± 0.3[a]	0.4 ± 0.5[a,b,c]
α-1 Antitrypsin deposit (visual assessment)	0.8 ± 0.7	1.8 ± 0.7[a]	1.6 ± 0.5[a]	1.2 ± 0.6

Note: Data are mean ± SD.
DC is of SPF 8, UVA-PF 7.
[a] $p \leq 0.05$ compared with control site.
[b] $p \leq 0.05$ compared with +SSR/+Veh site.
[c] $p \leq 0.05$ compared with +SSR site.
Abbreviations: AU, arbitrary unit; DC, day cream; Veh, vehicle; SSR, solar-simulated radiation.

Cumulative suberythemal exposure to DUVR-induced photodamage including significant p53 nuclear accumulation, decrease in Langerhans cell number, thickening of epidermis, and increase in melanin deposits associated with more numerous and larger active melanocytes (Table 2). In the dermis, significant increase in lysozyme deposits on elastin fibres were observed (Table 2). These alterations were fully prevented by the day cream (Table 2).

The data show significant biological damage after 19 exposures to 0.5 MED of DUVR. This suberythemal dose (individual 0.5 MED, which averages 7.6 ± 1.4 J.cm^{-2}) is representative of exposure at temperate latitudes. For example, 68 J.cm^{-2} of DUVR equivalent can be received on a horizontal surface during a day in mid-April in Paris, France, of which, it has been estimated that people receive about 10% on the face (8). Thus,

Table 2 Biological Effects Induced by 19 Repeated Exposures to 0.5 MED DUVR and Protection Afforded by a Broad-Spectrum Day Cream

Parameter ($n = 10$)	Control	+DUVR	+DUVR/+DC
Hydration (AU)	57 ± 3	58 ± 3	61 ± 3
Elasticity (Ur/Ue)	0.79 ± 0.02	0.77 ± 0.04	0.73 ± 0.04
Epidermal thickness (μm)	61.6 ± 5.2	73.6 ± 5.2^a	75.4 ± 5.0^a
Epidermal proliferation (Ki67, %)	4.8 ± 1.0	6.3 ± 0.8	5.5 ± 0.7
SBC(/cm)	0.0 ± 0.0	0.4 ± 0.2	0.3 ± 0.1
P53 positive cells (%)	0.3 ± 0.2	2.4 ± 0.8^a	0.2 ± 0.1^b
Number of HLA-DR positive cells (/mm²)	522 ± 55	308 ± 36^a	523 ± 68^b
Size of HLA-DR positive cells (μm²)	58 ± 6	52 ± 5	55 ± 6
Number of DOPA-positive cells (/mm²)	330 ± 59	726 ± 68^a	$516 \pm 72^{a,b}$
Size of DOPA-positive cells (μm²)	61 ± 6	$116 \pm 7^{a*}$	$92 \pm 14^{a,b}$
Melanin (score)	11.1 ± 0.7	12.6 ± 0.6^a	11.1 ± 0.6^b
Elastin (AU)	12.0 ± 0.6	11.2 ± 0.8	11.7 ± 0.8
Lysozyme/elastin	0.14 ± 0.02	0.21 ± 0.04^a	0.14 ± 0.04
Pro-collagen I (AU)	22.1 ± 1.9	19.9 ± 2.8	24.2 ± 1.9
Pro-collagen III/pro-collagen I	0.20 ± 0.02	0.23 ± 0.06	0.23 ± 0.06
GAG (score)	4.9 ± 0.6	3.2 ± 0.6^a	5.0 ± 0.7^b

Mean ± SEM.
DC is of SPF 8, UVA-PF 7.
[a] $p \leq 0.05$ compared with control site.
[b] $p \leq 0.05$ compared with + DUVR unprotected site.
Abbreviations: AU, arbitrary unit; DC, day cream; DUVR, daily UV radiation.

the daily exposure dose of 7.6 J.cm^{-2} was consistent with real life conditions. As previously described with SSR (23), the data confirm that daily suberythemal exposure to DUVR is also detrimental, and can induce DNA damage (p53 expression), and Langerhans cells alteration. A low SPF broad-spectrum daily care product prevents these effects and should in theory protect human skin against long-term effects if used on a regular basis.

CONCLUSION

These studies demonstrate that broad-spectrum protection in moisturizers or day care products can prevent the "silent" suberythemal cumulative effects of UVR from inadvertent sun exposure.

REFERENCES

1. Kaminer MS. Photodamage: Magnitude of the Problem. In: Gilchrest B, ed. Photodamage. Cambridge: Blackwell Science, 1995:1–11.
2. Bisset DL, Hannon DP, McBride JF, et al. Photoaging of skin by UVA. In: Urbach F, ed. Biological Response to Ultraviolet A radiation. Overland Park, KS: Valdenmar Publishing Cie, 1992:181–188.
3. Kligman AM, Lavker RM. Cutaneous aging: the differences between intrinsic aging and photoaging. J Cut Aging Cosmet Dermatol 1988; 1:5–11.

4. Lavker RM. Structural alterations in exposed and non exposed human skin. J Invest Dermatol 1979; 73:59–66.

5. Gilchrest BA, Szabo G, Flynn E. Chronologic and actinically induced aging in human facial skin. J Invest Dermatol 1983; 80:81s–85s.

6. Ortonne J-P, Marks R. The solar spectrum. In: Kligman AM, ed. Photodamaged Skin: Clinical Signs, Causes and Management. London: Martin Dunitz, 1999.

7. Tuchinda C, Srivannaboon S, Lim HW. Photoprotection by window glass, automobile glass and sunglasses. J Am Acad Dermatol 2006; 54:845–854. Erratum in 55:74.

8. Godar D. UV Doses worldwide. Photochem Photobiol 2005; 81:736–749.

9. Kullavanijaya P, Lim HW. Photoprotection. J Am Acad Dermatol 2005; 52:937–958.

10. Seité S, Moyal D, Richard S, et al. Effect of repeated suberythemal doses of UVA in human skin. Eur J Dermatol 1997; 7:204–209.

11. Lavker RM, Gerberick GF, Veres D, et al. Cumulative effects from repeated exposures to suberythemal doses of UVB and UVA in human skin. J Am Acad Dermatol 1995; 32:53–62.

12. Czernielewski JM, Masouye I, Pisani A. Effects of chronic sun exposure on human Langerhans cell densities. Photodermatolog 1999; 5:116–120.

13. Seité S, Zucchi H, Moyal D, et al. Alterations in human epidermal Langerhans cells by ultraviolet radiation: quantitative and morphological study. Br J Dermatol 2003; 148:291–299.

14. Trautinger F, Mazzucco K, Knobler RM, et al. UVA- and UVB-induced changes in hairless mouse skin collagen. Arch Dermatol Res 1994; 286:490–494.

15. Lavker RM, Kligman AM. Chronic heliodermatitis: a morphologic evaluation of chronic actinic damage with emphasis on the role of mast cells. J Invest Dermatol 1988; 90:325–330.

16. Seité S, Zucchi H, Igondjo-Tchen S, et al. Elastin changes during chronological and photo-ageing: the important role of lysozyme. J Eur Acad Dermatol Venereol 2006; 20:980–987.

17. Matsuoka LY, Uitto J. Alterations in the elastic fibers in cutaneous aging and solar elastosis. In: Balin AK, Kligman AM, eds. Aging and the Skin New York: Raven Press, 1989, 141–151.

18. Lavker RM, Gerberick GF, Veres D, et al. Quantitative assessment of cumulative damage from repetitive exposures to suberythemogenic doses of UVA in human skin. Photochem Photobiol 1995; 62:348–352.

19. Pathak MA, Dalle Carbonare M. Biological Response to Ultraviolet A radiation. In: Urbach F, ed. Overland Park, KS: Valdenmar Publishing Company, 1992:189–208.

20. Rougier A, Richard A. In vivo determination of the skin protection capacity of a day-cream by means of ICL-S. Eur J Dermatol 2002, 12:XIX–XX.

21. Chung J, Cho S, Kang S. Why does the skin age? Rigel DS, Weiss RA, Lim, HW, et al. eds. Photoaging. New York: Marcel Dekker, 2004:1–13.

22. Duteil L, Queille-Roussel C, Rougier A, et al. Chronic UVA exposure: protective effect on skin induced pigmentation by a daily use of a day care cream containing broad band sunscreen. Eur J Dermatol 2002; 12:XVII–XVIII.

23. Young AR, Orchard GE, Harrison GI, et al. The detrimental effects of daily sub-erythemal exposure on human skin in vivo can be prevented by a daily-care broad-spectrum sunscreen. J Invest Dermatol 2007; 127:975–978.

24. Seité S, Colige A, Piquemal-Vivenot P, et al. A Full-UV spectrum absorbing daily use cream protects human skin against biological changes occurring in photoaging. Photodermatol Photoimmunol Photomed 2000; 16:147–155.

25. Lavker RM. Cutaneous Aging: Chronologic Versus Photoaging Photodamage. In: Gilchrest B, ed. Cambridge: Blackwell Science, 1995:123–135.

26. Lavker RM, Kaidbey KH. The spectral dependence for UVA-induced cumulative damage in human skin. J Invest Dermatol 1997; 108:17–21.

27. Seite S, Christiaens F, Bredoux C, et al. A full-UVR spectrum skincare product protects human epidermis and dermis against the adverse effects of simulated daily ultraviolet radiation. Photodermatol Photoimmunol Photomed 2008, In press.

28. Seite S, Medaisko C, Christiaens F, et al. Biological effects of simulated ultraviolet daylight: a new approach to investigate daily photoprotection. Photodermatol Photoimmunol Photomed 2006; 22:67–77.

14

Photoprotection in Colored Cosmetics

Zoe Diana Draelos
Dermatology Consulting Services, High Point, North Carolina, U.S.A.

SYNOPSIS

- Cosmetics can be a useful adjunct to traditional sunscreens.
- Facial foundations can contain organic plus inorganic filters and camouflage the underlying facial skin while providing meaningful photoprotection.
- Face powder can be applied over sunscreen products to enhance the ability of a sunscreen film to remain on the skin surface while increasing broad-spectrum photoprotection.
- Many daily facial moisturizers contain sunscreen ingredients and provide an SPF of 15, which is suitable for brief casual sun exposure.
- Opaque lipsticks provide excellent photoprotection under normal-use conditions.

INTRODUCTION: COLORED COSMETICS AND PHOTOPROTECTION

Colored cosmetics have traditionally been viewed as items for adornment of the face, rather than functionality. While the primary goal of this skin care category is to highlight, accentuate, and camouflage, it is worthwhile looking at the value of colored cosmetics for photoprotection as a secondary attribute. Colored cosmetics can be divided into several categories: facial foundations, facial powders, facial moisturizers, eyelid cosmetics, and lipsticks. Each of these categories can impart broad-spectrum photoprotection, if properly formulated, with organic and inorganic filters. Some of the ingredients incorporated into cosmetics as pigments and camouflaging agents can function as inorganic filters while adorning the face.

Colored cosmetics can also increase the skin longevity, a quality also known as substantivity, of traditional sunscreens. Substantivity is the ability of a sunscreen to stay where placed on the skin surface. Dermatologists have recommended that sunscreen needed to be reapplied every two hours. This recommendation was based on the lack of photostability for some organic sunscreen ingredients, such as avobenzone, and the effect of sweat, humidity, and rubbing on the sunscreen film. Some sunscreen formulations labeled as water-resistant are designed to adhere to the stratum corneum and resist water removal. These products, designed for beach use and extended wear, contain polymers that adhere to the skin surface preventing removal. Colored cosmetics do not perform well over this type of sunscreen, but can enhance the longevity of all other sunscreen formulations by adding another layer of photoprotection and encouraging setting of the sunscreen on the skin. Facial foundations and powders can absorb sweat and humidity to prevent water dissolution of the sunscreen film, a function known as setting. Also, the application of a cosmetic layer over the sunscreen can prevent physical removal by rubbing, because there is another layer for removal.

This chapter investigates the role of colored cosmetics in photoprotection. As previously discussed, colored cosmetics can increase the UVB and UVA protective abilities of sunscreens and increase the longevity of the sunscreen on the skin surface. Both these attributes are worth discussing further, since colored cosmetics in many ways can fill the aesthetic and functional voids in current sunscreen formulations.

FACIAL FOUNDATIONS

Facial foundations are designed to camouflage underlying skin blemishes, improve the appearance of skin texture, and add color to the face. In addition, facial foundations can provide photoprotection, as will be demonstrated. The ability of a facial foundation to conceal the underlying skin is known as coverage. The coverage of a foundation is directly related to the amount of titanium dioxide, zinc oxide, talc, kaolin, and precipitated chalk it contains. These pigments and powders are translucent. They blend the underlying skin color with pigment combinations to create the illusion of smooth, even-toned, blemish-free skin.

The amount of pigment in the formulation determines the degree of photo-protection. For example, sheer coverage foundations with minimal titanium dioxide are almost transparent and have a sun protection factor (SPF) around 2, since the UV radiation is still striking the skin. Most facial foundations provide moderate coverage and are translucent with an approximate SPF of 6. By adding UVB and UVA organic filters, the SPF of these formulations can be increased to 15 without compromising the aesthetics of the product (Fig. 1). Most facial foundations obtain photoprotection by adding monographed filters along with the powders and pigments to achieve the desired SPF. Facial foundations are an excellent way to enhance sunscreen compliance in young adolescents and adult females.

Yet, facial foundations can accomplish what no sunscreen can deliver, an unlimited SPF. No sunscreen can contain enough zinc oxide and/or titanium dioxide to completely obscure the underlying skin without creating a white grotesque appearance. Facial foundations, on the other hand, can provide complete coverage of the underlying skin for individuals with severe polymorphous light eruption, systemic lupus erythematosus, and other photosensitive dermatoses. This is achieved by formulating an anhydrous high-coverage foundation with large amounts of titanium dioxide to create an opaque skin-colored cream. These formulations do not contain any water and thus cannot be removed by perspiration or high-humidity conditions; however, a special solvent is required for removal at night and facial cleansing. These foundations, known as camouflaging foundations or surgical foundations, act as a complete sunblock, preventing any visible light or UV radiation from striking the skin. They are available in a wide variety of colors, but require some artistry for application.

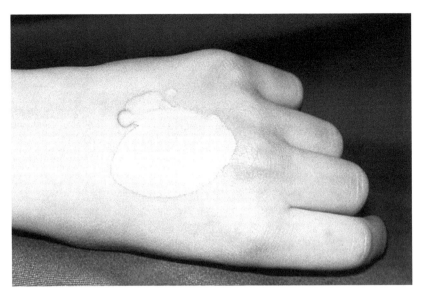

Figure 1 Facial foundations provide photoprotection because of the presence of both inorganic and organic filters.

We have already discussed the anhydrous facial foundations, but there are three other formulations worth mentioning: oil-based, water-based, and oil-free foundations. Oil-based foundations are water-in-oil emulsions containing pigments suspended in oil, such as mineral oil or lanolin alcohol. Vegetable oils (coconut, sesame, safflower) and synthetic esters (isopropyl myristate, octyl palmitate, isopropyl palmitate) may also be incorporated. The water evaporates from the foundation following application, leaving the pigment in oil on the face. This provides the facial skin with a moist feeling, especially desirable in dry-complected patients. These foundations are easy to apply, since the playtime, the time from application to setting, is prolonged, allowing manipulation of the pigment over the face for up to five minutes. These products can also contain increased concentrations of the organic oily filters to yield higher SPF photoprotection.

Water-based facial foundations are oil-in-water emulsions containing a small amount of oil, in which the pigment is emulsified, with a relatively large quantity of water. These are the most common facial foundations in the marketplace today. The primary emulsifier is usually a soap such as triethanolamine. The secondary emulsifier, present in smaller quantity, is usually glyceryl stearate or propylene glycol stearate. These facial foundations are appropriate for minimally dry to normal skin and usually have a maximum SPF of 15. More typically, they possess an SPF of 8, which is the maximum photoprotection that can be offered in a low oil formulation. These facial foundations cannot double as sunscreens in high-perspiration or high-humidity conditions as they are quickly removed from the face with water contact.

The final facial foundation category is oil-free facial foundations, containing no animal, vegetable, or mineral oils. These facial foundations are a variant of the water-based variety previously discussed; however, they contain dimethicone and/or cyclomethicone. These foundations are usually designed for individuals with acne or oily skin, since they emphasize the absence of oily substances believed to induce comedogenesis. The pigment is dissolved in water and other solvents, leaving the skin with a dry feeling resulting from the absence of oils. These facial foundations typically can only support an SPF of 8 and again are not good under moist conditions (1).

In addition to the availability of facial foundations in different formulations, there are also many different application forms. The method of application is important when considering photoprotection because the application technique determines the thickness of the protective film. Facial foundations are available in order of decreasing photo-protection in the following forms: water-based liquid, oil-based liquid, water-containing cream, anhydrous cream, stick, and cake (2). Liquid formulations are most popular because they are the easiest to apply, provide sheer-to-moderate coverage, and create a natural appearance. As discussed previously, oil-based liquids provide better photo-protection than water-based liquids. Creams deliver a thicker film to the skin surface and provide better photoprotection than liquids. Anhydrous creams and wax-based stick formulation are completely waterproof and deliver a thick light and UV radiation impervious film over the skin surface.

Finally, cake foundations, consisting of talc, kaolin, precipitated chalk, zinc oxide, and titanium dioxide compressed into a cake, provide excellent long-lasting photo-protection. They can be applied to the skin with a dry sponge in a powder form or with a moistened sponge to create a cream form. The newer mineral makeup facial foundations are of this type without the compression into a preformed cake. They have higher SPF ratings in the range of 20 to 30, but the delivered photoprotection is highly variable. These products are usually applied dry with an applicator brush attached to a tube containing the powder. If the foundation is lightly dusted over the face, the stated SPF will not be achieved. Also, these products tend to dust on and off the face easily, making product longevity an issue. Nevertheless, powders play an important role in enhanced photoprotection, which is the next topic of discussion.

FACIAL POWDERS

Facial powder is dusted over the face with a puff or a brush to provide the cosmetic benefits of coverage of complexion imperfections, oil control, a matte finish, and tactile smoothness to the skin. However, facial powders can provide additional photoprotection benefits. Facial powders contain predominantly talc, chemically known as hydrated magnesium silicate, and covering pigments. The covering pigments used in order of increasing photoprotection are titanium dioxide, kaolin, magnesium carbonate, magne-sium stearate, zinc stearate, prepared chalk, zinc oxide, rice starch, precipitated chalk, and talc (Fig. 2) (3). The more talc and covering pigments found in a powder, the higher the

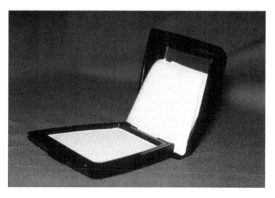

Figure 2 Facial powders contain titanium dioxide, kaolin, magnesium carbonate, magnesium stearate, zinc stearate, prepared chalk, zinc oxide, rice starch, precipitated chalk, and talc. All these ingredients function as inorganic filters.

SPF and the more opaque the powder appears to the eye. As might be expected, transparent powders offer an SPF of 2, translucent powders offer an SPF of 4 to 6, and opaque powders offer an SPF of 8 to 10, depending on the thickness of the application.

Face powder can be applied loose to the face, over a facial moisturizer or sunscreen, and on top of a facial foundation to increase product longevity and photoprotective abilities. They can absorb both perspiration and oil to increase the life of the originally applied sunscreen film. Many of the newer face powders, especially those in the mineral makeup lines, give the face a light shine, produced by nacreous pigments, such as bismuth oxychloride, mica, titanium dioxide–coated mica, or crystalline calcium carbonate. The increased shine is largely for cosmetic purposes and does not denote a powder with better photoprotection.

FACIAL MOISTURIZERS

Facial moisturizers were traditionally developed for the minimization of the appearance of dry skin; however, multifunctional products are now on the market. A new product category, known as sunscreen-containing facial moisturizers or antiaging facial moisturizers, provides excellent photoprotection in SPF ranges of 15 to 30. These products are designed for daywear only with casual sun exposure. They are aesthetically elegant and excellent for daily application before driving to work or shopping, but possess no water-resistant qualities, making them inappropriate for beachwear or extended outdoors activity. Their antiaging claim is based on the prevention of photodamage, which leads to wrinkling and dyschromia. As a matter of fact, the antiaging ingredient in most facial moisturizers making this claim is sunscreen.

There are two basic facial moisturizer formulations: oil-in-water emulsions in which water is the dominant phase and water-in-oil emulsions in which oil is the dominant phase. Oil-in-water formulations are used for the thinner daytime facial moisturizers and water-in-oil formulations are used for night creams or facial replenishing creams. Oil-in-water emulsions can be identified by their cool feel and nonglossy appearance, while water-in-oil emulsions can be identified by their warm feel and glossy appearance (4). Sunscreen-containing moisturizers are generally composed of mineral oil, propylene glycol, and water in sufficient quantity to form a lotion. The most popular organic sunscreen filter employed is octyl methoxycinnamate followed by octocrylene, oxybenzone, and metyl salicylate. Newer formulations are also using 1% to 3% micronized zinc oxide, which only slightly lightens the skin following application.

Sunscreen-containing facial moisturizers are the best product for increasing sun protection compliance in women and children. Using a multifunctional moisturizer that enhances skin barrier function, minimizes the appearance of dry skin, and provides photoprotection is a wise health decision. These products are more aesthetically pleasing, less sticky, spread to a thinner film, and are less prone to sting eyes than traditional sunscreens. Products with zinc oxide, ecamsule, octocrylene, avobenzone, and oxybenzone, or with diethylhexylnaphthalate (DEHN), avobenzone, and oxybenzone provide excellent UVA photoprotection, preventing photoaging and skin cancer.

EYELID COSMETICS

Most consumers will not apply sunscreens or the previously discussed sunscreen-containing moisturizers to the eyelid. Common reasons for missed application include eye stinging, stickiness, heaviness, and difficulty of application. One option for increasing

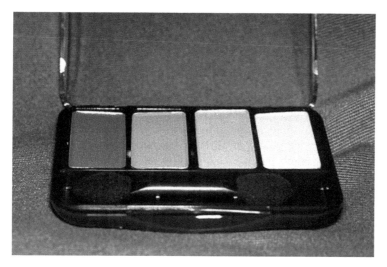

Figure 3 Eye shadows contain pigments and talc that can provide photoprotection to the often-neglected upper eyelid skin.

eyelid photoprotection in females is the use of eyelid cosmetics. Periorbital photoprotection is extremely important, especially with the increased incidence of basal cell carcinomas in the area. The most commonly used eyelid cosmetic is eye shadow, available as pressed powder, anhydrous cream, emulsion, stick, and pencil. All eye shadow formulations contain natural colors or inorganic pigments, functioning as inorganic filters that provide photoprotection (Fig.3). Only the following purified, natural colors or inorganic pigments listed in Table 1 can be used in the eye area as a result of the Food, Drug, and Cosmetic Act of 1938 (5).

Pressed powder eye shadows are the most popular formulations and are applied to the eyelid by lightly stroking a soft sponge-tipped applicator across the skin. They are predominantly talc with pigments and zinc or magnesium stearate used as a binder. Kaolin or chalk may be added to improve oil absorption and increase wearability. A water or oily binder system may also be used, with oily binder systems such as mineral oil, beeswax, or lanolin predominating. The amount of photoprotection afforded by these formulations depends on the thickness of the application. If the entire eyelid skin is obscured, excellent photoprotection is achieved. Thinner applications provide decreasing amounts of photoprotection. It is very difficult, however, to determine the photoprotection of an eye shadow, since they do not contain organic filters and are not labeled with an SPF.

Table 1 Eye Shadow Ingredients Providing Photoprotection

Iron oxides
Titanium dioxide (alone, or combined with mica)
Copper, aluminum, and silver powder
Ultramarine blue, violet, and pink
Manganese violet
Carmine
Chrome oxide and hydrate
Iron blue
Bismuth oxychloride (alone, or with mica or talc)
Mica

Better photoprotection is provided by anhydrous cream eye shadows, which contain inorganic pigments in petrolatum, cocoa butter, or lanolin. These formulations are waterproof, but have a short wearing time because of their tendency to migrate into the eyelid folds, especially in patients with oily complexions or redundant eyelid skin. The product is applied with the finger and gently rubbed across the eyelid skin. Anhydrous cream eye shadows have also been formulated as an emulsion applied with a sponge-tipped applicator or wand withdrawn from a cylindrical tube and stroked across the eyelid. These products, known as automatic eye shadows, are also waterproof, with increased wear duration over the creams. They contain beeswax, cyclomethicone, and pigments in a volatile petroleum distillate vehicle. They provide excellent photoprotection if applied as a thick film, and migration does not occur.

The most popular anhydrous eye shadows are eye shadow sticks and pencils. They are composed of pigments in petrolatum, but have added waxes, such as paraffin, carnauba, or ozokerite wax to allow extrusion of the product into a rod. Eye shadow sticks are in a roll-up tube and must be creamy to prevent drag as they are rubbed across the eyelid skin. For this reason, eye shadow sticks tend to migrate into eyelid creases in oily complected patients or those with redundant eyelid skin. A more modern packaging is to encase the rod in wood, thus forming an eye shadow pencil that is rubbed across the eyelid. The pencil form is not as creamy as the eye shadow stick. These waxy eye shadows provide the best photoprotection since they must be applied with the thickest film. If the eye shadow does not migrate into the folds of the eyelid, long-lasting photoprotection can be delivered.

Probably the best eyelid photoprotection is obtained by applying a sunscreen-containing facial moisturizer with zinc oxide to the eyelids and allowing the product to dry. Once drying has occurred, a colored powder eye shadow can be dusted over the skin. This will increase the wear time of the sunscreen-containing facial moisturizer, and the combination will possess a higher SPF than either product applied alone.

LIPSTICKS

The lips are similar to the eyes in that they are a frequently overlooked area for photoprotection. Perhaps some of the problems prevent sunscreen application. Lip photoprotection may taste bad, irritate the tender mucosa, require frequent application, and yield a poor cosmetic appearance. One way to increase the compliance of lip photoprotection is through the use of pigmented lip cosmetics, known as lipsticks. Lipsticks are mixtures of waxes, oils, and pigments in varying concentration to yield the characteristics of the final product. For example, a lipstick designed to remain on the lips for a prolonged period of time is composed of high wax, low oil, and high pigment concentrations. On the other hand, a product designed for a smooth creamy feel on the lips is composed of low wax and high oil concentrations (6). The former formulation will provide better photoprotection than the latter.

The photoprotection afforded by a lipstick is directly related to its ability to obscure the underlying lip mucosa. Products that have a high wax concentration produce a thicker film of pigment, which functions as an inorganic filter. Some lipsticks are available with added organic filters to increase the SPF of the formulation, which is listed on the packaging. It is very difficult, however, to produce a lipstick with an SPF over 30 because of the poor taste imparted by the higher-concentration organic photoprotectants.

The waxes commonly incorporated into lipstick formulations are white beeswax, candelilla wax, carnauba wax, ozokerite wax, lanolin wax, ceresin wax, and other synthetic waxes. Usually, lipsticks contain a combination of these waxes carefully selected and blended to achieve the desired melting point. Oils are then added, such as castor oil, white mineral oil, lanolin oil, hydrogenated vegetable oils, or oleyl alcohol, to form a film suitable for application to the lips. The oils are also necessary for dispersion of the pigments (7–9). These same waxes are used in lip balms, but pigments are not added. Both lipsticks and lip balms afford excellent lip photoprotection.

SUMMARY

Colored cosmetics can provide photoprotection to the face when used alone or in combination with sunscreens. The pigments found in all colored cosmetics, including facial foundations, powders, eye shadows, and lipsticks, function as inorganic filters delivering broad-spectrum photoprotection. The addition of organic filters serves to raise the SPF of the formulation. Sunscreen-containing moisturizers are essentially lower SPF sunscreens without water-resistant qualities that optimize aesthetics. Even though cosmetics are formulated with adornment as the primary goal, their ability to deliver or enhance photoprotection cannot be overlooked.

REFERENCES

1. Draelos ZD. Facial Foundations. In: Draelos ZD, ed. Cosmetics in Dermatology, 2nd ed. New York: Churchill Livingstone, 1995:1–14.
2. Fiedler JG. Foundation makeup. In: Balsam MS, Sagarin E, eds. Cosmetics, Science and Technology, Vol 1, 2nd ed. New York: Wiley-Interscience, 1972:317–334.
3. Wetterhahn J. Loose and compact face powder. In: deNavarre MG, ed. The Chemistry and Manufacture of Cosmetics, Vol IV, 2nd ed. Wheaton, IL: Allured Publishing Corporation, 1988:921–946.
4. Idson B. Moisturizers, emollients, and bath oils. In: Frost P, Horwitz SN, eds. Principles of Cosmetics for the Dermatologist. St. Louis: CV Mosby Company, 1982:37–44.
5. Lanzet M. Modern formulations of coloring agents: facial and eye. In: Frost P, Horowitz SN, eds. Principles of Cosmetics for the Dermatologist. St. Louis: CV Mosby Company, 1982:138–139.
6. Cunningham J. Color cosmetics. In: Williams DF, Schmitt WH, eds. Chemistry and Technology of the Cosmetics and Toiletries Industry. London: Blackie Academic & Professional, 1992:143–149.
7. Boelcke U. Requirements for lipstick colors. J Soc Cosmet Chem 1961; 12:468.
8. de Navarre MG. Lipstick, in The Chemistry and Manufacture of Cosmetics, 2nd ed. Wheaton, IL: Allured Publishing Corporation, 1975:778.
9. Poucher WA. Perfumes, Cosmetics and Soaps. Vol 3. 8th ed. London: Chapman and Hall, 1984:196–207.

15

Photoprotection and Products to Simulate or Stimulate UV Tanning

Zoe Diana Draelos
Dermatology Consulting Services, High Point, North Carolina, U.S.A.

SYNOPSIS

- Self-tanning products contain DHA, which is a semipermanent skin stain lasting for five to seven days.
- DHA is a 3-carbon sugar that reacts with skin protein to produce melanoidins, which are colored brown.
- Self-tanning products are nontoxic but impart minimal photoprotection to the skin possessing an SPF of 3 to 4.
- Tanning accelerators and tanning promoters lack proof of efficacy and may be dangerous.
- Self-tanning products may be a safe alternative to indoor and outdoor tanning.

INTRODUCTION

The desire to achieve tanned skin by fair-complected individuals is an interesting psychological phenomenon. There are many different explanations for this pursuit of skin darkening. One explanation focuses on differing work environments. When most individuals were engaged in agricultural pursuits, the farm owners sported fair skin, while the farmworkers sported tanned skin. Thus, tanned skin indicated a lower socioeconomic status. When lifestyles changed with the industrial revolution so that most persons worked indoors, only those who vacationed outdoors sported a tan, allowing tanned skin to be an indication of higher socioeconomic status. Some argue that Coco Chanel began the tanned skin revolution by popularizing the use of tanned women in her famous high-fashion advertisements. There can be no doubt after examining popular press images of women and men that tanned skin remains desirable, despite medical data to the contrary.

Tanning is a skin response to injury related to UVA exposure (1). The invention of indoor tanning has increased the opportunities for individuals in all latitudes to receive

UVA skin damage 24 hours daily regardless of season. A study of 3550 white females between the ages of 13 and 19 years reported that nearly one-third had used the tanning booth at least three times in their life (2). Thirty-seven percent of females and 11% of males reported using indoor tanning at least once. Indoor tanning was also positively correlated with other risk behaviors, such as alcohol, tobacco, and marijuana use. Adolescents who used two to three of these substances were more than three times as likely to use a tanning booth. Other factors that increased tanning booth use included a personal income or allowance, living in a nonurban locale, and physical maturity. Factors that correlated with decreased tanning booth use were greater cognitive ability, increased frequency of physical activity, and a mother with a college degree. This recognition has led many states to consider prohibiting minors from indoor tanning without parental consent (3).

The recognition that tanning is unsafe has led to an industry aimed at producing tanned skin without sun exposure. Products that stain the skin to mimic a tan are termed "self-tanning preparations" or "sunless tanners." Some argue that sunless tanning has led to a decrease in tanning booth use among frequent users (4). A survey found that 70% would decrease their tanning booth use, 26% would cut outdoor exposure, and 23% would increase sunscreen use after using self-tanning products. However, these numbers are controversial (5,6). It is interesting to note that 43% of tanning booths also offer the application of self-tanning products (7).

This chapter focuses on the use of products designed to simulate and stimulate a tan. The desire to stain the skin is not new, as ancient man used burnt ashes to blacken the skin. The products that simulate a tan are mostly based on dihydroxyacetone (DHA) lotions that produce staining of the skin. A variety of products, known as tanning accelerators and promoters, have also been introduced to enhance the ability of the skin to tan. This article examines the history, chemistry, formulation, and efficacy of these products.

HISTORY

Self-tanning creams are based on DHA as it induces darkening of the skin (8). This chemical was originally discovered in the 1920s as a possible artificial sweetener for diabetics by Procter & Gamble, Cincinnati, Ohio. Dr. Eva Wittgenstein noted that when the sweet, concentrated material splashed on the skin with chewing, the affected skin turned brown and the brown color could not be removed with rubbing or water contact. It was noted that the saliva turned the skin brown without staining clothing or the mouth. This side effect made the substance unsuitable as a glucose substitute, and DHA was not marketed until the 1950s when the first self-tanning cream was introduced into the marketplace. The first self-tanning creams were met with little enthusiasm, however, since the color was an unsightly orange.

CHEMISTRY

DHA ($C_3H_6O_3$) is a simple 3-carbon sugar that has no known oral toxicity. The sugar forms dimers when mixed in an aqueous solution, but it is the monomeric form that is used in self-tanning preparations (Table 1). Its activity is highest at pH 4 to 6, requiring storage in a cool, dry environment. DHA is chemically classified as a colorant or a colorless dye. It is actually an intermediate in carbohydrate metabolism in higher plants and animals and is a physiologic product of the body formed during glycolysis (9). The

Table 1 Chemistry of DHA

1. $C_3H_6O_3$
2. White crystalline hydroscopic powder
3. 3-carbon sugar
4. Stable at pH 4–6
5. Store in cool, dry environment
6. Reacts with proteins to produce brown color
7. Chromophore known as melanoidins

Abbreviation: DHA, dihydroxyacetone.

phosphate of DHA is found naturally as one of the intermediates of the Krebs cycle. Currently, DHA is manufactured as a white, crystalline hygroscopic powder by fermentation of glycerol using *Gluconobacter oxydans*.

TANNING REACTION

The tanning reaction occurs allowing the staining of the skin with DHA. The site of action of DHA is in the stratum corneum and involves the conversion of DHA to pyruvaldehyde with the elimination of water. The aldehyde reacts with the amine present in the skin keratin to form an imine. The remaining steps of the reaction are not known, but the result is cyclic and produces linear polymers that have a yellow or brown color known as melanoidins (10). Melanoidins structurally have some similarities to skin melanin (11). The browning reaction that occurs when DHA is exposed to keratin protein is known as the Maillard reaction, named after Louis-Camille Maillard who first described the reaction in 1912 (12). The Maillard reaction is currently defined as the reaction of the amino group of amino acids, peptides, or proteins with the glycosidic hydroxyl group of sugars to form brown products referred to as melanoidins.

Even though DHA is technically categorized as a colorant or colorless dye, the melanoidins impart a semipermanent color to the skin by linking to the side chains of proteins of the stratum corneum. The color similarity to melanin is due to the same absorption spectra of both substances. Maximal melanoidin formation and maximum color development occur at pH 5, which is the normal pH of healthy skin. Typically, the DHA is removed from the tube at pH 3 to 4, where it is most stable, but is rapidly raised to pH, following skin application.

SELF-TANNING PRODUCT USE

Self-tanning products can be formulated as creams, lotions, and sprays. DHA is usually added to a creamy base in concentrations of 3% to 5%; however, concentrations of 2.5% to 10% are possible (13) (Table 2). Lower concentrations of DHA produce mild tanning, while higher concentrations produce greater darkening (14). This allows self-tanning creams to be formulated in light, medium, and dark shades. Lower-concentration DHA products are easier to use, since they are less prone to streaking where uneven application leads to uneven brown staining. The addition of dimethicone improves the ability to spread the DHA and yields a more even natural appearance.

As might be expected, skin areas with more protein stain a darker color. For example, keratotic growths such as seborrheic keratoses or actinic keratoses will

Table 2 Application Technique for Self-Tanning Products

1. Wash skin thoroughly, soap residue can interfere with color development.
2. Do not apply any skin lotions or other products. If water-resistant products such as sunscreens or long-wearing moisturizers have been previously applied, clean the skin with rubbing isopropyl alcohol.
3. Exfoliate the skin with a scrub containing polyethylene beads to remove desquamating skin and the surface of seborrheic keratoses.
4. Remove a small amount of self-tanning product from the bottle, only enough to apply to one area at a time. Apply the product with a rubbing motion with long even strokes that do not overlap in one direction. Continue application until the entire skin has been coated. Apply a thin coat.
5. Wash hands thoroughly. Remove immediately from nails and hair.
6. Allow color to develop over the next 8–24 h.
7. If the depth of color desired is not achieved, better results are achieved with multiple thin coats on successive days.
8. Reapplication of the product is required every 5–7 days to maintain the color.

hyperpigment. Protein-rich areas of the skin, such as the elbows, knees, palms, and soles, also stain more deeply due to a thickened compact stratum corneum. For this reason, it is advisable to remove all dead skin through exfoliation before self-tanning cream application. This can be accomplished physically with an abrasive scrub containing polyethylene beads, a textured cloth, or a hydroxy acid moisturizer. It is important to immediately remove self-tanning products from the palms of the hands, or they too will stain brown with the application. DHA does not stain the mucous membranes, since a stratum corneum is not present, but will stain the hair and nails.

The chemical reaction is usually visible within 1 hour after DHA application, but maximal darkening may take 8 to 24 hours (15). The color lasts five to seven days as the stained stratum corneum is sloughed. Many self-tanning preparations contain a temporary dye to allow the user to note the sites of application and to promote even application, but this immediate color should not be confused with the Maillard reaction. Bronzers, which are water-based stains, may be added to produce a shorter-lived staining. Tan or brown powdered pigments and glitters can be added to produce immediate skin effects.

Self-tanning creams have enjoyed a renewed popularity since their original introduction in the 1950s. The original self-tanners produced a somewhat unnatural orange skin color. This problem has been corrected through the use of more purified sources of DHA that yield a more natural golden color. Yet, for persons with pink skin tones, the self-tanning creams may still appear unnatural. Self-tanning creams are most acceptable in persons with Fitzpatrick skin types II and III with golden skin undertones.

NEW DEVELOPMENTS IN SELF-TANNING TECHNOLOGY

There are several drawbacks to the currently marketed self-tanning products, which have been partially solved through new technology. One problem is the inability to achieve a rich dark brown color. Since DHA binds to protein, this challenge has been overcome by applying a protein-containing cream to the skin before application of the DHA. One proprietary formulation incorporates application of a sulfur-containing amino acid, such as methionine sulfoxide, to the skin just before applying the DHA. This protein interacts with the DHA, deepening the color of the skin stain.

Another problem is the immediate staining of the skin that does not mimic a gradual tan achieved with UV exposure. To give the appearance of a UV-acquired tan, many facial moisturizers and body lotions contain lower DHA concentrations that produce progressive darkening of the skin with repeated application. This allows gradual skin color acquisition providing more control over the final skin color. These products are more popular on the face where dramatic color changes are undesirable.

All DHA preparations impart a characteristic musty smell to the skin when the browning reaction occurs. The smell is not obnoxious, but undesirable, and is an indication that self-tanning products are being used. It is difficult to mask the odor with fragrance ingredients, since they can degrade or discolor the DHA formulation. One manufacturer has developed a self-tanning preparation that combines DHA and cyclodextrins to increase stability and reduce odor (16).

PROFESSIONAL DHA APPLICATIONS

Another challenge with self-tanning preparations is the difficulty in applying the cream or lotion evenly. While this problem has been overcome with addition of dimethicone to the formulation, it is still difficult to apply the product to the back or intertriginous areas. This need led to the development of proprietary DHA sprays that are applied in traditional UV-tanning salons as an alternative income source. This process has been given a variety of proprietary names, including the Parisian Tan and the Magic Tan. An industry guide to self-tanning suppliers is of 30 pages, indicative of the diversity in this market.

The customer enters a self-contained shower where a hand-held sprayer or spray heads mist the DHA-containing liquid over the entire body in an even film (17). Areas of the body where a tan is not desired, such as the palms, soles, between the toes, etc., are covered with petroleum jelly. These treatments cost approximately $40 to $80, depending on geographic location, and must be repeated every two weeks. The treatment is considered safe, since the DHA rapidly binds to skin keratin limiting systemic absorption. Even if some of the product did enter the mouth, it is nontoxic and can be safely consumed. Allergy to DHA is rare, but DHA-sensitive individuals must avoid all self-tanning preparations as they all contain DHA (18).

PHOTOPROTECTION AND SELF-TANNING PRODUCTS

Self-tanning products only stain the skin. They do not provide any meaningful photoprotection. DHA can only confer an SPF of 3 to 4, which is inadequate to be considered as a sunscreen filter. The brown skin color absorbs at the low end of the visible spectrum and minimally into the UVA spectrum (19). DHA has been added to some PUVA (psoralens plus ultraviolet A radiation) regimens to allow higher UVA doses to be delivered to the psoriatic plaques without damaging the surrounding normal skin. This technique is said to increase plaque clearing (20).

Some self-tanning preparations add organic filters, such as ethylhexyl methoxycinnamate, ethylhexyl salicylate, homosalate, benzophenone-3, or octocrylene, which are compatible with DHA. Inorganic filters, such as zinc oxide or titanium dioxide, must be avoided since they induce rapid degradation of the DHA. However, the majority of DHA products do not contain sunscreen, thus the consumer must not be lulled into a false sense of confidence that the skin stain can provide photoprotection. The major photoprotective effect of DHA products may be that they provide an alternative to outdoor and indoor UV-induced tanning.

TANNING ACCELERATORS AND PROMOTERS

A variety of products are marketed with the premise that they promote safe tanning. These products have been labeled tanning accelerators and tanning promoters. Tanning accelerators speed darkening of the skin by providing precursors to melanin, while tanning promoters increase skin photosensitivity, claiming that an equivalent tan can be achieved with less UV exposure. Tanning accelerators are based on tyrosine, but their efficacy is doubtful (21). Tanning promoters incorporate substances that create a phototoxic reaction, such as psoralens. Psoralens are dangerous in unskilled hands as eye sensitivity also increases and severe sunburns can occur. Since there is no such activity as safe tanning, the concept that psoralens can increase tanning safety and decrease photoexposure is unfounded. In the past, tanning pills were sold that contained canthaxanthin, which imparted a yellow color to the skin from carotenoids (22). However, they have been removed from the market because of the severe side effects of hepatitis, retinopathy, and aplastic anemia.

CONCLUSION

This chapter has examined self-tanning preparations, tanning accelerators, and tanning promoters. Tanning accelerators and tanning promoters are not useful or safe, but it may be worthwhile exploring the value of self-tanning products. Self-tanning products based on DHA confer limited UVA photoprotection and cannot be considered effective sunscreen filters, but the concept of sun avoidance from their use is worth investigating (Table 3).

Some argue that DHA staining of the skin is a safe alternative to the sun. Indeed, this is true. DHA provides an acceptable tan in many persons, which may decrease their desire to obtain a UV-induced tan. This may keep people out of the tanning booth and decrease the incidence of photodamage and skin cancer. However, it perpetuates the concept that light-complected persons should desire darker skin. I am not sure if this is desirable. The use of tanned models, with either UV-tanned skin or digitally altered tanned skin, in the media gives Caucasian youth the idea that dark skin is attractive. This concept should be changed. It is important that children grow up with the understanding that they must care for the skin color they received at birth. Failure to do so will ultimately result in disease. These ideas should be generalized for lifelong total health. Persons with a family history of diabetes should practice careful weight control and, persons with

---

Table 3 Advantages and Disadvantages of Self-Tanning Products

Advantages
1. Decreased outdoor tanning due to brown-stained appearance of the skin.
2. Alternative to indoor tanning offered at UV-tanning facilities.
3. Effective camouflage for lower extremity telangiectasias and cellulite.
4. Provides a safe method to achieve tanned skin in Caucasian individuals.

Disadvantages
1. Promotes the positive image of tanned skin.
2. Consumers may be deceived that stained skin is photoprotected.
3. Photoprotection is suboptimal at SPF 3–4.
4. Improper application may yield poor final appearance.

Abbreviations: UV, ultraviolet; SPF, sun protection factor.

coronary artery disease should watch their cholesterol levels from a young age. Skin health, or external health, should not be excluded from internal health.

A discussion of self-tanning products, tanning accelerators, and tanning promoters belongs in a sunscreen book, as these are products affecting the skin used in conjunction with sunscreens. Self-tanning products are the only semipermanent alternative to UV exposure for achieving skin darkening in Caucasian individuals. The active ingredient, i.e., DHA, has a proven safety profile, but tanning accelerators and promoters do not. Dermatologists can feel confident recommending the use of self-tanning preparations, but they should always be used in conjunction with a secondary sunscreen product.

REFERENCES

1. Gange RW. Tanning. Dermatol Clin 1986; 4(2):189–193.
2. Demko CA, Borawski EA, Debanne SM, et al. Use of indoor tanning facilities by white adolescents in the United States. Arch Ped Adolesc Med 2003; 157(9):854–860.
3. Dellavalle RP, Schilling LM, Chen AK, et al. Teenagers in the UV tanning booth? Tax the tan. Arch Pediatr Adolesc Med 2003; 157(9):845–846.
4. Sheehan DJ, Lesher JL. The effect of sunless tanning on behavior in the sun. South Med J 2005; 98(12):1192–1195.
5. Brooks K, Brooks D, Dajani Z, et al. Use of artificial tanning products among young adults. J Am Acad Dermatol 2006; 54(6):1060–1066.
6. Stryker JE, Yaroch AL, Moser RP, et al. Prevalence of sunless tanning product use and related behaviors among adults in the United States: results from a national survey. J Am Acad Dermatol 2007; 56(3):387–390.
7. Fu JM, Dusza SW, Halpern AC. Sunless tanning. J Am Acad Dermatol 2004; 50(5):706–713.
8. Maibach HI, Kligman AM. Dihydroxyacetone: a sun-tan-simulating agent. Arch Dermatol 1960; 82:505–507.
9. Chaudhuri RK, Hwang C. Self-Tanners: formulating with dihydroxyacetone. Cosmet Toilet 2001; 116:87–96.
10. Wittgenstein E, Berry KH. Reaction of dihydroxyacetone (DHA) with human skin callus and amino compounds. J Invest Dermatol 1961; 36:283–286.
11. Meybeck A. A spectroscopic study of the reaction products of dihydroxyacetone with aminoacids. J Soc Cosmet Chem 1977; 28:25–35.
12. Wittgenstein E, Berry KH. Staining of skin with dihydroxyacetone. Science 1960; 132:894–895.
13. Kurz T. Formulating effective self-tanners with DHA. Cosmet Toilet 1994; 109(11):55–61.
14. Maes DH, Marenus KD. Self-tanning products. In: Baran R, Maibach HI, eds. Cosmetic Dermatology. London: Martin Dunitz, 1994.
15. Goldman L, Barkoff J, Glaney D, et al. The skin coloring agent dihydroxyacetone. GP 1960; 12:96–98.
16. Lentini PJ, Tchinnis P, Muizzuddin N. US Patent 5 942 212. 1999.
17. Rogers CJ. Spray-on Tanning. Aesthetic Surg J 2005; 25(4):413–415.
18. Morren M, Dooms-Goosens A, Heidbuchel M, et al. Contact allergy to dihydroxyacetone. Contact Dermatitis 1991; 25:326–327.
19. Johnson JA, Fusaro RM. Protection against long ultraviolet radiation: topical browning agents and a new outlook. Dermatologica 1974; 175:53–57.
20. Taylor CR, Kwangsukstith C, Wimberly J, et al. Dihydroxyacetone-enhanced photochemotherapy for psorasis. Arch Dermatol 1999; 135:540–544.
21. Jaworsky C, Ratz JL, Dijkstra JW: Efficacy of tan accelerators. J Am Acad Dermatol 1987; 16(4):769–771.
22. Lober CW. Canthaxanthin the "tanning" pill. J Am Acad Dermatol 1985; 13:660.

16

Oral and Other Non-sunscreen Photoprotective Agents

Salvador González
Dermatology Service, Memorial Sloan Kettering Cancer Center, New York,
New York, U.S.A.; Ramon y Cajal Hospital, Alcalá University, Madrid, Spain

Yolanda Gilaberte-Calzada
Dermatology Service, Hospital San Jorge, Huesca, Spain

SYNOPSIS

- Oral photoprotective agents are a suitable complement for topical sunscreen protection.
- The effect of oral photoprotective agents is mainly systemic, preventing or reducing photoinduced oxidation, skin photodamage, and photoaging.
- Some oral photoprotective agents may be useful in skin cancer preventive strategy.
- Many botanical agents and formulations have antioxidant activity/properties and provide photoprotection at different levels.
- Evaluation of the photoprotective effect of oral agents includes erythema formation (SPF) and other parameters, including photoimmunoprotection, antimutagenic, and antioxidant activities.

INTRODUCTION

Sunscreen products are primarily designed to protect the skin from the harmful effects of solar ultraviolet (UV) radiation upon topical application. They contain molecules or molecular complexes that can absorb, reflect, or scatter UV photons. These are shielding sunscreens and are among the most efficient methods of protecting from solar erythema and sunburn caused by high-energy UV photons, but their potential efficacy in preventing photoaging depends on their ability to block low-energy UV light. In this regard, sunscreens that prevent local and systemic immunosupression are particularly useful to inhibit epidermal gene modifications like mutations on p53 gene, thymine dimers formation, and induction of apoptosis, or to restore the levels of collagen production (1–5). In addition, new substances with photoprotective capabilities, some of them after oral administration, have been recently developed that prevent, ameliorate, or even repair solar-induced skin damage. Furthermore, chemoprevention via non-toxic agents, especially botanical antioxidants constitutes a plausible strategy for prevention of acute and chronic photodamage, including photocarcinogenesis.

In this chapter, we provide an overview of the oral photoprotective agents and substances with photoprotective properties not included under conventional sunscreens, excluding DNA repair agents and DNA repair adjuvants, which are reviewed in another chapter. Finally a section will be dedicated to the evaluation of these agents in terms of photoprotection.

ORAL PHOTOPROTECTIVE AGENTS

The main method of use of photoprotective measures is pre-exposure topical application. However, they may be inconvenient, wear out fast, and are not very efficient providing global cutaneous protection. Therefore, additional measures, for example, oral treatments are promising tools to complement topical sunscreen use.

Recently, several oral photoprotective compounds have been commercialized that provide systemic coverage and are listed in Table 1. These products contain several active principles that enable different mechanisms to prevent cutaneous sun damage. Most of them possess antioxidant activities, which replenish the normal antioxidant capability of the body after systemic loss of endogenous antioxidants during UV exposure (6,7). These products include the following antioxidants:

Vitamin Derivatives

Carotenoids

Carotenoids are plant pigments that protect against photoinduced oxidative stress. They have been postulated to play a significant role on skin photoprotection after ingestion; however, most studies on carotenoid supplementation in healthy subjects showed no skin

---

Table 1 Oral Photoprotective Agents

Carotenoids
  Licopene
  Lutein and Zeaxanthin

Combination of antioxidants
  Mixture of tocopherol and ascorbate
  Mixture containing lycopene, β-carotene, α-tocopherol, and selenium
  Seresis: carotenoids (β-carotene and lycopene), vitamins C and E, selenium, and proanthocyanidins

Dietary botanicals: dietary flavonoids and phenolics
  PL extract
  Green tea
  Genistein
Omega-3 polyunsaturated fatty acid

Abbreviation: PL, *Polypodium leucotomos*.

photoprotection (8). A modest efficacy in systemic photoprotection has been shown to depend on the duration and dose of the supplementation before exposure to UV radiation, within the safety limits when administered in high (photoprotective) doses (9). More recently, oral ingestion of lycopene, the major carotenoid of the tomato and a very efficient singlet oxygen quencher, showed beneficial photoprotective effects. A significant decrease in the sensitivity toward UV-induced erythema has been observed in healthy human volunteers after 10 to 12 weeks of lycopene administration (10). Additionally, lutein and zeaxanthin, xanthophyllic carotenoids, commonly referred to as xanthophylls, have been assayed in a 12-week placebo-controlled, multicentered study where both xanthophylls were applied topically and orally administered (11). This study was designed to allow for direct comparisons of lutein and zeaxanthin efficacy between different routes of administration and to demonstrate the efficacy obtained when these two routes of administration were combined. The authors showed slight photoprotection at week 2 after ingestion, with greater efficacy when combined with topical application.

Combination of Antioxidants

Tocopherol and Ascorbate

In humans, oral administration of tocopherol and ascorbate showed no skin photoprotection when separately used (12,13). Therefore, the lack of effect of single-component compounds has justified the employment of combinations. Inclusion of vitamins C and E in photoprotective compounds increases the photoprotective effects compared with monotherapies (14). It seems that ascorbate regenerates tocopherol from its radical form and transfers the radical load to the aqueous compartment being eliminated by enzymatic antioxidant systems (15).

Antioxidant Complexes

An antioxidant complex containing lycopene, β-carotene, α-tocopherol, and selenium was administered orally, daily through 7 weeks in 25 healthy individuals to reduce UV-induced damages. A general reduction of the UV-induced erythema, a reduction of the UV-induced p53 expression, the number of sunburn cells, and a parallel reduction of the lipoperoxide levels have been probed. Additionally, the pigmentation increased. After the oral intake of this antioxidant complex, many parameters of the epidermal defense against UV-induced damages improved significantly (16).

Seresis

Seresis is an antioxidative combination containing physiological levels of lipid- and water-soluble compounds, including carotenoids (β-carotene and lycopene), vitamins C and E, selenium, and proanthocyanidins. A clinical, randomized, double-blind, parallel group, placebo-controlled study in young female volunteers (skin phototype II) demonstrated that Seresis slowed down the development of UVB-induced erythema and decreased UV-induced expression of MMP-1 and -9 (17).

In summary, oral intake of antioxidant complexes may supplement photo-protective measures provided by topical and physical agents and may also contribute to reduced DNA damage, leading to skin aging and skin cancers.

Dietary Botanicals

Dietary botanicals include dietary flavonoids and phenolics. Their photoprotective and anticarcinogenic properties are ascribed to their antioxidant and anti-inflammatory activities. The more scientifically studied of these botanicals are discussed.

Polypodium Leucotomos Extract

Polypodium leucotomos (PL) extract is a polyphenol-enriched natural extract from leaves of the fern *Polypodium leucotomos*. This plant extract has been used as adjuvant treatment for inflammatory skin conditions with no reported side effects. Besides its immunomodulatory properties, PL has antioxidant properties. Topically applied or orally administered PL leads to the quenching of free radicals, lipid peroxidation, and reactive oxygen species (ROS) such superoxide anion, singlet oxygen, hydroxyl radical, and hydrogen peroxide (18,19). These antioxidative properties are believed to be the main cause of the observed protection from oral PL against sun damage and psoralen plus UVA radiation (PUVA) phototoxicity. In this regard, topically applied or orally administered PL was shown to augment the UV doses required for immediate pigment darkening, minimal erythematogenic dose, and minimal melanogenic dose (17). Additionally, a low oral dose (7.5 mg/kg) of PL was shown to exert a significant photoprotective effect on human skin, reducing erythema, thymine dimer formation, and Langerhans cell depletion (20,21). The observed reduction in thymine dimers formation seems to be the result of enhanced base excision repair induced by its antioxidant effect. In addition, its beneficial effects also include (*i*) inhibition of *t*-UCA photoisomerization (22), and in vivo and in vitro cellular photoprotection (23–25), including abrogation of UV-induced TNF-α and nitric oxide (NO) production (26), (*ii*) enhancement of endogenous antioxidant systems (27), (*iii*) inhibition of photoinduced immunosupression (28), and (*iv*) modulation of cyclo-oxygenase 2 (Cox-2) expression and inflammation, preventing oxidative DNA damage (8-hydroxyguanine) and accelerating repair of thymine dimers (29). Approximately 30 minutes must be allowed following ingestion to observe the photoprotective effect, and the supplement must be repeatedly consumed to maintain the photoprotection.

Green Tea Polyphenols

Epigallocatechin-3-gallate (EGCG) is the major photoprotective polyphenolic component of green tea. While skin protection by green tea polyphenols (GTPPs) has not been proved in human intervention studies, their oral administration prevents UVB-induced skin tumor in mice, which is mediated through (*i*) the induction of immunoregulatory cytokine interleukin 12, (*ii*) IL-12-dependent DNA repair following nucleotide excision repair mechanisms, (*iii*) the inhibition of UV-induced immunosuppression through IL-12 DNA repair, and (*iv*) the inhibition of angiogenic factors and stimulation of cytotoxic T cells in a tumor microenvironment (30). Additionally, oral administration of GTPPs to mice remarkably inhibited UV-induced expression of skin MMPs, suggesting that GTPPs has a potential antiphotoaging effect (31).

Genistein

Genistein is a isoflavone first isolated from the fermented soybean, with potent antioxidant activity and low toxicity levels in animal studies (32). It is also a specific inhibitor of protein tyrosine kinases and a phytoestrogen. It has been shown that orally supplemented genistein inhibits UVB-induced acute and chronic skin photoaging and photocarcinogenesis in mice (33).

Omega-3 Polyunsaturated Fatty Acid

Omega-3 fatty acids have been reported to decrease UVB-induced sunburn and inflammation in a clinical trial; they also reduced UVA-dependent responses after three months of fish oil ingestion (34). However, fish oil is not widely used because large amounts must be consumed to achieve the desired effect, resulting in burping and gastric distress.

OTHER NON SUNSCREEN PHOTOPROTECTIVE AGENTS (TABLE 2)

Nonclassical Antioxidants

Skin damage due to UV light may also result from increased ROS production. Therefore, topical antioxidants are a successful strategy for diminishing UV-related damage of the skin. Classical antioxidants contained in sunscreen formulations include vitamin C, vitamin E and β-carotene, whose photoprotective effects against UVB and UVA are well characterized (35). In addition, there are new substances under investigation.

Vitamin-Related Compounds

Astaxanthin. Astaxanthin is a xantophilic pigment particularly efficient in the elimination of peroxilipidic radicals and inhibiting the concentration of free polyamines induced by UVA radiation, protecting fibroblasts from photoinduced damage (36).

Table 2 Other Non-sunscreen Photoprotective Agents

Nonclassical antioxidants
Vitamin-related compounds
Astaxanthin
Lutein and zeaxanthin
Polyphenolics
Ferulic and caffeic acids
Green tea polyphenols
Pomegranate
Resveratrol
Pycnogenol
PL extract
Flavonoids
Isoflavones
Genistein
Equol
Silymarin
Quercetin
Apigenin
Idebenone
Uncaria tomentose extract
PM thumb
N-(4-pyridoxylmethylene)-l- serine
Other photoprotective agents
Dihydroxyacetone
Caffeine and caffeine sodium benzoate
Pityriacitrin
Creatine
Cox-2 inhibitors

Abbreviations: PL, *Polypodium leucotomos*; PM, *Polygonum multiflorum*; Cox-2, cyclo-oxygenase 2.

Lutein and zeaxanthin. In humans, lutein and zeaxanthin showed increase in superficial skin lipids and decrease in lipid peroxidation after two weeks of topical application, which is beneficial in terms of photoprotection (11).

Polyphenolic Compounds

Polyphenolic compounds are an important part of human diet. Flavonoids and phenolic acids are the most abundant in food. Some of them have photoprotective properties, because they have antioxidative, anti-inflammatory and anticarcinogenic activities (37). They include the following:

Ferulic and caffeic acids. Ferulic and caffeic acids are hydroxycinnamic acids of vegetal origin. Topical application of a saturated aqueous solution of caffeic and ferulic acids in healthy humans afforded a significant protection to the skin against UVB-induced erythema (38). Ferulic acid is more frequently used in skin lotions and sunscreens than caffeic acids. Ferulic acid is a ubiquitous plant constituent that arises from the metabolism of phenylalanine and tyrosine. It occurs primarily in seeds and leaves both in its free form and when covalently linked to lignin and other biopolymers. Because of its phenolic nucleus and an extended side chain conjugation, it readily forms a resonance stabilized phenoxy radical that accounts for its potent antioxidant potential. UV absorption by ferulic acid catalyzes stable phenoxy radical formation and thereby potentiates its ability to terminate free radical chain reactions. By virtue of effectively scavenging deleterious radicals and suppressing radiation-induced oxidative reactions, ferulic acid may serve an important antioxidant function in preserving physiological integrity of cells exposed to UV radiation (39). Its maximal beneficial effect has been found by its incorporation into a topical solution of 15% L-ascorbic acid and 1% α-tocopherol improving chemical stability of these vitamins and doubled photoprotection to solar simulated irradiation of human skin from fourfold to approximately eightfold as measured by both erythema and sunburn cell formation. Inhibition of apoptosis was associated with reduced induction of caspase-3 and caspase-7. This antioxidant formulation efficiently reduces thymine dimer formation and provides significant synergistic protection against oxidative stress in skin and should be useful for protection against photoaging and skin cancer.

GTPP. Green tea extract is one of the most extensively studied antioxidants. The fresh leaves and bud of the tea plant *Cammelia sinesis* are steamed and dried in a process that preserves the polyphenolic antioxidants. Epigallocatechin-3-gallate (EGCC) is the most abundant and the most biologically active of the four major green tea polyphenolic catechins present in green tea extract. Green teas possess antioxidant, anti-inflammatory, and anticarcinogenic properties and appear to be beneficial when administered both orally and topically. As mentioned previously, an early study demonstrated that oral uptake of green tea induced a dose-dependent delay in tumor development following UV exposure in mice (40). Similar chemopreventive effects have been demonstrated following topical application of green tea polyphenolic catechins to hairless mice (41). ECGC appears to be an important component of green tea for its effect in suppressing UV-induced carcinogenesis (42). Additionally, green tea polyphenols have been shown to protect against other types of UV-induced damage, such as reduction in the number of sunburn cells and protection of epidermal Langerhans cells. Green tea extracts also reduced DNA damage that occurs after UV radiation. Thus it appears that topical application of green tea extract and some of its components are useful for mitigating the adverse effect of sunlight on human skin. ECGC induces a threefold reduction of UVB-induced lipid peroxide levels, prevented UVA-induced skin damage (roughness and sagginess), inhibited the expression of collagenase in cultured human epidermal fibroblasts as well as the activities of both activator protein 1 (AP1) and nuclear factor-kappa B (NF-κB) and reduced collagen cross-linking (43). Finally, the protective properties of GTPP against UV light pose potential value against photoaging. Despite the extensive body of scientific research on green tea extract, there is little clinical data on green tea–containing products. The main reason for this is that the GTPPs are highly reactive and sensitive to light and oxidation; they quickly lose activity if not used immediately after preparation. In addition, EGCG is highly hydrophilic, limiting its penetration in human skin. Because of these limitations, green tea extract is among the more difficult botanicals to formulate; standardized delivery systems for topical application of GTPPs are yet to be established (44). On the other hand, high concentrations of GTPPs or EGCGs can induce toxicity (45). It has been suggested that the addition of 0.1% butylated hydroxytoluene to 10% EGCG in a hydrophilic ointment significantly enhanced its stability (46). Despite all this, green tea–related products are favorites among consumers who have long believed in its health benefits.

Pomegranate. Pomegranate (*Punica granatum*, fam. *Punicaceae*) is a rich source of two types of polyphenolic compounds; anthocyanidins (such as delphinidin, cyanidin, and pelargonidin) and hydrolyzable tannins. It possesses strong antioxidant and anti-inflammatory properties (47). Pomegranate protects against the adverse effects of UVB radiation, inhibiting UVB-dependent activation of NF-κB and MAP kinase pathways. It also provides protection against the deleterious effect of UVA light.

Resveratrol. It is a polyphenolic phytoalexin found in the peels and seeds of grapes, nuts, fruits, and red wine. Topical application of resveratrol to hairless mice prior to UVB irradiation significantly inhibited edema and decreased the generation of hydrogen peroxide, leukocyte infiltration, and epidermal lipid peroxidation; therefore, resveratrol protects against the damages caused by acute UVB exposure, and these protective effects may be mediated via its strong antioxidant properties and significantly inhibited tumor incidence, delaying the onset of tumorigenesis Some studies have shown that NF-κB pathway plays a critical role in the chemopreventive effects of resveratrol against UVB radiation damages (48). On the other hand, the effect of resveratrol on photoaging remains to be examined. Additionally, resveratrol may be useful for enhancing the response of radiation therapies against hyperproliferative, precancerous, and neoplastic conditions (49).

Pycnogenol®. It is a standardized extract of the bark of the French maritime pine, *Pinus pinaster Ait*, which possesses potent antioxidant, anti-inflammatory, and anticarcinogenic properties. Topic application of Pycnogenol resulted in significant and dose-dependent protection from UV radiation-induced acute inflammation, immunosuppression, and carcinogenesis. Pycnogenol has photoprotective potential as a complement to sunscreens, possessing demonstrable activity when applied to the skin after, rather than before, UV exposure (50).

PL extract. Topical treatment with PL hydrophilic extract inhibits erythema and immediate pigment darkening reaction produced in vivo by UVB radiation and PUVA therapy (24). This effect is mediated not only by its antioxidant capability but also by its capability to inhibit the production of proinflammatory cytokines such as TNF-α or IL-6 (51). As mentioned previously, pretreatment of human keratinocytes with PL-inhibited solar-simulated-radiation-mediated increase of TNF-α and also abrogated NO production and the induction of inducible NO synthase elicited by UV radiation. In addition, PL inhibited the transcriptional activation of NF-jB and AP1 mediated by UV radiation. PL showed to be an inhibitor of UV-induced t-UCA photoisomerization and photo-decomposition and also in the prevention of the generation of oxidative metabolites catalyzed by TiO2. On the other hand, it also preserves the number and morphology of Langerhans cells during UV light exposure as well as during PUVA therapy (20,21,24). PL also appears to reduce elastosis and photoinduced skin tumors due to chronic exposure to UVB (52).

Flavonoids. Flavonoids are ubiquitous polyphenolic compounds; according to their chemical structure, they are divided into flavonols, flavones, flavanones, isoflavones, catechins, anthocyanidins, and chalcones. Over 4000 flavonoids have been identified, many of which occur in fruits, vegetables, and beverages (tea, coffee, beer, wine, and fruit drinks). The flavonoids have garnered interest because of their potential beneficial effects on human health, especially because of their anti-inflammatory, antitumor, and antioxidant activities.

Isoflavones. Isoflavones are one main group of phytoestrogens nonsteroid plant compounds with estrogen-like biologic reaction. Some of them have been shown to have important photoprotective activities

Genistein: Genistein has been shown to protect mouse skin from UVB-induced oxidative stress, UVB-induced photodamage, PUVA-induced photodamage, and UVB-induced carcinogenesis (53). In humans, genistein topically applied effectively blocked UVB-induced erytema and discomfort (33). Additionally, post-UVB application improved discomfort with minimal effect on erythema (33).

Equol: Red clover (*Trifolium pratense*) is a rich source of primary isoflavones like genistein and daidzein. Equol is a natural metabolite of the latter. It strongly protects against UV irradiation and inhibits tumor promotion during photocarcinogenesis (54) and photoaging (55). Its photoprotective action in mouse and human skin seems to be dependent on metallothionein, a cutaneous antioxidant that modulates UV photo-damage (56).

Although there is substantial evidence indicating that isoflavones are potentially useful topical agents for photoprotection in cellular or mouse studies, it is still questionable whether isoflavones really provide efficient photoprotection in humans, except for genistein. In a pigskin model, topical application of 0.5% solutions of three individual phytoestrogens, genistein, daidzein, and biochanin A, are better than similar solutions of equol in protecting pigskin from solar-simulated UV-induced photodamage. However, the protection was less than that provided by a topical combination of standard antioxidant solution containing 15% L-ascorbic acid, 1% α-tocopherol, and 0.5% ferulic acid (57).

Silymarin. Silymarin is a plant flavonoid isolated from the seeds of milk thistle (*Silybum marianum*). It consists of a mixture of three flavonoids, silybin, silydianin, and silychristin. Current experimental observations indicate that it protects against sunburn, DNA damage, nonmelanoma skin cancer, and immunosuppression (58). For some authors, silibinin is its bioactive component; topically applied in hairless mice, it showed a strong preventive efficacy against photocarcinogenesis, which involves the inhibition of DNA synthesis, cell proliferation and cell cycle progression, and induction of apoptosis (59). Further studies are required to determine the rate of cellular uptake, distribution, and long-term effect of silymarin on skin.

Quercetin. Quercetin is one of the promising flavonoids that possesses the higher antioxidant activity among them. Topical formulations containing quercetin successfully inhibit UVB-induced skin damage in mice (60).

Apigenin. Apigenin is a nonmutagenic bioflavonoid that prevents mouse skin carcinogenesis induced by UV exposure, which could be mediated in part by inhibition of Cox-2 protein expression induced by UVB (61).

Idebenone

Idebenone is a synthetic analog of coenzyme Q10. This low molecular–weight molecule is presumed to penetrate skin more efficiently than its parent compound. Both have been suggested as topical antioxidant ingredients for skin protection from oxidative damage caused by UV irradiation and pollution. Idebenone is a better antioxidant than other antioxidants like dL-tocopherol, coenzyme Q10, l-ascorbic acid, and alpha lipoic acid among others (44). Both 0.5% idebenone and 1% idebenone are available commercially. A clinical study using Prevage MD® by Allergan (Allergan, Irvine, CA) twice a day for six weeks has revealed a significant reduction in fine lines and wrinkles as well as an increase in skin hydration, resulting in a 30% global improvement in photodamage (62). Application of idebenone in the morning under sunscreen may provide additional protection from free-radical damage caused by the sun. Nevertheless, other studies found that idebenone does not increase the photoprotective value of an established antioxidant combination (63). This study showed that ubiquinone, idebenone, and kinetin offered little to no photoprotective value, talking in terms of UVR erythema response, in comparison to a topical antioxidant combination of vitamins C and E with ferulic acid. In summary, the information about the photoprotective effect of idebenone is, so far, controversial.

Uncaria Tomentosa Extract

The aqueous extract of *Uncaria tomentosa* (previously named *C-Med-100* and now renamed *AC-11*), an extract of cat's claw, appears to enhance the normal repair of cyclobutyl pyrimidine dimers following UVB exposure. The observed reduction in oxidative DNA damage (8-hydroxyguanine and strand breaks) is possibly the result of enhanced base excision repair or an inherent antioxidant effect, or both. In a single-blind, right side–left side beach sun exposure pilot study that included 42 healthy volunteers, there were dramatic and significant ($p < 0.0001$) reductions in erythema and blistering in volunteers who applied 0.5% topical AC-11 with an SPF-15 sunscreen when compared with the group that just applied an SPF-15 sunscreen (64).

Not all antioxidant substances have photoprotective effect despite being useful to prevent photoaging. CoffeeBerry® is the proprietary name for a mixture of antioxidants harvested from the fruit of the coffee plant *Coffea Arabica;* it contains potent polyphenols including chlorogenic acid, condensed proanthrocyanidins, quinic acid, and ferulic acid; it has been commercialized as a night and day cream to treat and prevent aging of the skin, the latter combined with octinate and oxybenzone (44). Another example is alpha lipoic acid, a naturally occurring antioxidant, that topically applied has failed to provide photoprotection in the animal model (pig) (65).

Polygonum Multiflorum Thumb

The root of *Polygonum multiflorum* (PM) *thumb* is used in Oriental medicine because it is supposedly endowed with antibacterial, antifungal, and antiaging properties. Topical administration of PM extracts after UVB irradiation sustained superoxide dismutase 1 immunoreactivity and protected against UVB-induced stress. These results indicate that topical application of PM extracts strongly inhibits oxidative stress induced by UVB irradiation and suggest that PM extract may have an antiphotoaging effect (66).

N-(4-pyridoxylmethylene)-l-serine

N-(4-pyridoxylmethylene)-l-serine (PYSer) is an antioxidant that suppresses iron-catalyzed ROS generation because of its iron-quenching activity. Topic application of PYSer significantly delayed and decreased formation of visible wrinkles induced by chronic UVB irradiation and inhibited UVB-induced increase in glycosaminoglycans (67). These results indicate that PYSer is a promising antioxidant in the prevention of chronic skin photoaging because of its iron-sequestering activity.

Topical application of antioxidants is limited by poor diffusion into the epidermis. Moreover, antioxidants tend to be unstable (68). Only when these formulation challenges are met can a topical antioxidant be effective. On the other hand, antioxidants are less potent than physical filters in preventing sunburn (69). In a search to overcome these problems, a new compound has been recently described. It is a combination of the UVB photon absorber 2-ethylhexyl-4-methoxycinnamate (OMC) and the antioxidant piperidine nitroxide TEMPOL. This de novo synthesized molecule has shown very promising preliminary results in photoprotection (70), but its applicability to human subjects still remains under scrutiny.

Other Photoprotective Agents

Dihydroxyacetone

Dihydroxyacetone produces temporary staining of the skin, but only offers a SPF of 3 to 4, conferring protection against long-wave UVA and visible light. In addition, the durability of this sunless tanning effect does not last for the duration of the tan (71) depending on the initial SPF provided. This ingredient has been removed from the U.S. Sunscreen Monograph because of its poor ability to provide photoprotection.

Caffeine and Caffeine Sodium Benzoate

Caffeine and caffeine sodium benzoate possess sunscreen properties and also enhance UVB-induced apoptosis when applied to the skin. Additional studies have shown that caffeine sodium benzoate strongly inhibited UVB-induced tumor formation (72). Another study revealed that caffeine applied topically after UV radiation resulted in a significant decrease in UV-induced skin roughness/transverse rhytides, and doubled the number of apoptotic keratinocytes, whereas other parameters, including epidermal hyperplasia, solar elastosis, and angiogenesis did not change (73). These findings suggest that topical application of caffeine to mouse skin after UV irradiation promotes the deletion of DNA-damaged keratinocytes and may partially diminish photodamage as well as photocarcinogenesis.

Pityriacitrin

Pityriacitrin (PIT) is a potent UV absorber indole compound naturally occurring in *Malassezia furfur*. PIT exhibits UV-protective activity on *Candida albicans* and staphylococci, with no detectable toxicity (74). Nevertheless, it has been shown in humans that the UV-protective effect of PIT is all in all very weak, suggesting that it is likely only an inferior cofactor in the development of hypopigmentation in pityriasis versicolor alba lesions following sun exposure (75).

Creatine

Exogenous creatine was readily up-taken by keratinocytes and increased creatine kinase activity, mitochondrial function, and protected against the effect of ROS, suggesting its efficacy against a variety of cellular stress conditions, including oxidative and UV damage in vitro and in vivo. This has further implications in other modulating processes involved in premature skin aging and skin damage (76).

Cox-2 Inhibitors

Cox-2 is an important metabolic enzyme upregulated in different types of cancer. Celecoxib, a selective inhibitor, decreased UVB-mediated inflammation, including edema, dermal neutrophil infiltration and activation, prostaglandin E2 (PGE$_2$) levels and the formation of sunburn cells (77). Moreover, celecoxib also inhibited acute oxidative damage and UVB-induced papilloma/carcinoma formation in long-term studies (78).

EVALUATION OF THE PHOTOPROTECTIVE CAPACITY OF A NON-SUNSCREEN PRODUCT

Although controversial, SPF is the most reliable indicator of the efficacy of sunscreen filters. However, Ery-PF (erythema protection factor) is more accurate than SPF because the test protocol only takes into account the erythematous response after 24 hours. Erythema measurement is an easy and noninvasive protocol that evaluates the efficacy of sunscreens. The question remains whether erythema induction as measured by SPF is a bona fide indicator of all UV damage. In fact, inflammation and loss of elasticity in photoaging is induced by suberythematous doses of UV radiation. Moreover, it has been recently reported that suberythematous UVB radiation not only alters Langerhans cell count and antigen-presenting function but also induces pyrimidine dimer formation and affects p53 expression (79,80). Therefore, there must be other methods to measure the capacity to protect from the sun damage for non-sunscreen substances. These methods are discussed next.

1. Photoimmunoprotection: Erythema is a poor indicator of immunosuppression. Current methods rely to determine immunosupression include the sunscreen ability to inhibit UV-induced local suppression of contact- or delayed-type hypersensititivy responses, using either the induction or the elicitation arms of these responses. The induction arm of the contact hipersensitivity response is sensitive to a single suberythemal exposure of solar-simulating radiation, which enables direct comparison with SPF, but it requires a large number of volunteers and is not cost-effective (81). On the other hand, the elicitation arm exploits prior sensitization to contact or recall antigens and can be applied to small groups of volunteers. Some protocols, however, require repeated solar simulation exposures, invalidating direct comparisons with SPF, which is based on a single exposure. In conclusion, candidate sunscreens should not substantially alter the relationship between UVR-induced erythema and immune modulation.
2. Antimutagenic activity: The mutation protection factor is defined as the ability of a sunscreen to inhibit p53 mutations, i.e., induced by UVB irradiation (82). Standardized techniques to calculate the mutation protection factor as well as the immune protection factor are yet to be developed.
3. Antioxidant activity: It has been suggested that a standardized protocol of tests including photochemiluminescence, prooxidative systems with measurement of

primary and secondary oxidation products, UVB-irradiated keratinocytes stained for thymine dimer formation, and sunburn cell assays as measures of antioxidant capacity might be useful as tools to compare the environmental protection factor (EPF) of various antioxidants (83).

CONCLUDING REMARKS AND FUTURE PERSPECTIVES

This chapter has provided an overview of several different compounds that highlight the potential beneficial effects of oral photoprotective agents and other dietary supplements in the prevention of photodamage and subsequent photocarcinogenesis and photoaging. The mechanisms of photoprotection of most of these compounds are not fully defined yet; many possess antioxidant activity, but others are completely unknown, and this remains a very active area of both basic and clinical research.

Antioxidants and other nonstandard photoprotective agents may be used together with conventional sunscreens in topical formulations to widen their photoprotective spectrum. In this regard, oral photoprotective agents show promise for several reasons: they are easy to use and they potentially provide enhanced skin photoprotection, particularly in high-risk groups. In addition, some of these compounds have shown the ability to delay or even decrease the frequency of skin cancer.

Adjuvant treatments to standard sunscreens have become a focus of interest to the scientific community, particularly in public health and preventive medicine. In this regard, some of the components with a botanic origin and a verified safety profile have been successfully assayed against UV damage and in the prevention of skin cancer, using in vitro techniques, animal models, and emerging clinical studies employing suitable biomarkers such as erythema formation. Some compounds are already available as oral supplements and others have been incorporated to topical products, including sunscreens. Nevertheless, further clinical trials will be required to validate the preventive and therapeutic value of these products.

In summary, oral sunscreens have demonstrated therapeutic value in the prevention of sun damage and other deleterious alterations associated to skin aging. It will be interesting to assess their efficacy in preventing photoaging in humans in long-term clinical trials.

REFERENCES

1. Seite S, Colige A, Piquemal-Vivenot P, et al. A full-UV spectrum absorbing daily use cream protects human skin against biological changes occurring in photoaging. Photodermatol Photoimmunol Photomed 2000; 16(4):147–155.
2. Moyal D. Immunosuppression induced by chronic ultraviolet irradiation in humans and its prevention by sunscreens. Eur J Dermatol 1998; 8(3):209–211.
3. van der Pols JC, Xu C, Boyle GM, et al. Expression of p53 tumor suppressor protein in sun-exposed skin and associations with sunscreen use and time spent outdoors: a community-based study. Am J Epidemiol 2006; 163(11):982–988.
4. Al Mahroos M, Yaar M, Phillips TJ, et al. Effect of sunscreen application on UV-induced thymine dimers. Arch Dermatol 2002; 138(11):1480–1485.
5. Bernerd F, Vioux C, Asselineau D. Evaluation of the protective effect of sunscreens on in vitro reconstructed human skin exposed to UVB or UVA irradiation. Photochem Photobiol 2000; 71 (3):314–320.

6. Pattison DI, Davies MJ. Actions of ultraviolet light on cellular structures. EXS 2006; (96):131–157.

7. DeBuys HV, Levy SB, Murray JC, et al. Modern approaches to photoprotection. Dermatol Clin 2000; 18(4):577–590.

8. Garmyn M, Ribaya-Mercado JD, Russel RM, et al. Effect of beta-carotene supplementation on the human sunburn reaction. Exp Dermatol 1995; 4(2):104–111.

9. Biesalski HK, Obermueller-Jevic UC. UV light, beta-carotene and human skin–beneficial and potentially harmful effects. Arch Biochem Biophys 2001; 389(1):1–6.

10. Stahl W, Heinrich U, Aust O, et al Lycopene-rich products and dietary photoprotection. Photochem Photobiol Sci 2006; 5(2):238–242.

11. Palombo P, Fabrizi G, Ruocco V, et al. Beneficial long-term effects of combined oral/topical antioxidant treatment with the carotenoids lutein and zeaxanthin on human skin: a double-blind, placebo-controlled study. Skin Pharmacol Physiol 2007; 20(4):199–210.

12. Fuchs J, Kern H. Modulation of UV-light-induced skin inflammation by D-alpha-tocopherol and L-ascorbic acid: a clinical study using solar simulated radiation. Free Radic Biol Med 1998; 25(9):1006–1012.

13. McArdle F, Rhodes LE, Parslew R, et al. UVR-induced oxidative stress in human skin in vivo: effects of oral vitamin C supplementation. Free Radic Biol Med 2002; 33(10):1355–1362.

14. Eberlein-Konig B, Ring J. Relevance of vitamins C and E in cutaneous photoprotection. J Cosmet Dermatol 2005; 4(1):4–9.

15. Wefers H, Sies H. The protection by ascorbate and glutathione against microsomal lipid peroxidation is dependent on vitamin E. Eur J Biochem 1988; 174(2):353–357.

16. Cesarini JP, Michel L, Maurette JM, et al. Immediate effects of UV radiation on the skin: modification by an antioxidant complex containing carotenoids. Photodermatol Photoimmunol Photomed 2003; 19(4):182–189.

17. Greul AK, Grundmann JU, Heinrich F, et al. Photoprotection of UV-irradiated human skin: an antioxidative combination of vitamins E and C, carotenoids, selenium and proanthocyanidins. Skin Pharmacol Appl Skin Physiol 2002; 15(5):307–315.

18. Gonzalez S, Pathak MA. Inhibition of ultraviolet-induced formation of reactive oxygen species, lipid peroxidation, erythema and skin photosensitization by *Polypodium leucotomos*. Photodermatol Photoimmunol Photomed 1996; 12:45–56.

19. Gomes AJ, Lunardi CN, Gonzalez S, et al. The antioxidant action of Polypodium leucotomos extract and kojic acid: reactions with reactive oxygen species. Braz J Med Biol Res 2001; 34 (11):1487–1494.

20. Middelkamp-Hup MA, Pathak MA, Parrado C, et al. Orally administered Polypodium leucotomos extract decreases psoralen-UVA-induced phototoxicity, pigmentation, and damage of human skin. J Am Acad Dermatol 2004; 50(1):41–49.

21. Middelkamp-Hup MA, Pathak MA, Parrado C, et al. Oral Polypodium leucotomos extract decreases ultraviolet-induced damage of human skin. J Am Acad Dermatol 2004; 51(6): 910–918.

22. Capote R, Alonso-Lebrero JL, Garcia F, et al. Polypodium leucotomos extract inhibits trans-urocanic acid photoisomerization and photodecomposition. J Photochem Photobiol B 2006; 82 (3):173–179.

23. Gonzalez S, Joshi PC, Pathak MA. *Polypodium leucotomos* extract as an antioxidant agent in the therapy of skin disorders. J Invest Dermatol 1994; 102:651–659.

24. Gonzalez S, Pathak MA, Cuevas J, et al. Topical or oral administration with an extract of *Polypodium leucotomos* prevents acute sunburn and psolaren-induced phototoxic reactions as well as depletion of Langerhans cells in human skin. Photodermatol Photoimmunol Photomed 1997; 13:50–60.

25. Alonso-Lebrero JL, Domínguez-Jiménez C, Tejedor R, et al. Photoprotective properties of a hydrophilic extract of the fern *Polypodium leucotomos* on human skin cells. J Photochem Photobiol B 2003; 70:31–37.

26. Janczyk A, Garcia-Lopez MA, Fernandez-Peñas P, et al. A Polypodium leucotomos extract inhibits solar-simulated radiation-induced TNF-alpha and iNOS expression, transcriptional activation and apoptosis. Exp Dermatol 2007; 16(10):823–829.

27. Mulero M, Rodriguez-Yanes E, Nogues MR, et al. Polypodium leucotomos extract inhibits glutathione oxidation and prevents Langerhans cell depletion induced by UVB/UVA radiation in a hairless rat model. Exp Dermatol 2008.

28. Siscovick JR, Zapolanski T, Magro C, et al. Polypodium leucotomos inhibits ultraviolet B radiation-induced immunosuppression. Photodermatol Photoimmunol Photomed 2008; 24 (3):134–141.

29. Zattra E, Coleman C, Acad S, et al. Oral Polypodium leucotmos extract decreases UV-induced COX-2, accelerates removal of CPDs and 8-ox-dG in Xpc+/- mice. J Invest Dermatol 2008; 128(suppl 1):s34.

30. Katiyar S, Elmets CA, Katiyar SK. Green tea and skin cancer: photoimmunology, angiogenesis and DNA repair. J Nutr Biochem 2007; 18(5):287–296.

31. Vayalil PK, Mittal A, Hara Y, et al. Green tea polyphenols prevent ultraviolet light-induced oxidative damage and matrix metalloproteinases expression in mouse skin. J Invest Dermatol 2004; 122(6):1480–1487.

32. Messina MJ, Persky V, Setchell KD, et al. Soy intake and cancer risk: a review of the in vitro and in vivo data. Nutr Cancer 1994; 21(2):113–131.

33. Wei H, Saladi R, Lu Y, et al. Isoflavone genistein: photoprotection and clinical implications in dermatology. J Nutr 2003; 133(11 suppl 1):3811S–3819S.

34. Rhodes LE, O'Farrell S, Jackson MJ, et al. Dietary fish-oil supplementation in humans reduces UVB-erythemal sensitivity but increases epidermal lipid peroxidation. J Invest Dermatol 1994; 103(2):151–154.

35. Pinnell SR. Cutaneous photodamage, oxidative stress, and topical antioxidant protection. J Am Acad Dermatol 2003; 48(1):1–19.

36. Goto S, Kogure K, Abe K, et al. Efficient radical trapping at the surface and inside the phospholipid membrane is responsible for highly potent antiperoxidative activity of the carotenoid astaxanthin. Biochim Biophys Acta 2001; 1512(2):251–258.

37. Lambert JD, Hong J, Yang GY, et al. Inhibition of carcinogenesis by polyphenols: evidence from laboratory investigations. Am J Clin Nutr 2005; 81(1 suppl):284S–291S.

38. Saija A, Tomaino A, Trombetta D, et al. In vitro and in vivo evaluation of caffeic and ferulic acids as topical photoprotective agents. Int J Pharm 2000; 199(1):39–47.

39. Graf E. Antioxidant potential of ferulic acid. Free Radic Biol Med 1992; 13(4):435–448.

40. Wang ZY, Agarwal R, Bickers DR, et al. Protection against ultraviolet B radiation-induced photocarcinogenesis in hairless mice by green tea polyphenols. Carcinogenesis 1991; 12 (8):1527–1530.

41. Elmets CA, Singh D, Tubesing K, et al. Cutaneous photoprotection from ultraviolet injury by green tea polyphenols. J Am Acad Dermatol 2001; 44(3):425–432.

42. Gensler HL, Timmermann BN, Valcic S, et al. Prevention of photocarcinogenesis by topical administration of pure epigallocatechin gallate isolated from green tea. Nutr Cancer 1996; 26 (3):325–335.

43. Rutter K, Sell DR, Fraser N, et al. Green tea extract suppresses the age-related increase in collagen crosslinking and fluorescent products in C57BL/6 mice. Int J Vitam Nutr Res 2003; 73(6):453–460.

44. Farris P. Idebenone, green tea, and Coffeeberry extract: new and innovative antioxidants. Dermatol Ther 2007; 20(5):322–329.

45. Hsu S. Green tea and the skin. J Am Acad Dermatol 2005; 52(6):1049–1059.

46. Dvorakova K, Dorr RT, Valcic S, et al. Pharmacokinetics of the green tea derivative, EGCG, by the topical route of administration in mouse and human skin. Cancer Chemother Pharmacol 1999; 43(4):331–335.

47. Afaq F, Mukhtar H. Botanical antioxidants in the prevention of photocarcinogenesis and photoaging. Exp Dermatol 2006; 15(9):678–684.

48. Adhami VM, Afaq F, Ahmad N. Suppression of ultraviolet B exposure-mediated activation of NF-kappaB in normal human keratinocytes by resveratrol. Neoplasia 2003; 5(1):74–82.

49. Reagan-Shaw S, Mukhtar H, Ahmad N. Resveratrol imparts photoprotection of normal cells and enhances the efficacy of radiation therapy in cancer cells. Photochem Photobiol 2008; 84 (2):415–421.

50. Sime S, Reeve VE. Protection from inflammation, immunosuppression and carcinogenesis induced by UV radiation in mice by topical Pycnogenol. Photochem Photobiol 2004; 79 (2):193–198.

51. Brieva A, Guerrero A, Pivel JP. Immunomodulatory properties of an hydrophilic extract of *Polypodium leucotomos*. Inflammopharmacol 2002; 9:361–371.

52. Alcaraz MV, Pathak MA, Rius F, et al. An extract of *Polypodium leucotomos* appears to minimize certain photoaging changes in a hairless albino mouse animal model. Photodermatol Photoimmunol Photomed 1999; 15:120–126.

53. Shyong EQ, Lu Y, Lazinsky A, et al. Effects of the isoflavone 4',5,7-trihydroxyisoflavone (genistein) on psoralen plus ultraviolet A radiation (PUVA)-induced photodamage. Carcinogenesis 2002; 23(2):317–321.

54. Widyarini S, Husband AJ, Reeve VE. Protective effect of the isoflavonoid equol against hairless mouse skin carcinogenesis induced by UV radiation alone or with a chemical cocarcinogen. Photochem Photobiol 2005; 81(1):32–37.

55. Reeve VE, Widyarini S, Domanski D, et al. Protection against photoaging in the hairless mouse by the isoflavone equol. Photochem Photobiol 2005; 81(6):1548–1553.

56. Widyarini S, Allanson M, Gallagher NL, et al. Isoflavonoid photoprotection in mouse and human skin is dependent on metallothionein. J Invest Dermatol 2006; 126(1):198–204.

57. Lin JY, Tournas JA, Burch JA, et al. Topical isoflavones provide effective photoprotection to skin. Photodermatol Photoimmunol Photomed 2008; 24(2):61–66.

58. Katiyar SK. Silymarin and skin cancer prevention: anti-inflammatory, antioxidant and immunomodulatory effects (Review). Int J Oncol 2005; 26(1):169–176.

59. Mallikarjuna G, Dhanalakshmi S, Singh RP, et al. Silibinin protects against photocarcinogenesis via modulation of cell cycle regulators, mitogen-activated protein kinases, and Akt signaling. Cancer Res 2004; 64(17):6349–6356.

60. Casagrande R, Georgetti SR, Verri WA Jr., et al. Protective effect of topical formulations containing quercetin against UVB-induced oxidative stress in hairless mice. J Photochem Photobiol B 2006; 84(1):21–27.

61. Tong X, Van Dross RT, Abu-Yousif A, et al. Apigenin prevents UVB-induced cyclooxygenase 2 expression: coupled mRNA stabilization and translational inhibition. Mol Cell Biol 2007; 27 (1):283–296.

62. McDaniel D, Neudecker B, Dinardo J, et al. Clinical efficacy assessment in photodamaged skin of 0.5% and 1.0% idebenone. J Cosmet Dermatol 2005; 4(3):167–173.

63. Tournas JA, Lin FH, Burch JA, et al. Ubiquinone, idebenone, and kinetin provide ineffective photoprotection to skin when compared to a topical antioxidant combination of vitamins C and E with ferulic acid. J Invest Dermatol 2006; 126(5):1185–1187.

64. Emanuel P, Scheinfeld N. A review of DNA repair and possible DNA-repair adjuvants and selected natural anti-oxidants. Dermatol Online J 2007; 13(3):10.

65. Lin JY, Lin FH, Burch JA, et al. Alpha-lipoic acid is ineffective as a topical antioxidant for photoprotection of skin. J Invest Dermatol 2004; 123(5):996–998.

66. Hwang IK, Yoo KY, Kim DW, et al. An extract of Polygonum multiflorum protects against free radical damage induced by ultraviolet B irradiation of the skin. Braz J Med Biol Res 2006; 39 (9):1181–1188.

67. Kitazawa M, Ishitsuka Y, Kobayashi M, et al. Protective effects of an antioxidant derived from serine and vitamin B6 on skin photoaging in hairless mice. Photochem Photobiol 2005; 81 (4):970–974.

68. Kullavanijaya P, Lim HW. Photoprotection. J Am Acad Dermatol 2005; 52(6):937–958.

69. Hamanaka H, Miyachi Y, Imamura S. Photoprotective effect of topically applied superoxide dismutase on sunburn reaction in comparison with sunscreen. J Dermatol 1990; 17(10): 595–598.

70. Damiani E, Astolfi P, Cionna L, et al. Synthesis and application of a novel sunscreen-antioxidant. Free Radic Res 2006; 40(5):485–494.

71. Draelos ZD. Self-tanning lotions: are they a healthy way to achieve a tan? Am J Clin Dermatol 2002; 3(5):317–318.

72. Lu YP, Lou YR, Xie JG, et al. Caffeine and caffeine sodium benzoate have a sunscreen effect, enhance UVB-induced apoptosis, and inhibit UVB-induced skin carcinogenesis in SKH-1 mice. Carcinogenesis 2007; 28(1):199–206.

73. Koo SW, Hirakawa S, Fujii S, et al. Protection from photodamage by topical application of caffeine after ultraviolet irradiation. Br J Dermatol 2007; 156(5):957–964.

74. Machowinski A, Kramer HJ, Hort W, et al. Pityriacitrin–a potent UV filter produced by Malassezia furfur and its effect on human skin microflora. Mycoses 2006; 49(5):388–392.

75. Gambichler T, Kramer HJ, Boms S, et al. Quantification of ultraviolet protective effects of pityriacitrin in humans. Arch Dermatol Res 2007; 299(10):517–520.

76. Lenz H, Schmidt M, Welge V, et al. The creatine kinase system in human skin: protective effects of creatine against oxidative and UV damage in vitro and in vivo. J Invest Dermatol 2005; 124(2):443–452.

77. Fischer SM, Lo HH, Gordon GB, et al. Chemopreventive activity of celecoxib, a specific cyclooxygenase-2 inhibitor, and indomethacin against ultraviolet light-induced skin carcinogenesis. Mol Carcinog 1999; 25(4):231–240.

78. Wilgus TA, Koki AT, Zweifel BS, et al. Inhibition of cutaneous ultraviolet light B-mediated inflammation and tumor formation with topical celecoxib treatment. Mol Carcinog 2003; 38 (2):49–58.

79. Hanneman KK, Cooper KD, Baron ED. Ultraviolet immunosuppression: mechanisms and consequences. Dermatol Clin 2006; 24(1):19–25.

80. Lavker RM, Gerberick GF, Veres D, et al. Cumulative effects from repeated exposures to suberythemal doses of UVB and UVA in human skin. J Am Acad Dermatol 1995; 32(1):53–62.

81. Fourtanier A, Moyal D, Maccario J, et al. Measurement of sunscreen immune protection factors in humans: a consensus paper. J Invest Dermatol 2005; 125(3):403–409.

82. Maier T, Korting HC. Sunscreens - which and what for? Skin Pharmacol Physiol 2005; 18 (6):253–262.

83. McDaniel DH, Neudecker BA, Dinardo JC, et al. Idebenone: a new antioxidant - Part I. Relative assessment of oxidative stress protection capacity compared to commonly known antioxidants. J Cosmet Dermatol 2005; 4(1):10–17.

17
Photoprotection by Fabric

Kathryn L. Hatch
*Department of Agricultural and Biosystems Engineering, The University of
Arizona, Tucson, Arizona, U.S.A.*

Linda Block
UA Cooperative Extension, The University of Arizona, Tucson, Arizona, U.S.A.

Peter Gies
Australian Radiation Protection and Nuclear Safety Agency, Yallambie, Victoria, Australia

SYNOPSIS

- The most important determinants of how photoprotective a fabric is are (*i*) percentage cover (or its opposite, % porosity) and (*ii*) the type and concentration of chemicals comprising the fabric.

- Percentage cover is the percentage of fabric surface area occupied by yarn/fiber. Percentage porosity is the percentage of fabric surface area not occupied by yarn or fiber. These are areas referred to as fabric interstices. UV rays pass directly through a fabric interstice, striking the skin under the fabric without ever striking a fiber, which might deter its passage.

- Percentage cover is the most important factor, as it determines how much of incident UV will strike a fiber as the ray moves from the face of the fabric to the skin surface under the fabric.

- Any fabric that has a percentage cover of 94% or less will have a UPF less than 15, the lowest value permitted for a fabric with a claim of UV protection. This statement holds true no matter what the fiber content of the fabric is and what chemicals have been applied.

- Other fabric features that influence how photoprotective a fabric is are yarn openness and fabric thickness, as these structural features determine the path of scattered radiation from the fabric face to the fabric back.

- Chemicals in fabrics that can alter UV rays that strike them include the fiber polymers, pigments, dyes, optical whitening agents, and specially designed UV-absorbing compounds (often called UV-cutting agents). Specific chemicals within each of these classifications will have different interactions with solar UV radiation.

INTRODUCTION

Long before the advent of sunscreens, products developed for the sole purpose of protecting human skin from harmful solar ultraviolet (UV) rays, people wore clothes for the specific purpose of protecting their skin when outdoors under the summer sun. Notable examples include head-to-toe garments worn by men, women, and children living in Middle Eastern countries and in the Sahara Desert in Africa and by Victorian women in England and the United States. About 1990, clothing for protection from UV radiation became a topic of considerable interest in the scientific community because of rapidly increasing skin cancer rates. The interest centered on how to (*i*) assess photoprotection, primarily sunburn protection, provided by fabric, the material from which garments are made, and (*ii*) engineer fabric to provide excellent photoprotection, particularly protection from sunburn. Reviews of the subject began to be published in 1993 (1). Recently, three lengthy reviews on the topic of fabrics as solar UV protection materials were published (2–4), adding further to information summarized in 2000 (5), 2003 (6), and 2004 (7). Today, there are at least nine documents that specify how to prepare and test fabric for photoprotection and how to use data collected to provide a singular value on labels of garments sold with a claim to UV protection and about garment style requirements (8–16).

This review does not repeat what has been previously summarized. Rather, this review focuses on the two most fundamental concepts that must be clearly understood for anyone to understand how fabric must be engineered to provide photoprotection. The first concept centers on fabric structure, which plays a key role in how much incident UV radiation passes though the fabric unchanged. The second concept centers on fabric chemistry, which determines whether incident UV rays reach the skin beneath the fabric. Specific chemistries are briefly discussed.

FABRIC ARCHITECTURE

A brief introduction to fabric architecture is necessary to ensure that textile terminology used in this chapter is understood, as aspects of fabric architecture (also called structure or construction) play critical roles in fabric as a photoprotective material. For detail beyond what is offered below about fabric architecture, refer to the book by Hatch (17).

Fiber

Fabrics are manufactured products whose fundamental unit is fiber. Fibers are always much longer than they are wide and usually nearly round. The smallest usable fibers are 0.5 in (15 mm) long and approximately 0.0004 in (10 μm) wide. While there is not an upper limit to length, the upper limit to width is approximately 0.002 in (50 μm), because yarn and garment fabric made from wider fibers are too coarse to be comfortably worn next to the skin. Fibers are classified by length as either *staple* or *filament*. Natural fibers—for example, cotton, flax (linen), and wool—are only available as staple. Manufactured fibers (such as rayon, acetate, polyester, nylon, acrylic, and olefin) and silk (a natural fiber) are available as both filament and staple. Filament fibers are often miles long, while staple fibers are so short that length is specified in inches: for example, wool fibers are 0.5 to 15 in, cotton fibers 0.5 to 2.5 in, and flax (linen) fibers 1 to 14 in. Most summertime garments are made from fabrics made entirely or partially from cotton fiber, a combination (i.e., blend) of polyester fiber in staple form and cotton fiber. Many garments sold with a claim of sunburn protection are made from polyester or nylon fiber.

Yarn

Fibers are manufactured into yarns, which are cylindrical structures extremely long in comparison with their width. Most yarns in garment fabrics are spun yarns (yarns made from staple-length fibers), but some are made from filament yarns (yarns made from filament fibers). Figure 1 shows a short section of a spun yarn made with cotton fiber (left) and a short section of a filament yarn composed of polyester filaments (right). Here, the polyester fiber filaments have been textured, i.e., changed from being absolutely straight, so the filaments do not pack tightly together. Texturing helps water vapor emitted from the skin to pass through the yarn structure and improves the feel of the fabric on the skin, thus improving the comfort of the fabric.

Fabric Construction

Yarns are used to manufacture fabric, which are structures "having substantial surface area in relation to thickness and sufficient mechanical strength to give the assembly inherent cohesion." The categories of fabric constructions are woven, knit, nonwoven, twisted, and compound. The two construction classes of interest to the subject of this chapter are knit and woven, as these are the constructions primarily found in garment fabrics (Figs. 2 and 3).

Knit fabrics are those that are composed of intermeshing loops of yarn. The major classes of knit fabrics are weft and warp knits, but it is the weft-knit fabrics (the jerseys and rib weft knits) that are primarily used in the manufacture of the popular summertime T-shirts, golf shirts, and "lightweight "running pants (Fig. 2). Woven fabrics are those that have two or more sets of yarns interlaced at right angles to each other. Since nearly all woven fabrics

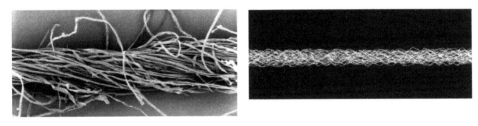

Figure 1 Photomicrographs of a spun (*left*) and filament (*right*) yarn. *Source*: From Ref. 17.

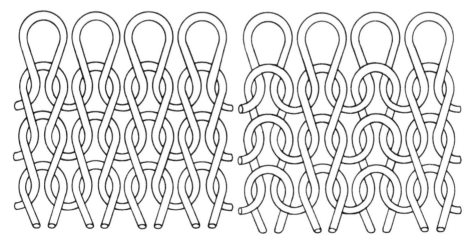

Figure 2 Jersey-weft knit (*left*) and single rib weft knit (*right*). *Source*: From Ref. 17.

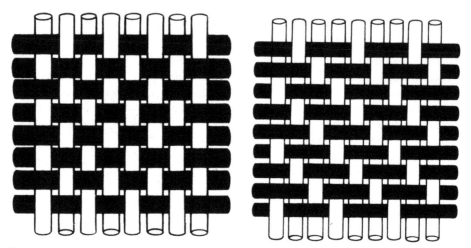

Figure 3 Plain weave (*left*) and twill weave (*right*) woven fabrics. *Source*: From Ref. 17.

of interest are those with two sets of yarns (lengthwise yarns called warp yarns and crosswise yarns called weft yarns) and have either plain or twill weave structure, only those structures are illustrated in Figure 3. Jeans, dresses, and sport shirts as well as many slacks and skirts are made from woven fabrics. Usually, the easiest way to differentiate the type of fabric, knit or woven, is to see if it stretches when pulled in the direction of the yarns. Knit fabrics elongate easily and considerably in relation to woven fabrics.

FEATURES IMPORTANT TO PHOTOPROTECTION

The photoprotectiveness of fabrics is expressed as UV protection factor (UPF; see next section). Three features of fabric that have a major impact on photoprotection are percentage cover, yarn "openness," and fabric thickness or yarn size (Table 1).

Presence of Interstices

Unlike sunscreens, which form continuous films on the skin surface, fabrics have areas where there is no fiber. There are "holes or pores"—more properly called interstices— through the fabric (from the face to the back of the fabric). The presence of interstices is obvious in Figures 2 and 3 as these are the areas between the yarns. Radiation that is perpendicularly incident to the fabric surface at an interstice passes directly though the fabric. This radiation is called *directly transmitted radiation*.

Of major interest is to know how much of the fabric's volume is unoccupied by yarn or fiber. The reason is that where there is no fiber, incident UV rays will pass directly through. Actually a volume measurement is not made. Rather, the approach is to determine what percentage of a fabric's surface area is not occupied by fiber or, oppositely, to determine the percentage of fabric surface area occupied by yarn or fiber. The first determination is called percentage porosity, and the latter, percentage cover or percentage cover factor.

In Figure 4, percentage cover data are provided for nine woven fabrics (18). In all the fabrics, the yarns are spun yarns of the same size. What differs in each set of three fabrics is the type of fiber composing the fabric: cotton, modal (a type of rayon fiber), and modal Sun (a rayon fiber modified during fiber production by introducing a compound to reduce the transmittance of UV radiation through it). As one looks across from left to right on each row of fabrics, the black area increases and the white space lessens,

Table 1 Factors that Affect Photoprotectiveness of a Fabric

Fabric architecture	Determines the pathway and/or the length of the pathway for a UV ray to pass from the fabric face to the fabric back.
% cover factor: the percentage of fabric surface area occupied by yarn/fiber. Oppositely, % porosity is percentage of fabric surface area not occupied by yarn/fiber	Related to the closeness of the yarns in the fabric; called fabric count (formerly called yarn count). Fabrics with % cover < 94% will always have UPF values < 15, no matter what the fabric chemistry is or what the structural features of the fabric are. The interstices in the fabric, empty spaces between yarns, allow radiation that strikes the fabric perpendicularly in these areas of the fabric surface to pass directly through the fabric without ever striking a fiber.
Yarn openness/density of fibers with the yarn	Comparing two fabrics with identical cover factor and chemistries but differing in the spacing of fibers with the fabric's yarns; the fabric made with yarns having more space between fibers within the yarns would probably be less protective than a fabric made with yarns with less space between the fibers as there is less chance for a scattered UV ray to be stopped before reaching the other side of the fabric. There is no research that documents this, however. In other words, the arrangement of the fibers in the yarn changes the pathway of the ray through the yarn.
Yarn size/fabric thickness	The thicker the fabric, all other fabric structural features and chemistry being the same, the more likely that an incident UV ray will not emerge on the opposite side of the fabric.
Fabric chemistry	Determines which UV rays striking a fiber will be blocked from passing through the fabric. With the exception of fiber polymers, the higher the concentration of these compounds on fiber surfaces or within the fiber itself, the higher the UPF of the fabric.
Fiber polymers	Some fiber polymers strongly convert UV wavelengths to wavelengths outside the UV range.
Fiber additives	
Dyes	Some dyes strongly block UV wavelengths and thus help to increase the fabric photoprotection.
Pigments	Generally, the presence of pigments within fibers is known to enhance photoprotection.
OWAs	Overall, the addition of OWAs to fabric improves the measured UPF.
Compounds designed to enhance photoprotection	These UV cutting agents can be applied to fabrics during laundering or applied in the textile mill. As long as they stay bound to the fabrics, they provide an increase in photoprotection.

Abbreviations: UPF, UV protection factor; OWA, optical whitening agents.

corresponding to the increasing percentage cover from left to right. The technique used to determine the percentage cover was image analysis, which involves dividing the total number of black pixels by the total number of pixels to determine percentage cover.

Figure 5 shows the most important concept of all (18). According to this concept, until percentage cover is at least 94%, the UPF value for a fabric remains below UPF 15

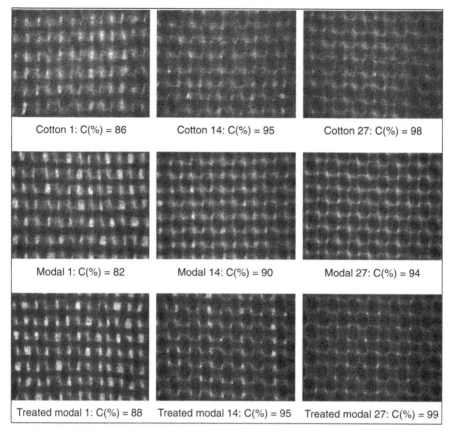

Figure 4 Effect of percentage cover [C(%)] for three sets of fabrics. Note that the black area increases and the white area lessens, corresponding to increasing percentage of cover from left to right. *Source*: From Ref. 18.

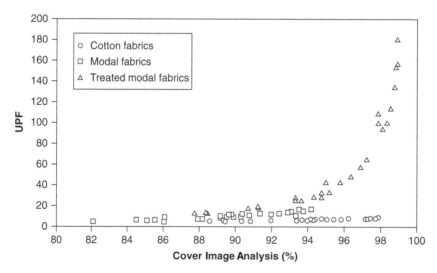

Figure 5 The combined effect of percentage cover and fibers to offer high photoprotection. *Source*: From Ref. 18.

(the accepted minimum value) even when the fibers in the fabric (modal Sun) have the capability of capturing a broad range of the UV radiation directed at the fabric. Another way to explain this concept is that UPF only increases when percentage cover is greater than 94% and the fibers in the fabric are highly photoprotective. Only the fabrics made from modal Sun fibers (i.e., fiber modified to inhibit transmittance of UV through it) have significantly increased UPF values as percentage cover increases above 94%.

Percentage cover of a fabric is not necessarily constant over the lifetime of the garment. When garments are laundered, the fabric from which they are made may shrink. Percentage cover would increase because in the shrinkage process the yarns move closer together. One hundred percent cotton and rayon fabrics, especially those which have not been finished to control shrinkage, are more likely to shrink than 100% nylon, 100% polyester, and polyester/cotton blend fabrics. Some 100% cotton fabrics, especially those with a knit construction may have high shrinkage percentages. When shrinkage results in a fabric that has a percentage cover of 94% or greater, then photoprotection of that fabric would be expected to increase, because shrinkage leads to an increase in percentage cover. Percentage cover may decrease when a fabric stretches, as is often the case with knit fabrics. The tighter a knit garment fits, the greater the potential for percentage cover to decrease (i.e., % porosity to increase).

Density of Fibers Within Yarns

How closely packed the fibers are in a yarn structure will influence degree of photoprotection provided by the fabric. UV rays that strike a fiber at the fabric surface, rather than "empty space" between fibers in the yarn, may be *backscattered* and then poses no harm to the skin under the fabric. Also, UV rays that do strike a fiber right at the fabric surface may be altered to wavelengths outside the UV region (e.g., visible light) or possibly to UV region wavelengths that are less damaging to the skin. Unfortunately, there have been no studies on UV transmission of fabrics of different yarn densities while maintaining all other aspects of a fabric's architecture to be identical.

Yarn Size/Fabric Thickness

Yarn size, the diameter of the yarn, and fabric thickness, the distance between fabric face and back, are thought to influence photoprotection. There are no data, however, that demonstrate their contribution. Theoretically, the greater the distance UV rays have to travel through the fabric, the greater the number of opportunities they will have to strike a fiber that has the capability to change their wavelengths to ones outside of the UV portion of the electromagnetic spectra. This would be most true in fabrics that are composed of two or more fibers such as cotton (which does not alter the wavelength of UV rays) and polyester (which does change the wavelength of incident UV to wavelengths outside the UV range).

DETERMINATION OF FABRIC PHOTOPROTECTION

Fabrics can provide photoprotection against several types of UV-induced changes: sunburn response, tanning reaction, precancerous skin lesion development, photoaging, and skin moisture retention. Each type requires different testing protocols, all of which have been recently described in detail by Hatch and Osterwalder (2). Because fabrics used in almost every research study are described in terms of UPF value, a brief description of this in vitro sunburn protection assessment is given here. A review of in vivo sunburn protection determination has been provided by Hatch and Osterwalder (2).

The first step in determining sunburn protection is to place a swatch of the fabric in a spectrophotometer equipped with an integrating sphere, which is essential for collecting UV rays passing directly through the fabric (through the fabric interstices) and those passing through the fibrous part of the fabric and emerging as scattered radiation. This instrument has the capability of directing UV rays toward a fabric placed in the instrument, so that its surface is perpendicular to the source of the UV rays; this instrument also has the capability of detecting scattered as well as directly transmitted UV radiation. The reason for mounting the swatch perpendicular to incident radiation is to make sure that UV transmission is maximal and the measured UV protection is the least. Therefore, the UV protection provided by clothing in actual wear situation when the incident UV rays are not at right angles is usually higher than that determined in the laboratory (19). The instrument then directs one wavelength at a time toward the fabric surface. If rays of that wavelength pass through the fabric (face to back), they will be detected by a photodetector under the fabric. The data collected are number of transmitted rays. The instrument then cycles to the next wavelength in the UV range (or it might be programmed to skip to every other wavelength or every 5th wavelength). The photodetector records how many rays pass through the fabric. Usually, the first swatch is removed, another swatch taken from an area some distance from where the first swatch was cut from the fabric is then mounted in the spectrophotometer, and the above process is repeated. Testing at least two swatches, often more, is done to obtain a better estimate of the photoprotection of the fabric. Once the data have been collected, percentage transmittance and/or fabric UPF value is calculated.

Percentage Transmittance/Blocking

Percentage transmittance is the ratio of the amount of radiation transmitted through the fabric to the amount of radiation directed perpendicular to the fabric surface. While total percentage transmittance can easily be calculated and reported, this is not usually done because the information that is more valuable is to calculate percentage of the UVB radiation transmitted and percentage of UVA radiation transmitted or conversely, percentage of UVB blocked and percentage UVA blocked. Results might be 10% UVB and 20% UVA transmitted, which would be 90% UVB and 80% UVA blocked. This information is useful to the extent that one knows how much UVB is being directly transmitted (through the fabric interstices) and how much is being reflected off fiber surfaces as it makes its way unchanged through the yarn structures.

While percentage transmittance/blocking information is useful, it does not communicate an important difference that may exist among a group of fabrics. To explain, consider just two fabrics, each blocking 90% of incident UV rays using transmittance testing. However, when human subjects wore swatches of these two fabrics on their arms and the same solar radiation (the same dose of radiation) was directed at the swatch surfaces, the skin was much redder under one swatch than the other. The explanation for this difference lies in the fact that each UV ray is not equal in its skin-burning potential.

UPF Value of Fabrics

A better indication of sunburn photoprotection is UPF. In this system, any individual wearing swatches of two fabrics—side by side—with the same UPF value will observe the same degree of skin reddening when the swatches are removed. This is because the transmittance data collected in the spectrophotometer are combined with erythemal action spectra data in the determination of UPF (16). Erythemal action spectra data are data collected using human subjects (in vivo data). These data give the relative differences among the UV rays to cause cutaneous erythema. Each wavelength has been assigned a weight on the basis of the length of time it takes to observe just perceptible redness to the skin of the subject being irradiated. Weights are assigned on the basis of length of time to just perceptible redness—the shorter the time, the higher the weight.

The equation below (3) is used to calculate the UPF value of a fabric.

$$UPF = \frac{\sum_{\lambda=290}^{400} E(\lambda) \cdot S(\lambda) \cdot \Delta\lambda}{\sum_{\lambda=290}^{400} E(\lambda) \cdot T(\lambda) \cdot S(\lambda) \cdot \Delta\lambda}$$

where:

$E(\lambda)$ = solar spectral irradiance (W m^{-2} nm^{-1})
$S(\lambda)$ = relative erythemal spectral effectiveness
$\Delta\lambda$ = measured wavelength interval (nm)
$T(\lambda)$ = average spectral transmittance of the specimen

By definition, UPF is the ratio of average effective UV irradiance transmitted through air to the average effective UV irradiance transmitted through fabric. For example, if percentage cover is approximately 94%, then approximately 6% of incident UV is transmitted; therefore, the UPF will be 100% (without the fabric) divided by 6% (with the fabric) or approximately UPF 15. The UPF value calculated therefore indicates how much longer a person can stay in the sun when fabric covers the skin as compared with the length of time without fabric covering to obtain the same erythemal response, with the endpoint being "just perceptible skin reddening." Therefore, similar to sun protection factor (SPF) of sunscreens, UPF is also heavily weighted to reflect protection against the biological effects of UVB, and less so of the UVA.

In Figure 6, the spectral transmissions of UV through five fabric swatches are shown. It should be noted that the lower the transmission in the UVB region, the higher is the UPF value of the tested fabric. Specific details on how to conduct transmittance testing and use the transmittance data to calculate a UPF value for the fabric tested can be found in standard documents that were developed by committees within national, regional, or international standard setting organizations (8,9,11,12,14). Fabrics with UPF values above 40 are classified as protective in Europe (14) In locations with high intensity solar radiation, UPF values of 50+ may be required for clothing to protect sufficiently against solar UV (20).

FABRIC CHEMISTRY

Fabric chemistry that is important in this discussion is the presence of chemicals that have the capability of interacting with UV rays. Another way to say this, actually the most common way to say this, is "the presence of chemicals that *absorb* UV rays." In this paper, the term "absorb" is not used because it can be and unfortunately is inferred to mean that UV radiation is being absorbed like water into a sponge and held at the skin surface. Of course, this is not the correct picture and is a picture that that places harmful "substances" near the skin. Various mechanisms are at work within a fabric; two such mechanisms are (*i*) conversion of incident UV wavelengths to heat wavelengths and (*ii*)

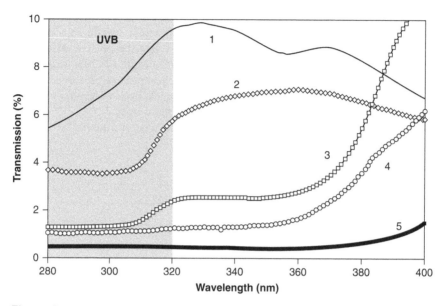

Figure 6 Spectral transmittances of five fabrics of differing UPF. Fabric 1 (mean UPF 12, no rating), fabric 2 (mean UPF 24, UPF rating 20), fabric 3 (mean UPF 60, UPF rating 50+), fabric 4 (mean UPF 86, UPF rating 50+), and fabric 5 (mean UPF 240, UPF rating 50+).

conversion from a UV wavelength with high sunburn potential to a UV wavelength of lesser sunburn potential, but these mechanisms are not discussed here.

The fabric chemistries that are of primary interest are

1. polymers that compose fibers,
2. chemicals added to fiber during manufacture (called fiber additives),
3. dyes and pigments used to color the fabric,
4. optical whitening compounds, and
5. compounds designed to capture or alter UV rays.

Fiber Polymers

How fibers rank relative to each other in regard to photoprotection has been reported by Crews and colleagues (21). They found that fibers could be classified in three distinct groups given here in decreasing order of photoprotectiveness:

Group 1: polyester (best photoprotection)
Group 2: wool, silk, and nylon
Group 3: cotton and rayon (cellulosic fibers) (least photoprotection)

It is not surprising to find polyester fiber at the top of the list as polyester fiber is made from polymers containing benzene rings, structures known to convert UV wavelengths to wavelengths outside the UV range.

The grouping shown above is based on fibers without any compounds added that would alter photoprotection. These results should not be confused with or compared to results of those studies in which *fabric of various fiber contents* were judged best for photoprotection and ranked. In these cases, wool fabrics were judged best for photoprotection, a ranking they achieved easily as wool fabrics tend to be thicker than fabrics made from other fibers.

Dyes

Dyes are organic chemicals that are able to selectively capture certain wavelengths of light and reflect certain wavelengths of light within the visible range of the electromagnetic spectrum. Dye molecules may also capture wavelengths in the UV range and those that do would be expected to contribute to the photoprotection of the individual wearing the fabric to which they are applied. Also, dyes with the strongest ability to capture wavelengths in the UVB region would be expected to produce fabrics with greater photoprotection. As fabric is dyed to a deeper shade using the same dye, photoprotection provided to the wearer of the fabric should increase because of greater dye concentration in the darker fabric.

Srinivasan and Gatewood (22) studied the effect of dyeing a bleached cotton fabric with dyes of various colors (hues) known to interact differently with UV radiation (Table 2). Fourteen direct dyes, most often used to color cotton fabrics, were chosen. The dyes selected differed in chemical classification (monoazo, disazo, triazo, polyazo, stilbene, and phthalocyanine). Dyes were applied to 5-g fabric swatches at theoretical concentrations of 0.5% and 1.0% on weight of fiber (owf); 1% owf represents a medium depth of shade typical of summertime fabrics.

Direct dyes were chosen because dyes from this class are most often used to color cotton fabrics. The 14 dyes selected differed in chemical classification (monoazo, disazo, triazo, polyazo, stilbene, and phthalocyanine). The hues were yellow (4 dyes), red (3 dyes), violet (1 dye), blue (3 dyes), green (1 dye), brown (1 dye), and black (1 dye). After prescouring the print cloth, dyes were applied to 5-g fabric swatches at theoretical concentrations of 0.5% and 1.0% on owf. A control sample was prepared by subjecting the bleached print cloth to a blank dyeing process with all ingredients except the dye to eliminate the effect of fabric shrinkage on percentage transmittance and therefore on calculated UPF. Specimens of dyed fabric were submitted for UV transmittance assessment using American Association of Textile Chemist and Colorist (AATCC) test

Table 2 UPF of Fabrics That Contain the Same Concentration of Various Direct Dyes

Direct dye used to dye fabric	Fabric UPF after 0.5% owf dyeing process	Fabric UPF after 1.0% owf dyeing process	Adjusted 1.0% dyed fabric UPF
None			4.1
Yellow 12	13.1	18.6	17.8
Yellow 28	19.9	29.3	21.6
Yellow 44	18.4	28.6	25.3
Yellow 106	19.3	27.6	25.0
Red 24	27.6	37.1	31.3
Red 28	38.7	50.7	41.3
Red 80	17.3	24.7	20.3
Violet 9	20.9	28.8	23.5
Blue 1	21.5	30.2	25.5
Blue 86	16.2	18.6	24.0
Blue 218	13.1	19.0	16.6
Green 26	22.3	29.2	26.2
Brown 154	22.8	30.6	24.7
Black 38	29.8	40.2	33.7

Abbreviations: UPF, UV protection factor; owf, weight of fiber.
Source: From Ref. 22.

method 183-2000 (11). The mean UV, UVA, UVB percentage transmittance values were calculated from each scan and averaged for 16 scans (4 specimens × 2 scans × 2 replications). UPF values were then calculated.

Analysis of variance was conducted on the UPF data to determine if application of dye changed UPF values of the cotton print cloth and whether greater owf application led to higher UPF. The dyed fabric UPF values are shown in columns 2 and 3 of Table 2.

These data show that increasing the concentration of the dye in the fabric leads to increased UPF. For each dye, the fabric UPF value is higher after the 1.0% owf application of dye than after the 0.5% owf application; namely, the darker fabric of each pair would afford greater sunburn protection.

To determine the specific-dye effect on UPF of the fabric, the concentration of dye in each fabric needed to be the same. This was not the case because the dyes had different exhaust rates. To determine the percentage exhaustion from the dye bath, the absorptiometric measurements of the residual dye bath solution were compared with calibration curves prepared from dye solutions at known concentrations based on the weight of the commercial dye.

Having the dye exhaust rate data made it possible for the researchers to use an analysis of covariance, treating concentration as a covariable. Fisher's least significant difference test was then used to determine which of the dyed fabrics differed in their UPF values. The adjusted UPF values are as shown in column 4 of Table 2.

The adjusted results show that fabric color (hue) is not a reliable indicator of UV protection provided by dyed fabrics because dyes of the same hue produced fabrics with varying UPF at identical concentration level. This study also showed that black fabric does not necessarily provide the best sunburn protection, as one of the red dyes (Red 28) produced a fabric having a higher UPF value than the black fabric. Here it is critical to remember that color seen is due to one's brain interpreting the *visible* rays that reach one's eyes. Color is not the result of "seeing" invisible UV radiation. No conclusions were drawn about the relationship between dye chemical constitution (class) and UV protection because of the limited number of dyes in each of the chemical classes.

Srinivasan and Gatewood (22) also devised an equation similar to that used in calculating the UPF of fabrics for evaluating dyes in solution on the basis of their transmittance values. This equation calculates the effective UV transmittance, which is the relative effectiveness of dyes in improving the UV protection of a fabric, on the basis of the transmittance of dyes in solution weighted for solar spectral irradiance and relative erythemal spectral effectiveness. Because this method takes into consideration the effectiveness of both UVA and UVB transmittances and because the concentrations of the dyes in the solutions can be more easily controlled than in fabric, it led the researchers to conclude that determining the effective UV transmittance of dyes in solution would probably be an excellent procedure to screen dyes before going through the expense of applying them to fabrics to investigate UPF effectiveness.

Pigments

Pigments in textiles are inorganic microscopic-sized particles, some of which are colored. In textiles, pigments

1. are naturally present in conventional cotton fibers, making the fibers brownish;
2. are present in naturally pigmented (colored) cotton fibers, making the fibers green, pink, brown, or tan;
3. may be incorporated into manufactured fibers to reduce luster and/or color them;

4. are used to dye fabrics of any fiber composition to yield solid-colored fabrics;
5. are used in printing fabric to yield either a solid-colored or patterned fabric;
6. are purposefully added to manufactured fibers to enhance the photoprotection of the fabric; and
7. are applied to cotton fabric in finishing to form a layer of photoprotective chemical over the cotton fiber surface.

The presence of pigments *within* fibers is known to enhance the photoprotection of fabrics containing them. Pailthorpe (23), observing that unbleached conventional cotton fabrics had a higher UPF than bleached cotton fabrics, speculated that the presence of pigments in the unbleached cotton fabric was the reason. Crews and colleagues (21) showed this was true when they found that the UV transmission of bleached conventional cotton (white because the pigment was removed from the cotton fiber) was nearly twice that of unbleached conventional cotton containing pigment. Further, Hustvedt and Crews (24) showed that naturally pigmented (also called naturally colored) cotton fabrics had UPF values far superior to conventional, bleached, or unbleached cotton. The values reported for naturally pigmented cotton fabrics were: green, UPF 30 to 50+; tan, UPF 20 to 45; and for unbleached conventional cotton fabric, UPF 8. Additionally, the UPF values of the naturally pigmented cottons, even after 80 AATCC fading units of xenon lamp light exposure, merited sun protection ratings of "good" (UPF 15 to 24) to "very good" (UPF 25 to 39) according to ASTM 6603 voluntary labeling guidelines for UV-protective textiles (9).

Wedler and Hirthe (25) showed that when ultrafine TiO_2 particles are added to the polymer solution of manufactured fibers in low concentration and those fibers are made into very thin, lightweight fabrics, then high photoprotection to human skin can be achieved. Manufactured fibers to which these particles are added include rayon (modal), polyester, and nylon.

Three recent research studies explore ways to improve the photoprotection of cotton fabrics (26–28). Briefly, Xin and colleagues (26) developed a method to apply a thin layer of titania film to the surface of cotton fibers and showed that the UPF rating of the treated fabrics were 50+. Further, they showed that films adhered fast to the fabric even after 55 launderings, as the UPF remained to be 50+. Xu and colleagues (27) were able to form an inorganic network consisting of Ti-O-repeating units, $(Ti-O)_n$ Because UVA was not effectively blocked by the treatment, they also used an optical whitener (see below). This treatment increased the UPF of the cotton fabric from 6.5 to 79. Zheng-Rong and colleagues (28) applied ZnO nanosol as a finishing agent during pigment dyeing of cotton fabric, which included the usual adhesive to adhere the pigment to the cotton surface. UPF of the cotton fabric reached 50+, the fastness of the treatment to washing was excellent, and the comfort of wearing the treated fabric was the same as wearing the cotton fabric without the treatment.

Optical Whitening Agents

Optical whitening agents (OWAs), also known as florescent whitening agents and brighteners, are included in almost every heavy duty detergent product sold in the United States and Europe because they whiten and brighten fabrics. These compounds are also commonly applied to cotton and cotton blend fabrics during mill finishing for the same reason.

OWAs convert a portion of the incident UV to a visible blue wavelength and reflect this as visible blue light. Therefore, a person will perceive a fabric with OWA to be whiter and brighter than an identical fabric that does not contain OWA.

Although most OWA compounds have weak absorbance at the UVB spectrum, studies have been done to evaluate what improvement in fabric UPF could be achieved with the addition of these compounds to cotton fabric in the textile finishing mill (29), or during laundering of fabrics which were and were not mill finished with OWA (30). Overall, the addition of OWAs to fabric did improve the UPFs. In the laundering studies, UPF value tended to increase with each laundering of the fabric, partly because of the deposition of OWA onto the fabric and partly because of fabric shrinkage. However, the UPF increase, even after multiple launderings, usually did not reach 30. Readers interested in more detailed summaries are referred to review articles by Hatch (7), Hatch and Osterwalder (2), and CIE (3).

Compounds Designed to Enhance Photoprotection

Compounds designed (developed) specifically to enhance photoprotection provided to the skin by fabrics are called UV-cutting agents (UVCAs) or UV-absorbing agents in the literature. These compounds have chromophore systems that absorb UV radiation very effectively while in situ on textiles. Of importance is that these compounds stay on the fabric through multiple washings (i.e., are substantive to the fabric), and their photoprotective property does not decrease with fabric wetting (5). UVCAs also contribute to fabric whiteness and brightness. It should be noted that UVCAs should not be confused with compounds whose purpose is to slow the solar degradation of fibers.

UVCAs Applied to Fabric in the Finishing Mill

When UVCAs are applied in the textile mill to cellulosic fabrics, cellulosic-blended fabrics, 100% polyester fabrics, or 100% nylon fabrics, the finished fabrics are usually made into garments for which a claim of UV protection will be made. However, the presence of these chemicals on mill-finished fabrics is often not revealed in labeling. Details of the research undertaken to establish the increases in UPF of fabrics to which these compounds were applied are provided in various studies (31–35). For summaries of these studies please refer to review articles by Hatch and Osterwalder (2), CIE (3), and Hatch (6).

UVCAs Applied to Fabric During Laundering

A few laundry product manufacturers add the specially designed photoprotection compounds to detergents and fabric softeners, or use these compounds to make a dedicated laundry product whose sole intent is to enhance the UPF values of cotton and cotton blend fabrics laundered with it. At the present time, laundry detergents and fabric softeners containing UVCAs are only available for purchase in Europe, Asia, and Australia. Rinse cycle fabric softeners (conditioners) containing UVCAs are currently only available in Switzerland and Japan. A laundry additive, Rit SunGuard, manufactured by Phoenix Brands (Indianapolis, Indiana) and distributed primarily to grocery stores, is only available in the United States. It has been shown that these products led to significant improvement in UPF values of cotton fabrics, which initially have little sunburn protection capability (36–41). Summaries of these studies are available in recent reviews (2,3,7).

Of particular interest are two studies conducted by researchers outside the product development arena to determine differences in the amount of UPF enhancement that would result by home-laundering fabrics with different laundry products (42,43). Wang and colleagues (42) laundered a jersey fabric (initial UPF 4.7) and a print cloth fabric (initial UPF 3.1). They found that after five cycles of laundering in water only, the UPF of their jersey fabric increased to 7.1 and UPF of their print cloth increased to 4.2, which they attributed to fabric shrinkage. After five cycles of washing in AATCC detergent with OWA, the UPF value was 6.0 for jersey and 4.4 for print cloth. After washing the swatches once with detergent containing UVCA, the UPF for jersey was 11 and 7 for print cloth. By the fifth wash cycle, the jersey fabric had a UPF value of 23, and the print cloth had a value of about 12.

Using different products, Kim and colleagues (43) laundered two white knit fabrics: a 100% cotton jersey (initial UPF of 14.2) and a 60% cotton-40% polyester pique (initial UPF of 23.4). After one laundering cycle with the Rit SunGuard product, UPF values were 81.4 ± 23.0 (jersey) and 39.6 ± 8.3 (pique). With Rit Whitener and Brightener product, values were 30.5 ± 6.1 (jersey) and 36.6 ± 6.1 (pique). UPF values above 30 were obtained by the conclusion of the fifth laundering with Tide (Proctor and Gamble, Cincinnati, Ohio) and with Wisk® (Unilever, Englewood Cliffs, New Jersey). The authors concluded that adding only the Rit SunGuard product to laundry water resulted in the most rapid achievement of a UPF of 30+.

Sprays

Several UVCA-containing products are available in spray cans: Puraderm (http://www.puraderm.com/products_sunsafe.htm), UV Block by Atsko (http://www.atsko.com/products.html#uvprotection), and Grainger's (http://www.grangersusa.com/products/spray-on-uv-waterproofing.html). No research information was found on improvement of UPF of fabric to which they were applied.

PURCHASING CLOTHING FOR PHOTOPROTECTION

Clothing has always been understood to be a means to shade the skin from the sun. There are currently two major classifications of photoprotective garments: (*i*) garments sold with a specific claim for sunburn protection and (*ii*) cover-up garments. UV-protective garments are excellent and necessary choices for individuals who are prone to sunburn and for those with photosensitivity diseases. Fabrics used in these garments have the required percentage cover of 94%. Most garments are made from 100% cotton fabric, a blend of cotton and polyester fiber, 100% nylon fabric, or 100% polyester fabric. The 100% cotton fabric garments are usually treated with a specially designed UV compound; however, it is usually not possible to know how the nylon or polyester fabrics have been treated. Garments made with nylon and polyester fiber will most likely be designed to allow water vapor from the skin to pass through the garment. Mesh fabric is commonly used as part of the garment in the underarm area, in pleats across the back of a shirt, or on the leg of pants because water vapor otherwise has difficulty passing though these fabrics with high percentage cover. One hundred percent cotton photoprotective garments do not need, and usually do not have, these design elements; water vapor can easily pass through, as there is space between the fibers in the yarns. Water vapor can also pass directly through fabrics made of rayon fibers. Sporting goods shops are an excellent place to find these UV-protective garments. For a listing of companies based in the United States, which offer these garments for sale, log into http://cals.arizona.edu/research/uv-protective-clothing.

For various reasons, people wanting to protect their skin may not choose to purchase UV-protective clothing because of the cost and not finding a preferred garment style or a fabric they wish to have next to their skin. For this group of people, the task becomes one of making the "wisest" choices of cover-up garments among those in the retail marketplace or hanging in their closets. Let's say the person prefers cotton garments. Wise choices would be garments made with naturally pigmented cotton fiber/ fabric and garments that have been pigment dyed. Labeling on the garment, in catalog descriptions, or at point of sale in a retail store will usually reveal these garment fabric "features" because the garment manufacturer wants the consumer to know what is distinctive about this product choice. Other 100% cotton garments, even those made from white (bleached) cotton fabric, can be good choices provided they have been or will be immediately laundered using laundry products containing dedicated photoprotection chemicals. Garments made from 100% cotton fabric that have been repeatedly laundered would also offer good photoprotection because of the buildup of OWA and fabric shrinkage. Threadbare garments would not be good choices.

An erroneous piece of advice in selecting photoprotective fabric is to hold fabrics up to a visible light source, view the fabric surface, and decide through which fabric one sees the most distinctive pinpoints of light; that fabric is then judged as the least photoprotective. This popular advice is scientifically incorrect for the following reason. The most distinctive points of light will occur when the black fabrics are held up to the light because black means that the visible light striking the fibers is all captured, hence none goes through the fabric (Fig. 7A). There are no scattered visible rays emerging from the side of the fabric being viewed by the human eye, hence the fabric might be judged as not photoprotective. On the other hand, shining visible light to a fabric made with fibers that allow *visible* radiation to pass through will not only result in visible rays passing through the fabric interstices (pores, holes), but through the fibrous area as well (Fig. 7B). With white fabric, all the incident *visible* radiation passes through, some as direct radiation and some as scattered radiation. The scattering "softens" or "blurs" the directly transmitted *visual* rays, resulting in less-distinctive pinpoints of light. The white fabric might be then judged to be photoprotective. However, one has to remember that it is the capturing of the *invisible UV rays,* rather than the *visible light,* that determines the UPF of the fabric. So, if the black and white fabrics capture the same invisible UV rays, the UPF of the fabrics will be the same regardless of the amount of visible light passing through

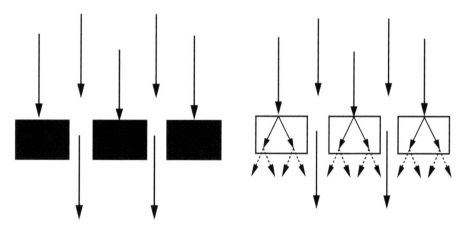

(A) Incident light makes interstices distinctive

(B) Incident rays scattered, so interstices not distinctive

Figure 7 Transmittance of *visible* radiation though a black fabric and a white fabric with identical percentage cover. *Source*: Adapted from Ref. 5.

them. If the white fabric captures more of the incident UV rays than the black fabric, particularly the most erythemogenic UVB rays, then the white fabric will be more photoprotective than the black fabric.

SUMMARY

Photoprotection by fabrics is highly dependent on the construction of the fabric. Fabric may appear to form a continuous covering on the skin surface, but a close look at a fabric reveals that the fiber, its fundamental unit, is not present everywhere. This feature of fabrics makes them different from sunscreens, a product in which the UV compounds are uniformly distributed over the skin surface to form a continuous photoprotection barrier.

Fabrics must have a percentage cover of 94% before the minimum acceptable amount of sunburn photoprotection (UPF 15) can be achieved. This level of protection is only possible when the fabric's fibers have some capability of preventing incident UV rays from passing though the fibrous matrix. Once fiber covers the skin in an almost continuous "film," then it is the chemistry of the fibers (meaning the polymers from which they are composed) and all the other chemicals present on the surface of the fibers or within the fiber (between the polymers), such as colorants and pigments, OWAs, and compounds designed to stop UV rays that determine how photoprotective the fabric will be to the skin underneath it.

The fabrics that are popular in the summer are those made from 100% cotton and rayon fibers, or fabrics made with a blend of these fibers with polyester fiber. Unfortunately, cotton and rayon fibers, composed of cellulosic polymers, have little ability to prevent UV radiation from passing though them. Therefore, for these fabrics, the presence of UV-absorbing or UV-reflecting chemicals within and on the surface of the fibers is critical. In many ways, wearing of garments that cover the arms and legs and torso has advantages over the use of sunscreens. These include the fact that garments do not have to be reapplied during the day, they last for months to years, UVA as well as UVB protection is provided by the chemistry of most fabrics, garments do not have to be put on 30 minutes before going outside as the protection is immediate, and there are no known skin reactions to any of the compounds used to enhance the photoprotection of fabrics. The downside of photoprotection by fabrics is that the wearer may not know the level of protection afforded unless he or she has purchased clothing bearing a label stating the photoprotection provided by the garment fabric. It is inadvisable for consumers to make judgments, even comparative ones, about the percentage cover of fabrics in garments, because there is no simple and reliable way to do so outside of testing laboratories.

REFERENCES

1. Textiles and Sun Protection Mini-Conference Proceedings. The Society of Dyers and Colourists of Australia and New Zealand (New South Wales section), May 20, 1993.
2. Hatch KL, Osterwalder U. Garments as solar ultraviolet radiation screening materials. Dermatol Clin 2006; 24(1):85–100.
3. CIE (International Commission on Illumination) Technical Report. UV Protection and Clothing, CIE 172:2006, CIE Central Bureau, Vienna, Austria, 2006.
4. Gies P. Photoprotection by clothing. Photodermatol Photoimmunol Photomed 2007; 23(6):264–274.
5. Osterwalder U, Schlenker W, Rohwer H, et al. Facts and fiction on ultraviolet protection by clothing. Radiat Prot Dosimetry 2000; 91(1):255–259.

6. Menter JM, Hatch KL. Clothing as solar radiation protection. Curr Probl Dermatol 2003; 31:50–63.

7. Hatch KL. Fabrics as UV radiation filters. In: Shaath NA, ed. Sunscreens: Regulations and Commercial Development. 3rd ed. New York: Karger Publishing, 2004:557–572.

8. Standards Association of Australia, Standard AS/NZS 4399: Sun protective clothing: evaluation and classification. Australian/New Zealand Standards. Homebush, Australia, 1996. Available at: www.standards.com.au.

9. American Society for Testing and Materials (ASTM International). Standard D 6603 – 00, Standard guide for labeling of UV-protective textiles. In: ASTM Standards, Vol. 7:03, 2004. Available at: www.astm.org.

10. American Society for Testing and Materials. ASTM D6544 – 00: Standard practice for preparation of textiles prior to ultraviolet (UV) transmission testing. In: ASTM Standards, Vol. 7:03, 2004. Available at: www.astm.org.

11. American Association of Textile Chemists and Colorists. Test method 183: Transmittance or blocking of erythemally weighted ultraviolet radiation through fabrics. In: AATCC Technical Manual, AATCC, Research Triangle Park NC, 2000.

12. British Standards Institute. Standard 7914-1998: Method of test for penetration of erythemally weighted solar ultraviolet radiation through clothing fabrics. Available at: www.bsi.org.uk.

13. British Standards Institute. Standard 7949-1999: Children's clothing, requirements for protection against erythemally weighted solar ultraviolet radiation. Available at: www.bsi.org.uk.

14. European Committee for Standardization. Standard EN 13758-1: textiles – solar UV-protective properties – part 1: method of test for apparel fabrics. Available at: www.cenorm.be/.

15. European Committee for Standardization. Standard EN 13758-2: textiles – solar UV-protective properties – part 2: classification and marking of apparel. Available at: www.cenorm.be/.

16. McKinley AF, Diffey BL. A reference spectrum for ultraviolet induced erythema in human skin. CIE J 1987; 6:17–22.

17. Hatch KL. Textile Science. Apex NC: Millennium Print Group, 2006.

18. Algaba, I, Riva A, Crews PC. Influence of fiber type and fabric porosity on the UPF of summer fabrics. AATCC Rev 2004; 4(2):26–31.

19. Ravishanker J, Diffey BL. Laboratory testing of UV transmission through fabrics may underestimate protection. Photodermatol Photoimmunol Photomed 1997; 13:202–203.

20. Gies P, Roy C, Javorniczky J, et al. Global solar UV index: Australian measurements, forecasts and comparison with the UK. Photochem Photobiol 2004; 79(1):32–39.

21. Crews PC, Kachman S, Beyer AG. Influences on UVR transmission of undyed woven fabrics. Text Chem Colorist 1999; 31(6):17–26.

22. Srinivasan M, Gatewood BM. Relationship of dye characteristics to UV protection provided by cotton fabric. Text Chem Colorist Am Dyestuff Reporter 2000; 32(4):36–43.

23. Pailthorpe MT. Textile parameters and sun protection factors. In: Proceedings of the Textile and Sun Protection Mini-conference, University of New South Wales; 1993 May 20; Society of Dyers and Colourists of Australia and New Zealand (New South Wales Section), Kensington, NSW; p 32–53.

24. Hustvedt, G, Crews PC. The ultraviolet protection factor of naturally-pigmented cotton. J Cotton Sci 2005; 9(1):47–55.

25. Wedler M, Hirthe B. UV-absorbing micro additives for synthetic fibers. Chem Fibers Intl 1999; 49:72.

26. Xin JH, Daoud WA, Kong YY. A new approach to UV-blocking treatment for cotton fabrics. Textile Res J 2004; 72(2):97–100.

27. Xu P, Wang W, Chen S-L. UV blocking treatment of cotton fabrics by titanium hydrosol, AATCC Rev 2005; 5(6):28–31.

28. Li Zheng-Rong, Xu H-Y, Fu K-J, et al. ZnO nanosol for enhancing the UV-protective property of cotton fabric and pigment dyeing in a single bath. AATCC Rev 2007; 7(6):38–41.

29. Reinehr D, Eckhardt C, Kaufmann W. Skin protection against ultraviolet light by cotton textiles treated with optical brighteners. In: the Fourth World Surfactants Congress, Asociacion Espanola de Productores de Sustancias para Aplicaciones Tensioactivas; Barcelona Spain 1996; 264–276.

30. Zhou Y, Crews PC. Effect of OBAs and repeated launderings on UVR transmission through fabrics. Text Chem Colorist 1998; 30(11):19–24.

31. Hilfiker R, Kaufmann W, Reinert G, et al. Improving sun protection factors of fabrics by applying UV-absorbers. Text Res J 1996; 66(2):61–70.

32. Reinert G, Fuso F, Hilfiker R, et al. UV-protecting properties of textile fabrics and their improvement. Text Chem Colorist 1997; 29(12):36–43.

33. Jöllenbeck M. New UV absorbers for sun protective fabrics. In: Altmeyer P, Hoffmann K, Stücker M, eds. Skin cancer and UV Radiation. Berlin Heidelberg: Springer, 1997:382–387.

34. Jöllenbeck M, Härri H-P, Schlenker W, et al. UV protective fabrics. In: UV-protective Fabrics. In: Proceedings of AATCC Functional Finishes and High Performance Textiles Symposium; 2000 Jan 27–28.

35. Eckhardt C, Rohwer H. UV protector for cotton fabrics. Text Chem Colorist Am Dyestuff Reporter 2000; 32(4):21–23.

36. Eckhardt C, Osterwalder U. Laundering clothes to be sun protective. In: Cahn A, ed. Proceedings 4th World Conference of Detergents: Strategies for the 21st Century. Montreux: 1998; p. 317–322.

37. Rohwer H, Eckhardt C. Laundry additive for the sun protection of the skin. SÖFW J 1998; 11:1241–1244.

38. Rohwer H, Osterwalder U, Dubini M. Enhanced textile sun protection within a few washes. 39th International Detergency Conference, Luxembourg, Sept 1999.

39. Rohwer H, Kvita P. Sun protection of the skin with a novel UV absorber for rinse cycle application. SÖFW J 1999; 125:1–5.

40. Spillmann N. Sun protection via laundry products – Innovative science and creative effects to complete the circle of sun protection. Proceedings of the 5th World Conference on Detergents, Montreux 2002:42.

41. Schaumann M, Rohwer H. UV absorbers for fabrics. Happi 2003; 36(2):59–61.

42. Wang SQ, Kopf AW, Marx, J, et al. Reduction of ultraviolet transmission through cotton t-shirt fabrics with low ultraviolet protection by various laundering methods and dyeing: clinical implications. J Am Acad Dermatol 2001; 44(5):767–774.

43. Kim J, Stone J, Crews P, et al. Improving knit fabric UPF using consumer laundry products: a comparison of results using two instruments. Fam Consumer Sci Res J 2004; 33(2):141–158.

18
Photoprotection by Glass

Chanisada Tuchinda
Department of Dermatology, Faculty of Medicine Siriraj Hospital, Bangkok, Thailand

Henry W. Lim
Department of Dermatology, Henry Ford Hospital, Detroit, Michigan, U.S.A.

SYNOPSIS

- Presently, most of the glass manufactured is float glass.
- Advances in glass manufacturing technology have resulted in the availability of a wide variety of glass—from clear glass that allows most visible light to go through to glass that can reflect heat, insulate, and filter a large portion of UV rays.
- Windshield of automobile is made from laminated glass, which has excellent UV-filtering property. Side and rear windows are made of tempered glass, which is less effective at filtering UV, hence accounting for eruption occurring on side-window-exposed body sites in patients with photosensitivity.
- Aftermarket window films decrease transmission of UV, visible light, and infrared radiation. In the United States, federal and state regulations specify the minimal amount of visible light transmittance through these films (for windshield, 70% minimum; for side and rear windows, 20% to 35% minimum).

INTRODUCTION

The hazardous effect of ultraviolet radiation (UVR) is now well recognized; public education is ongoing. People are recommended to seek shade during the peak UVB period (10 a.m.–4 p.m.), seek shade when outdoor, regularly use sunscreen, wear protective clothing, and use hat and sunglasses (1–6). However, people may not be aware that overexposure to the sun can occur even if they are indoors.

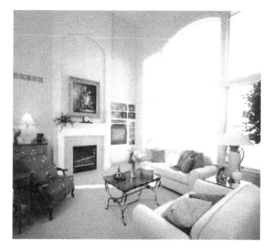

Figure 1 A common residential window configuration is likely to have substantial UV exposure. *Source*: From Ref. 9, with permission from Elsevier.

Eighty percent of the average day of Americans is spent indoors (7). Although not as high as the outdoor workers, a study in 2000 demonstrated that homeworkers still receive high ultraviolet (UV) exposure between 7 and 10 standard erythema dose (SED) per day in spring and 2 or more SED in winter and on cloudy summer days (1 SED is equivalent to an erythemal effective radiant exposure of 100 J/m^2) (8).

Compared with all exterior building components, windows provide the least amount of insulation. It is known that standard glass filters out ultraviolet B (UVB), but ultraviolet A (UVA), visible light, and infrared radiation are still transmitted. Current residential and commercial architectural designs incorporate more and larger window areas for a better view (Fig. 1). This design trend is supported by the evolution of energy-efficient glazing; however, with larger windows, more UV rays are transmitted into the buildings. There are new developments in the glass industry, resulting in additional efficient filters for UVA and infrared radiation that can now be incorporated to the glass. Most of these glasses are indistinguishable to the human eyes but provide different degrees of UV and infrared protection. This chapter will review an update on the role of photoprotection by glass.

WINDOW GLASS AND PHOTOPROTECTION

History of Glass

The origin of glass began almost 5000 years ago. Archaeologists have discovered evidence of glass objects as early as 3000 B.C. (10). There were records that demonstrated that the ancient Greeks used glass in their buildings for baths and rooms. Window glass is believed to originate in Rome at the end of the third century; it was very thick and translucent, so it could let the light in, but people could not see out. In 1921, on the Italian island, Murano, workers developed clear, almost transparent glass called "cristallo"; this is where the word "crystal" comes from (10).

In the Middle Ages, glass making was a hand-made process. Window glass was made by blowing the molten glass into a flat disc, which was then spun to thin and flatten it out. Over hundreds of years, technical methods have been developed to make clear glass in large quantity, resulting in glass manufacturing as we know it today (10).

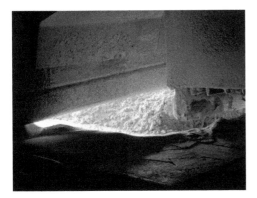

Figure 2 "Batch" is a mixture of very high-quality silica sand and other materials such as salt cake, limestone, dolomite, feldspar, soda ash, and powdered cullet. Glass is made by melting and cooling the batch. *Source*: From Ref. 9, with permission from Elsevier.

What is Glass?

Glass is a mixture of sand: very high-quality silica sand added with other materials such as salt cake, limestone, dolomite, feldspar, soda ash, and cullet. Cullet is broken glass, adding cullet helps the batch melt more easily (10). The resulting mixture is called a batch (Fig. 2). Melting and later cooling of the batch makes a solid glass without forming crystals, thereby making glass transparent. In the past, most of the glass manufactured in the United States was plate glass, which was made by a process of grinding and polishing. Now, plate glass has been almost totally replaced by float glass (10).

Presently, 90% of flat glass is manufactured as float glass. The term "float" glass, derived from the production method, was introduced in the United Kingdom by Sir Alastair Pilkington in 1959 (11). Float glass refers to glass made by melting the batch in a furnace at 1500°C; then the molten batch is poured from a furnace into a controlled chamber that contains a bed of molten tin. The glass floats on the tin and takes the shape of the container (10). After leaving the chamber, the molten glass is put in an oven. Here it is slowly cooled. This process, called "annealing," produces a long ribbon of high-quality flat glass that will be later cut into smaller pieces for fabrication.

Types of Glass

Common types of architectural glass used in residential and commercial buildings are summarized in Table 1, and discussed in the following paragraphs.

Clear Glass

Clear glass is generally described as transparent and colorless (10). Majority of the glasses are produced by the float glass process. The primary characteristic of glass in architectural applications is to provide protection from the outside elements, while providing a view and enabling visible light transmittance to the interior. Depending upon its thickness, a single pane of clear glass allows up to 90% of the visible light (assessed from 400 to 780 nm), up to 72% of UV (assessed from 300 to 380 nm), and up to 83% of solar heat to pass through (9).

Table 1 **Common Types of Glass Used in Residential and Commercial Buildings**

Clear glass
Tinted glass
Reflective glass
Low-E glass
Tempered glass
Laminated glass
Insulating glass
UV-blocking coated glass

Abbreviation: Low-E, low-emissivity.
Source: Modified from Ref. 9, with permission from Elsevier.

Tinted Glass

Tint glass is made by adding coloring agents to the batch mix. These coloring agents include bronze, green, blue, and gray. The tint is typically specified for its aesthetic and solar-radiation absorption properties (12). Tinted glass also transmits less UV compared with clear glass.

Reflective Glass

This type of glass is designed to reflect light and heat, commonly used in commercial buildings. Reflective glass is a clear or tinted glass that has very thin layer of metal or metal oxide on the surface. The use of these coatings gives the glass a mirrorlike appearance (10). Commonly used coatings include silver, copper, gold, and earth tone. Reflective glass minimizes unwanted solar heat gain and reduces UV transmission. It eliminates the ability to see the interior of a building from the outside; observers will only see their own reflection during daylight. At night, however, because of the higher light intensity inside than the outside, the mirroring effect is reversed. An outside observer may see in, but an interior observer may only see his or her own image (9).

Low-Emissivity Glass

Low-emissivity (Low-E) glass is the type of glass that is gaining in popularity and is broadly used in residential and commercial building. It is a clear glass that comprised microscopically thin, optically transparent layers of silver sandwiched between layers of antireflective metal oxide coatings. Most low-E coated glass will significantly reduce the loss of generated heat. The most common low-E products also minimize undesirable solar heat gain through a window without the loss of color neutrality and visible light transmission (13). These coatings reflect from 40% to 70% of the solar heat that is normally transmitted through clear glass, while allowing the full amount of visible light to pass through. If the windows are designed to let in the heat from winter sun while retaining the heat generated from inside the building, such as those needed in northern area of the United States, the low-E coatings are applied to the inside pane of glass. In southern areas or hot climates, low-E coatings are applied to outside pane of the glass and are usually applied to bronze-, green-, or gray-tinted glass to reduce glare and to reflect the sun's heat away from the building (10). Different types of low-E coatings have been designed to allow for high, moderate, or low solar gain applications, so attention to product-specific performance attributes is necessary to achieve the desired effect.

Tempered Glass (Toughened Glass)

Tempered glass is the type of glass that is two or more times stronger than annealed glass. When broken, it shatters into many small fragments, preventing major injury (14,15). This type of glass is intended to be used when strength, thermal resistance, and safety are important considerations, such as for glass facades, sliding door, building entrances, and bath and shower enclosures (14). It is also used for side and rear windows of automobiles.

Laminated Glass

Laminated glass, sometimes called "lami" is made by permanently bonding two pieces of glass together with a tough plastic interlayer [polyvinyl butyral (PVB)] under heat and pressure (10,13). Once bonded together, the glass sandwich acts as a single unit and generally appears very similar to standard clear glass, and the interlayer is virtually invisible. The benefit of laminated glass is that if broken, glass fragments will adhere to the PVB interlayer rather than falling free, thereby reducing the risk of physical injury and property damage. It provides a characteristic "spider web" cracking pattern when the impact is not enough to completely pierce the glass (15). Laminated glass effectively filters over 99% of UV up to approximately 375 nm without sacrificing visible light transmission; with new developments, new types of laminated glass has become more transparent to wavelengths above 380 nm. Laminated glass also provides sound insulation. It is commonly used in automobiles (for windshields), airports, museums, sound studios, schools, greenhouses, and large public spaces. To enhance the quietness of the ride, laminated glass is now used for side and rear windows of high-end cars.

Insulating Glass

It is a glass made in insulated glazing unit (IGU). IGU is a set of two or more panes of glass enclosing a hermetically sealed air or gas space (10,16) (Fig. 3). In the United

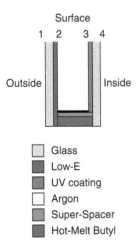

Figure 3 An IGU is a combination of two or more panes of glass with a sealed airspace between panes. Inert gas, e.g., argon or krypton, is commonly filled between panes of glass in IGUs to enhance insulation. These gases are less heat conductive than air. The UV-blocking coated glass is designed for use in an IGU configuration. Hot-melt-butyl is a type of sealant in IGU. *Abbreviation*: IGU, insulating glass unit. *Source*: Guardian Industries Corp (Auburn Hills, Michigan, US).

Kingdom, this is often called "double glazing." The most important function of insulating glass is for heat insulation. Glass itself has no insulative property but the air space between glass layers does. Argon is the gas commonly used in IGU as it is economical. Krypton, considerably more expensive, is not generally used except for a very thin double-glazing or high-performance triple-glazing units (3 pieces of glass) (17). Today, insulating glass units (IGUs) are included in over 95% of all windows sold in the United States. Although still a small percentage of total window sales, for very cold climates areas, triple-glaze IGUs are growing in popularity (9).

UV-Blocking Coated Glass

This type of glass has a very thin, special coating that makes it nearly distinguishable from standard clear glass (9). The coating blocks nearly all UV but maintain visible light transmission. UV-blocking coated glass is designed for use in an IGU; it is commonly used in windows and framing of museum quality artwork.

Spectrally Selective and UV-Blocking Insulating Glass

This glass package provides the highest degree of UV protection. It is made of one piece of spectrally selective low-E-coated glass and one piece of UV blocking–coated glass. It blocks more than 99% of UV transmission (assessed from 300 to 380 nm) and 70% of unwanted solar heat gain, while allowing nearly 70% visible light to pass through (9).

The transmissions of visible light and UV through different types of glass are shown in Table 2, Table 3, Figure 4A, and Figure 4B. It should be noted that the glass performance data referenced throughout this document have been generated by Guardian Industries Corp. (Auburn Hills, Michigan, U.S.) by using the Lawrence Berkeley National Laboratory (LBNL) Window 5 software program. Spectral performance data contained in

Table 2 **Typical Residential Architectural Window Glass Configurations with Properties of Solar, Visible Light, and Ultraviolet Transmission[a]**

Type of glass	Thickness (mm)	Tsol[b] (%)	Tvis[b] (%)	Tuv[b] (%)
Monolithic[c] clear glass	3.0 mm	83%	90%	72%
Monolithic tint glass	3.0 mm	61%	62%	40%
Monolithic laminated glass	6.0 mm	74%	88%	0.6%
Double glazed[d] clear glass	3.0 mm/3.0 mm IGU[e]	72%	82%	57%
Double-glazed tint glass	3.0 mm/3.0 mm IGU	52%	56%	33%
Double-glazed spectrally selective low-E glass	3.0 mm/3.0 mm IGU	36%	71%	20%
Double-glazed laminated glass	6.0 mm/3.0 mm IGU	63%	80%	0.5%
Double-glazed spectrally selective UV-blocking glass	3.0 mm/3.0 mm IGU	34%	69%	0.1%

[a]Data provided by Guardian Industries Corp. (Auburn Hills, Michigan, U.S.).
[b]Tsol: transmission of solar radiation, Tvis: transmission of visible light (assessed from 400–780 nm), Tuv: transmission of ultraviolet radiation (assessed from 300–380 nm).
[c]Monolithic glass: a single pane of uncoated glass.
[d]Double glazed: an insulating glass unit formed using two layers of glass separated by a sealed airspace.
[e]IGU: Insulating glass unit.
Source: From Ref. 9, with permission from Elsevier.

Table 3 Typical Commercial Architectural Window Glass Configurations with Properties of Solar, Visible Light, and UV Transmission[a]

Type of glass	Thickness (mm)	Tsol[b] (%)	Tvis[b] (%)	Tuv[b] (%)
Double-glazed tint glass	6.0 mm/6.0mm IGU	35%	40%	20%
Double-glazed spectrally selective low-E glass	6.0 mm/6.0 mm IGU	32%	68%	28%
Double-glazed reflective glass	6.0 mm/6.0 mm	13%	19%	17%
Double-glazed spectrally selective reflective glass	6.0 mm/6.0 mm	24%	43%	25%
Double-glazed laminated glass	6.0 mm/6.0 mm IGU	58%	79%	0.5%
Double-glazed spectrally selective UV-blocking glass	6.0 mm/6.0 mm IGU	32%	67%	0.2%

[a]Data provided by Guardian Industries Corp. (Auburn Hills, Michigan, U.S.).
[b]Tsol: transmission of solar radiation, Tvis: transmission of visible light (assessed from 400 to 780 nm), Tuv: transmission of ultraviolet radiation (assessed from 300 to 380 nm).
Source: From Ref. 9, with permission from Elsevier.

the Window 5 program have been submitted by the individual product manufacturers and verified by LBNL staff and a peer review process.

Thickness of Glass

Float glass is commonly produced in a wide range of thickness depending on the application requirements. The most common thickness of residential and commercial window glass is between 2.3 and 6 mm. Examples of common glass thickness and the associated application are demonstrated in Table 4. Effect of thickness of glass on UV transmission is demonstrated in Table 5.

Color of Glass

Glass is produced in a wide range of color depending on the application requirements. Examples of common glass colors and the associated applications are demonstrated in Table 6. Effect of glass colors on the properties of solar, visible light, and UV transmission is demonstrated in Figure 5.

Testing Methods for Quantitative Assessment of UV Protection of Glass

Several factors affect UV transmission of a finished window glass. Some of the main factors are glass type, glass color, interleave between glass, and coating on glass (9). Thickness of glass has little effect on UV transmission. Spectrometry is a method used in determining UV transmission of the glass. The tested glass sample is placed in a specimen holder of spectrophotometry in alignment to illuminating beam. The wavelength from 280 to 780 nm is scanned with 5 nm intervals. In this chapter, the relative transmission in the range of 300 to 380 nm is used to calculate transmission of UV (Tuv, %). The relative transmission in the range of 400 to 780 nm is used to calculate transmission of visible light (Tvis, %).

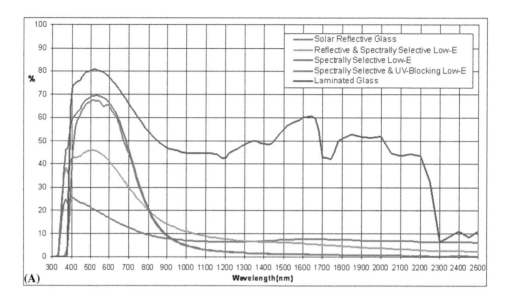

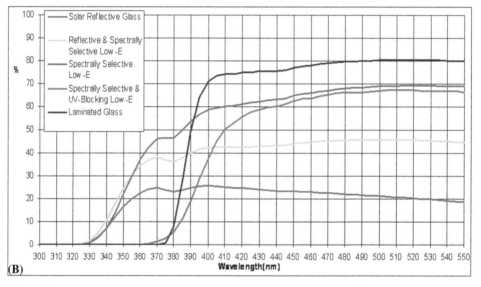

Figure 4 (**A**) Ultraviolet, visible light, and near infrared transmittance (300–2500 nm) of different types of architectural glass. *Source*: Data are provided by Guardian Industries Corp. Auburn Hills, Michigan, U.S. (**B**) Ultraviolet and short-wavelength visible light transmittance (300–550 nm) of different types of architectural glass. *Source*: Data are provided by Guardian Industries Corp. Auburn Hills, Michigan, U.S. Modified from Ref. 9, with permission from Elsevier.

AUTOMOBILE GLASS AND PHOTOPROTECTION

It has been estimated that a person spends an average of 80 to 107 min/day exposed to sunlight while driving or traveling by car (7,18). UVA exposure inside a car was shown to be high enough when calculating a person's lifetime UV exposure (7). Transmission of UVR through automobile glass depends on the type and tint of glass (9). For safety reasons, all windshields are made from laminated glass, which can filter most of the UVA.

Table 4 Common Architectural and Automotive Glass Thickness and Applications[a]

Application	Monolithic glass thickness	Application configurations
Residential architecture	2.3 mm, 3.0 mm, 4.0 mm, 5.0 mm, 6.0 mm	IGU comprised two pieces of equal-thickness glass
Commercial architecture	5.0 mm, 6.0 mm, 8.0 mm, 10.0 mm	IGU typically comprised two pieces of equal-thickness glass
Automotive (monolithic tempered glass)	3.1 mm, 4.0 mm, 5.0 mm	Monolithic tempered glass used primarily for side and rear windows in passenger vehicles
Automotive (laminated glass)	4.0 mm, 5.0 mm, 6.0 mm	Laminated glass used primarily for front windshield and some side windows

[a]Data provided by Guardian Industries Corp. (Auburn Hills, Michigan, U.S.).
Abbreviation: IGU, insulating glass unit.
Source: From Ref. 9, with permission from Elsevier.

Table 5 Percentage of UV Transmission Through Different Types and Thickness of Glass[a]

Glass type	Thickness	Tuv (%)[b]
Clear glass	2.3 mm	75
Clear glass	6.0 mm	63
Tinted green	2.3 mm	47
Tinted green	6.0 mm	28
Tinted bronze	2.3 mm	46
Tinted bronze	6.0 mm	24
Low-E	2.3 mm	21
Low-E	6.0 mm	19

[a]Data provided by Guardian Industries Corp. (Auburn Hills, Michigan, U.S.A.).
[b]UV transmission measured between 300 and 380 nm.
Abbreviations: UV, ultraviolet; Tuv, transmission of UV; Low-E, low-emissivity.

However, side and rear windows are usually made from tempered glass (non-laminated glass); therefore, a significant level of UVA can pass through. Individuals traveling by car can be exposed to considerable amount of UVA through side and rear windows. Several studies demonstrated that signs of chronic UV exposure such as photoaging and premalignant skin cancers are more prevalent among those to the driver's side (19–21). Photosensitive patients such as those with polymorphous light eruption also present with skin lesions that flare on the arm on the driver's side. It was shown that parts of the drivers' bodies closest to a window such as driver's arm or driver's head received the most radiation (22). UV exposure was two to three times greater in a smaller car compared with a larger car (23).

A study was conducted on UV transmission through samples of windshields, side windows, rear windows, and sunroofs of Mercedes-Benz cars (22). Windshields were found to effectively block UV of wavelengths shorter than 375 to 385 nm. For insulative

Table 6 Common Architectural and Automotive Glass Colors and Types and Their Applications[a]

Application	Glass types
Residential architecture	Clear, bronze, gray, spectrally selective low-E, spectrally selective UV-blocking low-E, laminated glass
Commercial architecture	Clear, low iron clear, bronze, gray, green, blue green, reflective, spectrally selective low-E, spectrally selective reflective low-E, laminated glass
Automotive (monolithic tempered and laminated)	Solar green, solar gray, solar control coated glass

[a]Data provided by Guardian Industries Corp. (Auburn Hills, Michigan, U.S.).
Abbreviations: Low-E, low-emissivity; UV, ultraviolet.
Source: From Ref. 9.

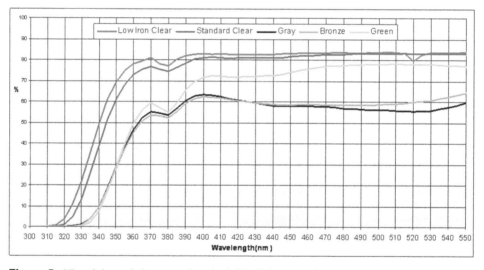

Figure 5 Ultraviolet and short-wavelength visible light transmittance (300–550 nm) of common glass with different colors. *Source*: Data are provided by Guardian Industries Corp. Auburn Hills, Michigan, U.S. Modified from Ref. 9, with permission from Elsevier.

green glass, significant UV transmission through the glass started at 385 nm, reaching 11% at 390 nm. Back and side windows were less effective in filtering UV than the windshield. For back-window glass, UV transmission started at 335 nm rising with a minor decrease between 370 and 385 nm to a maximum of 63% at 390 nm. Sunroof glass filters UV shorter than 335 nm. In this study, simulated UV exposure during driving was done by placing dummies with attached dosimeters in the car. On the arm, the averages of UVA exposure when the windows were shut and opened were 3 to 4% and 25 to 31% of ambient radiation, respectively. In an open convertible car, the most intense UV exposure was found on the driver's vertex, and the relative personal dose reached 62% of ambient radiation (22).

   Hampton et al. assessed the percentage of UVA transmission through a range of automobile glass types coated with different color tints (24). The most important factor in reducing penetration of UVA through automobile glass is lamination. Clear

Table 7 Percent of UV and Visible Light Transmission Through Different Types of Automobile Glass[a]

Application	Glass type	Tvis[b] (%)	Tuv[b] (%)
Vision glass			
Windshield	Standard green tint laminated glass	75%	3%
Windshield	Solar management laminated glass	71%	2%
Tempered side window	Standard green tint	79%	48%
Tempered side window	Solar management glass[c]	73%	33%
Tempered rear window	Standard green tint	79%	48%
Tempered rear window	Solar management glass	73%	33%
Privacy glass			
Tempered side window	Gray privacy glass[d]	18%	8%
Tempered rear window	Gray privacy glass	18%	8%
Moon or sun roof	Laminated, dark gray privacy glass	6%	2%

[a]Data provided by Guardian Industries Corp. (Auburn Hills, Michigan, U.S.A.).
[b]Tvis: transmission of visible light, Tuv: transmission of ultraviolet radiation (assessed from 300 to 380 nm).
[c]Solar management glass: tinted glass with enhanced solar control characteristics that is designed to block infrared radiation, thereby reducing the solar heat transmitted into the car.
[d]Privacy glass: monolithic, tempered tinted glass with enhanced solar control characteristics and very low visible light transmission, thereby significantly reducing solar heat transmission and visibility through the glass.
Source: From Ref. 9, with permission from Elsevier.

non-laminated glass provided the lowest UVA protection, followed by non-laminated light green, non-laminated dark green, and laminated clear glass. Gray-tinted laminated glass provided the highest UV protection. Only 0.6% of UVA and 0.8% of UVA1 was transmitted through gray-tinted laminated glass compared with 62.8% of UVA and 80.5% of UVA1 by non-laminated clear glass. Clinical relevance of UV exposure in automobile in the photosensitive patient was also assessed. A 5 J/cm^2 dose of UVA, which is sufficient to induce cutaneous eruption in patients with severe photosensitivity, could be obtained when the arm is placed near a non-laminated clear window for 30 minutes, or non-laminated light green window for 1 hour. If a laminated gray window were used as a substitute, at least 50 hours of UV exposure would be required to produce skin lesions in those patients. In addition to lamination and tinting, UVA exposure in automobiles can be influenced by non-glass-related factors such as position of the individual in a vehicle, direction of travel with respect to the sun, and time of the day.

Percent of UV and visible light transmission through different types of automobile glass is shown in Table 7. It should be noted that as UV transmission decreases, it is the long-wave UV, predominantly UVA1, which continues to be transmitted.

ENHANCED PHOTOPROTECTION THROUGH THE USE OF WINDOW FILM

Window film is transparent plastic film or metallic laminate, which is applied to glass windows. Because significant UVA can transmit through side and rear windows of the cars, it is now possible for automobile owners to further darken the tint on side and rear windows. Window film reduces the transmission of UV rays, visible light, and infrared radiation; permits reduction of interior heat gain; and minimizes the fading of interior components. Because window film can restrict the driver's vision especially in dark condition, in the United States, aftermarket tints are not allowed to go below the federally mandated 70% minimum visible light transmittance of automobile windshields, except for the top 4 in (10.2 cm) of the windshield (25). Most states in the United States do allow aftermarket tinting of side and rear windows. The minimum allowable visible light transmission levels for side and rear windows are determined by each state, most of them do allow tint with no less than 35% visible light transmittance (25), while some states allow window tint as dark as 20% visible light transmittance (26). It has been reported that window film with 35% and 20% visible light transmittance filtered UVA below 370 and 380 nm, respectively (27).

The benefit of window film in photoprotection was supported by an in vitro study (28). Mouse fibroblasts were subjected to four conditions: exposure to solar simulating radiation (SSR) alone, SSR filtered through automobile glass (tempered glass), SSR filtered through UV-absorbing film, and SSR filtered through automobile glass coated with UV-absorbing film. Capability for photoprotection was measured by 3T3 neutral red uptake assay. Cells exposed to SSR alone had significant cell death with survival rate of only 11%. Cells exposed to SSR filtered with automobile glass had 37% survival rate, while those irradiated through window film and the combination of automobile glass with film had survival rates 90% and 93%, respectively. In this study, the authors also measured UVR through a car window. They measured UVR from the driver's side window glass, the driver's side window glass with UV-absorbing film applied and through the windshields. The side window with UV-absorbing film blocked most of the UVR, allowing only 0.4% UV transmission, followed by the windshield that allowed 2% UV transmission. Side-window glass without film allowed UVR transmission as high as 79% of solar UVR (28).

Because of a wide variety of films and the ease of installation, aftermarket automobile window tinting has become popular. However, automobile tint is best installed by professionals; without the proper tools and techniques, amateur filming is prone to bubbling and separation from the glass.

CONCLUSION

In addition to outdoor UV exposure, UV exposure through architectural window glass and automobile glass while being indoor and in a car is a topic that should be addressed. Nowadays, new glass technologies can give us options to choose the glass that provide high UV protection. Awareness of photoprotection by glass is an important component of the total photoprotection strategy.

REFERENCES

1. Kullavanijaya P, Lim HW. Photoprotection. J Am Acad Dermatol 2005; 52(6):937–958.
2. Sliney DH. Photoprotection of the eye-UV radiation and sunglasses. J Photochem Photobiol B 2001; 64(2–3):166–175.
3. Parisi AV, Kimlin MG, Wong JC, et al. Diffuse component of solar ultraviolet radiation in tree shade. J Photochem Photobiol B 2000; 54(2–3):116–120.
4. Turnbull DJ, Parisi AV. Spectral UV in public shade settings. J Photochem Photobiol B 2003; 69(1):13–19.
5. Hoffmann K, Laperre J, Avermaete A, et al. Defined UV protection by apparel textiles. Arch Dermatol 2001; 137(8):1089–1094.

6. Menter JM, Hollins TD, Sayre RM, et al. Protection against UV photocarcinogenesis by fabric materials. J Am Acad Dermatol 1994; 31(5 pt 1):711–716.

7. McCurdy T, Graham SE. Using human activity data in exposure models: analysis of discriminating factors. J Expo Anal Environ Epidemiol 2003; 13(4):294–317.

8. Parisi AV, Meldrum LR, Kimlin MG, et al. Evaluation of differences in ultraviolet exposure during weekend and weekday activities. Phys Med Biol 2000; 45(8):2253–2262.

9. Tuchinda C, Srivannaboon S, Lim HW. Photoprotection by window glass, automobile glass and sunglasses. J Am Acad Dermatol 2006; 54(5):845–854.

10. NGA (National Glass Association). Available at: http://www.glass.org/indres/info.htm. Accessed March 2008.

11. Production of glass. Available at: http://www.glassonweb.com/glassmanual/topics/index/production.htm. Accessed March 2008.

12. Body-tinted glass. Available at: http://www.glassonweb.com/glassmanual/topics/index/tinted.htm. Accessed March 2008.

13. Guardian Industries. Available at: www.guardian.com/en/na/index.html. Accessed March 2008.

14. Tempered glass. Available at: http://www.glassonweb.com/glassmanual/topics/index/tempered.htm. Accessed March 2008.

15. Architectural glass. Available at: http://en.wikipedia.org/wiki/Architectural_glass. Accessed March 2008.

16. Insulating glass. Available at: http://www.glassonweb.com/glassmanual/topics/index/insulating.htm. Accessed March 2008.

17. Insulated glazing. Available at: http://en.wikipedia.org/wiki/insulated_glazing. Accessed March 2008.

18. Edlich RF, Winters KL, Cox MJ, et al. The use of UV-protective windows and window films to aid in the prevention of skin cancer. J Long Term Eff Med Implants 2004; 14(5):415–430.

19. Foley P, Lanzer D, Marks R. Are solar keratoses more common on the driver's side. Br Med J (Clin Res Ed) 1986; 293(6538):18.

20. Singer RS, Hamilton TA, Vooorhees JJ, et al. Association of asymmetrical facial photodamage with automobile driving. Arch Dermatol 1994; 130(1):121–123.

21. Moulin G, Thomas L, Vigneau M, et al. A case of unilateral elastosis with cysts and comedones Favre-Racouchot syndrome. Ann Dermatol Venereol 1994; 121(10):721–723.

22. Moehrle M, Soballa M, Korn M. UV exposure in cars. Photodermatol Photoimmunol Photomed 2003; 19(4):175–181.

23. Parisi AV, Wong JC. Quantitative evaluation of the personal erythemal ultraviolet exposure in a car. Photodermatol Photoimmunol Photomed 1998; 14(1):12–16.

24. Hampton PJ, Farr PM, Diffey BL, et al. Implication for photosensitive patients of ultraviolet a exposure in vehicles. Br J Dermatol 2004; 151(4):873–876.

25. LaMotte J, Ridder W III, Yeung K, et al. Effect of aftermarket automobile window tinting films on driver vision. Hum Factors 2000; 42(2):327–336.

26. Automotive film state laws. http://www.iwfa.com/PreProduction_copy(1)/consumer_info/auto_statelaws.html. Accessed March 2008.

27. Johnson JA, Fusaro RM. Broad-spectrum photoprotection: the roles of tinted auto windows, sunscreens and browning agents in the diagnosis and treatment of photosensitivity. Dermatology 1992; 185(4):237–241.

28. Bernstein EF, Schwartz M, Viehmeyer R, et al. Measurement of protection afforded by ultraviolet-absorbing window film using an in vitro model of photodamage. Lasers Surg Med 2006; 38(4):337–342.

19

Sun, Eye, Ophthalmohelioses, and the Contact Lens

Minas Coroneo

Department of Ophthalmology, University of New South Wales at Prince of Wales Hospital, Sydney, New South Wales, Australia

INTRODUCTION

Sight, our highest bandwidth sense, mediates via optic nerve fibers that provide the majority of the fibers of sensation to the human brain, is on the one hand totally dependent on visible light energy, and on the other, can be damaged by it and the contiguous ultraviolet (UV) and infrared wavelengths.

Our understanding of the effects of sunlight on the eye has improved over time. There is a realization that the pathogenesis of a large number of ocular conditions could be attributable in large measure to UV radiation. These conditions have been grouped and named "the ophthalmohelioses," from the Greek ophthalmos (eye) and helios (sun), to refer collectively to diseases of the eye caused by sunlight. Table 1 is a list of the ophthalmohelioses—ocular conditions in which sunlight has been postulated to play a role in pathogenesis.

Much of the UV light that strikes the eye is reflected, indirect light (albedo). Although it is commonly known that one can be sunburned while under the shade of an umbrella, the elegant studies of Urbach (1) demonstrated that reflected light struck the regions of the orbits. It was therefore not surprising that the ophthalmohelioses were prevalent in places of high ground reflectance or in individuals exposed under these conditions. Because of the indirect and geometrical nature of this exposure, individual exposure was inaccurately estimated from the standard questionnaires used in epidemiological studies—individual exposures and factors peculiar to individuals could result in underestimation of exposure.

Another source of underestimation by individuals of levels of exposure is that UV levels can be high on cloudy days or under certain weather conditions and that peak exposure occurs in the middle of the day. Whereas peak UV exposure is widely believed to occur in the middle of the day (reflected in the well-known advice to avoid the midday sun), recently high ocular exposure has been recorded in mornings and evenings (2). In this study, peak ocular exposures were recorded at 9 a.m. and 3 p.m. when the solar zenith angle was $50°$ (Fig. 1) during spring and autumn (latitude 36 degrees, 39 minutes north).

Table 1 A List of the Ophthalmohelioses

Eyelid	Wrinkles; sunburn; photosensitivity reactions; cicatricial ectropion; dermatochalasis; premalignant changes; malignancies, such as basal cell carcinoma, squamous cell carcinoma, and melanoma
Ocular surface	Vernal catarrh, pinguecula, pterygium, climatic keratopathy (labrador keratopathy), actinic granuloma, keratitis (flash, snow blindness), arcus/transparency, band keratopathy, corneal endothelial polymorphism, reactivation of herpetic keratitis, scleritis in porphyria, senile scleral plaques, post-photorefractive keratectomy (PRK) haze, malignancy of the cornea or conjunctiva
Uvea	Melanoma, miosis, pigment dispersion, uveitis, blood-ocular barrier incompetence
Crystalline lens	Cataract, anterior capsular herniation, early presbyopia, capsular pseudoexfoliation, subluxation in Marfan syndrome, intraocular lens dysphotopsia
Vitreous	Liquification
Retina	Photic maculopathy, erythropsia, macular degeneration, choroidal melanoma, visual loss with photostress in carotid stenosis
Glaucoma	Experimental
Ocular posture	Intermittent exotropia
Systemic	Xeroderma pigmentosum, basal cell carcinoma, basal cell nevus syndrome, porphyria cutanea tarda, polymorphous light eruption, drug-induced photosensitivity, uremia, immunosuppression, myopia

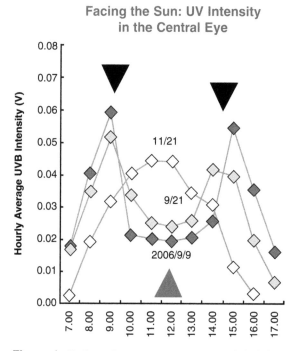

Figure 1 Peak ocular exposures were recorded during morning and afternoon hours, in sharp contrast to the commonly held belief that the greatest UV exposure occurs during midday.

Unlike the skin, the eye is less exposed to direct light and is largely insolated by scattered, reflected light. This type of exposure increases the likelihood of peripheral light-focusing (PLF) effects and would be expected to maximize ocular damage (Table 1).

In addition to the potentially harmful effects of normal levels of sunlight on the eye, there are also concerns about the ozone hole and the ophthalmic consequences of increased ocular UV insolation (3). There is a unique exposure of the human eye, and in particular the exposure of the human limbus, as well as the fact that a large temporal visual field not only aids survival but acts as a large collecting zone for UV light incident on the temporal limbus. There is also a growth in knowledge of ocular stem cell populations from initial findings in the limbus (4) and a gradual realization that peripheral light foci coincide with certain ocular stem cell populations. As there is no animal model of pterygium, researchers relied on cell culture studies and were able to culture epithelial cells typical of pterygium. This has enabled scientists to explore the role of UV-induced inflammatory events and in particular the role of matrix metalloproteinases in the pathogenesis of pterygium and cortical cataract. It is likely that similar pathways are involved in the pathogenesis of several of the ophthalmohelioses. As the eye provides the only substantial lens-focusing system of the body, the ophthalmohelioses would be expected to develop earlier than the dermatohelioses, and so eyes are exposed to increasing amounts of UV radiation. The increased pterygium prevalence may be an early consequence of this exposure.

The ophthalmohelioses have a tremendous impact on patients' quality of life and have significant implications to the cost of health care. While cataract is not entirely due to insolation, it now seems certain that sunlight plays a contributory role—cataract is one of the most, if not the most, commonly performed surgical procedure in many societies. Pterygium, typically afflicting a younger population, adds a tremendous burden, both human and financial, in sunny countries (5).

There has been great interest in prevention of these diseases as well as identifying at-risk individuals. There is also a large variation in the protection afforded by sunglasses and hats. Standard-setting groups are just starting to recognize that lateral protection afforded by sunglasses is of considerable importance. Yet even with the best of intentions, in certain environments (surfing), sunglass and hat wear are inconvenient and consequently are seldom used. It is in this setting that UV-blocking contact lenses may play a particularly limited but important role. As they typically span the limbus, they are currently the most effective means of reducing, if not eliminating, peripheral light foci.

UV-blocking contact lenses have been available for many years, but their use as ocular protectants has been limited. While they do not provide protection to the facial skin and eyelids, protection by this means may be a pragmatic and reliable solution in certain situations offering advantages over sunglasses, the efficacy of which has raised concerns.

Populations at increased risk of ocular UV damage include those that have high exposure—both outdoors (sailors, surfers) and indoors (welders)—and in patients who may be photosensitized by genetic factors or drugs. Ground reflectance of UV light can be a critical determinant of ocular exposure. The best natural reflector is snow, explaining why goggles are usually necessary for adequate protection on the snowfields (6). This explains why ocular UV exposure can be similar in vastly different climates. Thus, pterygium can occur under vastly different climatic conditions—two cases of pterygium blindness have been reported in an indigenous Australian (7) and an Alaskan native (8). Short wavelength UV radiation is scattered and reflected, terrain reflectance being more important than terrain elevation. Cloud cover and haze may actually increase ocular UV exposure (9,10).

There was early understanding of the importance of the role reflected UV light plays in the etiology of the dermatohelioses. Urbach (1) performed a series of experiments using a chemical dosimeter system and mannequin heads, which were irradiated under different conditions. On exposure to UV light, the heads turned from yellow to deep red and the change quantified by reflection photometry. These experiments demonstrated that terrain reflectance was a key determinant of ocular UV exposure. Many conventional spectacles/sunglasses offer little side protection from albedo, as much of the lateral conjunctiva and limbus remain exposed. Such glasses reduce glare from direct, visible light and may encourage wearers to increase their exposure to UV albedo. This would result at the very least in increased UV insolation of the ocular surface and perhaps even of intraocular structures as a result of pupil dilatation (because of shading from direct visible light by sunglasses). Hedblom (11) pointed out that wearing conventional sunglasses was frequently associated with the development of photokeratoconjunctivitis ("snow blindness") on Antarctic missions.

INITIAL STUDIES ON PERIPHERAL LIGHT-FOCUSING EFFECT

Initial studies (12–14) have determined the pathways by which the anterior eye, acting as a side-on lens, focuses light onto the opposite side of the eye, most noticeably to the distal (nasal) limbus, the usual location of pterygium and pinguecula (called the type 1 phenomenon). Light proceeds across the anterior eye via transcameral pathways and not by so-called sclerotic scatter. The degree of limbal focusing is determined in part by the corneal shape and anterior chamber depth, and this may explain why particular individuals in a particular environment are afflicted. Using computer-assisted optical ray-tracing techniques (15–17), the transcameral light pathways were confirmed.

It has been calculated that the peak light intensity at the distal limbus is approximately 20 times that of the incident light intensity (14)—this has further been refined in subsequent studies to take into account corneal shape (15,16) as well as focusing on the crystalline lens (17). The limbal effect peak intensity was found at an incident angle of 104° (17). Furthermore, it seems that the light focus is actually not a spot, but a complex arc shape—explaining why it is difficult to appreciate when viewing along the path of incident light.

The earliest report of PLF is from the work of von Helmholz (18). By asking a subject to accommodate, he was able to observe a movement of the light focus anteriorly, neatly demonstrating that the anterior crystalline lens surface (and iris) move forward during accommodation. Graves (19) described a method of corneal illumination, termed "sclerotic scatter," in which light was presumed to pass horizontally across the cornea by total internal reflection within the corneal stroma. Although this is considered as a possible pathway in initial observations (12), initial ray-tracing studies (13) determined that this mechanism could not occur. Another early report from Mackevicius (20) linked the observation of a limbal focus to pterygium pathogenesis. Rizzuti (21) used a penlight in keratoconus patients to illuminate the temporal limbus and noticed distal limbal focusing. He claimed that this was not seen in normal corneas.

Calculations would predict (15) that a steeply curved cornea (as is seen in keratoconus) would be expected to produce an intense distal limbal focus. Furthermore "normal" corneas also produce such foci. It was noticed in cattle (22) that limbal foci occurred and coincided with the sites of precursor lesions for squamous carcinoma— ironically bovine eyes were used (14) to work out the optical pathways involved in conjunction with ray-tracing experiments. Light focusing was again implicated in pterygium pathogenesis (23), but the pathway was thought to be by sclerotic scatter (transcorneal) and the mechanism of pathogenesis to involve damage to subconjunctival tissue, dellen formation, and subsequent pterygium formation.

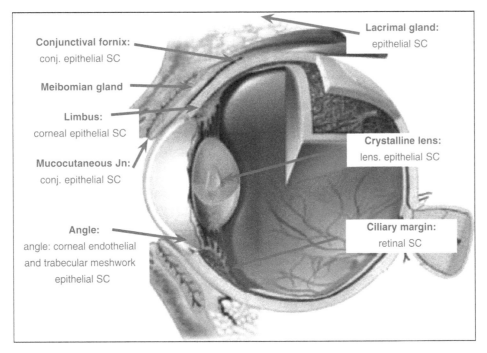

Figure 2 The location of stem cells (SC) at the sites of the principal peripheral-focusing phenomena.

These previous studies failed to define the precise optical pathways, the intensity of the limbal focus, the potential to damage stem cells, and the pathophysiological mechanisms involving matrix metalloproteinase activation (24,25).

They also failed to recognize that limbal focusing was one of a series of foci induced by the anterior eye's peripheral optics. As the PLF phenomena were being elucidated, the location and importance of ocular stem cell populations were becoming evident. Perhaps the earliest report of the critical nature of the limbus in renewal of the corneal epithelium was published in 1971 (4). A recent review of ocular stem cells (26) confirms the location of stem cells at the sites of the three principal PLF phenomena (Fig. 2).

1. The limbus
2. The nasal crystalline lens equator
3. The eyelid margin

Figure 3 is a schematic diagram (27) of the hypothesis of corneal epithelial replacement. Basal limbal stem cells generate transient amplifying cells, and these give rise to centripetally directed postmitotic cells suprabasally and terminally differentiated cells superficially. Apart from renewal of corneal epithelium, the limbus maintains a barrier so that normally conjunctival and corneal epithelium remains separated. Ordinarily, little direct UV light strikes the ocular surface. With PLF, a beam of 20× the incident intensity crosses the anterior chamber, little altered by aqueous humor (28) and strikes the basal and relatively unprotected stem cells. This circumvents the normal protection of this corneal stem cell niche by the more superficial limbal cells that normally absorb directly incident light (29). As stem cells are pluripotent and capable of division, alteration by UV light can conceivably result in a tissue mass of a number of cell types that break the limbal barrier and invade the cornea. Of interest is the recent finding

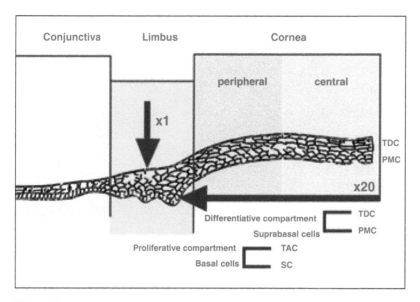

Figure 3 A schematic diagram of the hypothesis of corneal epithelial replacement.

(30) that the presence of a pterygium can be associated with deep corneal changes at the level of the endothelium, and Descemet's membrane and that endothelial cell density may be lower in these eyes. This is consistent with damage induced by PLF.

Pterygium Pathophysiology and Peripheral Light-Focusing Effect

A hypothesis that explains pterygium pathophysiology by postulating an alteration of limbal stem cells may also help to explain the characteristic wing shape of the pterygium. Early observations (31) of pigmentary patterns in the corneal epithelium suggest that areas of limbus contribute pie-shaped areas of the corneal epithelium. These patterns have recently been elegantly demonstrated by UV photography (32).

Using this concept and a population balance model of corneal and limbal epithelial production (33), we were able to model the expected wing shape of a pterygium (34). Further indirect evidence that PLF plays a role in disease pathogenesis is the observation that iris melanoma occurs more frequently in the horizontal aspects of the iris (Fig. 4) (35).

Pterygium can be located temporally—in some series, this is seen in only 2% of cases. However, in one study of sawmill workers (36), 15% had temporal pterygium alone and 11% had both temporal and nasal pterygia together (36). In an Arabic population, temporal pterygium was reported in 2.4% of cases, whereas in a Chinese population, in 6.7% of cases (37). There was an early suggestion that a large nose would protect the eye from sunlight (38), and this appears to be true for peripheral light crossing the midline in the direction of the temporal limbus.

There is further indirect evidence that pterygium pathogenesis is related to PLF phenomena. In the upper panel of Figure 5A, a patient with a right divergent strabismus has a nasal pterygium affecting his left orthophoric eye. If pterygium was due to UV radiation striking the eye axially, the right nasal bulbar conjunctiva is more exposed and would be expected to be afflicted by pterygium ahead of the left eye. This phenomenon was first noted by Saad (39). Recently, pterygium has been reported in the sighting eye of a marksman (40), consistent with previous observations of the dominant eye being

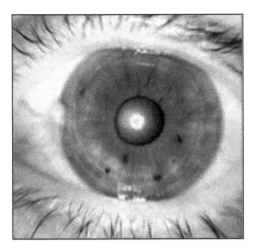

Figure 4 An iris melanoma is present underlying a nasal pterygium.

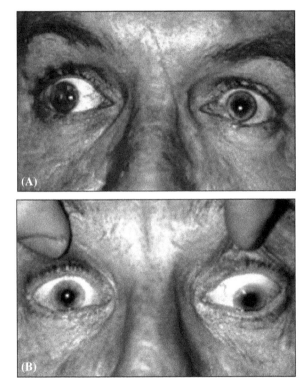

Figure 5 (**A**) Upper, a patient with a right divergent strabismus has a nasal pterygium affecting his left orthophoric eye. (**B**) Lower, a patient that has a pterygium in his hypotropic left eye.

predominantly affected by pterygium (41). In the lower panel of Figure 5B, a patient has a pterygium in his hypotropic left eye. The pterygium is displaced superiorly, again consistent with transcameral light pathway as a causative factor.

Recently, we developed a method that may detect early (preclinical) ocular surface sunlight-induced damage using UV fluorescence photography (UVFP) (42,43). Figure 6A, B

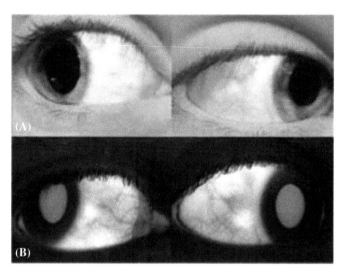

Figure 6 (**A, B**) Images from an 11-year-old girl. The areas of fluorescence are seen only on ultraviolet photography, and in these areas the ocular surface is clinically normal.

Table 2 **Evidence of Ocular Damage in Children at Various Ages: Evidence of Ocular Sun Damage in Children Stratified by Age Group, as Determined by Using Standard Visible Light Photography (Control) and UV Florescence Photography**

Age group (years)	Number of children with changes consistent with pingueculae on control photography	Number of children with fluorescent areas on UV fluorescence photography
3–8	0/27 (0%)	0/27 (0%)
9–11	0/23 (0%)	6/23 (29%)
12–15	7/21 (33%)	17/21 (81%)

demonstrates areas of nasal limbal fluorescence in eyes that are otherwise clinically normal. These areas of fluorescence are consistent with focal damage induced by PLF. In a study in school-aged children, we were able to detect these changes in children aged nine years and more (Table 2). The prevalence of these changes increased with chronological age, with clinical changes (pinguecula) being noted from age 13. We were surprised to find that in the 12- to 15-year-old group, 81% of children had evidence of damage (clinical and preclinical).

The possible causes of fluorescence include cross-linking of collagen induced by UV irradiation, the presence of metabolites such as reduced NADH or derivatives of amino acids such as tryptophan, or evidence of altered corneal epithelial stem cells (42,43). Since exposure to UV radiation in childhood increases the risk of subsequent development of pterygium (44), effective preventive strategies at this time of life may prove to be crucial. A number of studies (45–47) have found that children lack understanding and awareness of UV damage to the eyes and that sun protection practices among adolescents are not only suboptimal but appear to have declined (47). During the

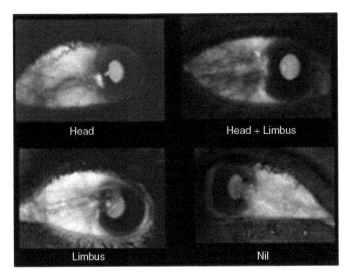

Figure 7 Fluorescence patterns in established pterygia.

course of these studies, we found that both the children and their parents were very interested in the changes that we could demonstrate. It may be that this graphic demonstration of early preclinical and clinical changes of sun damage will reinforce the important health message to reduce sun exposure and adopt preventive measures. In fact, there has been an acknowledgment that future educational programs will require an innovative approach to modify adolescent behaviors in relation to sun exposure and sun protection (47).

Using UVFP, we went on to investigate the patterns of fluorescence in established pterygia. Four patterns were seen (Fig. 7), with 80% of patients demonstrating fluorescence at the leading edge of the pterygium, at the limbus, or both. We postulated that the areas of fluorescence represented areas of cellular activity within the pterygium. Lack of fluorescence was thought to occur in pterygia that are "burned out" and represent disease that is no longer active.

We have previously pointed out (14) that pterygia have been found to develop about a decade before UV-induced skin conditions and thus may be an early indicator of increased UV insolation. Changes detected on UVFP may prove to be the earliest indicator of UV changes in the body.

Cataract and Peripheral Light-Focusing Effect

A second type of light-focusing effect was originally noticed if the light source was moved more anteriorly (than the location required to produce a limbal focus). Light is focused by the anterior eye, through the pupil (circumventing the protective effect of the iris), and onto the crystalline lens equator stem cells (Fig. 8).

Subsequently, light exits the eye through the vascular ciliary body and appears as a red spot on the ocular surface—this phenomenon was most easily observed in lightly pigmented eyes. Recently, we (17) have completed ray-tracing studies that demonstrate that the peak intensity of visible light varied between $3.7\times$ and $4.8\times$. Focusing of UVA showed attained higher peak intensities of $4.6\times$ to $8.6\times$ with maximum peak intensities occurring at angles of incidence of $82°$ to $86°$.

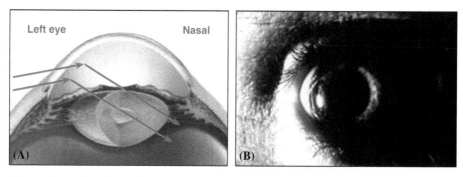

Figure 8 (**A, B**) Light is focused by the anterior eye, through the pupil, and onto the crystalline lens equator stem cells.

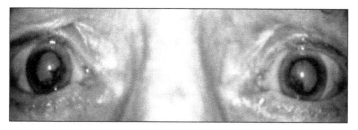

Figure 9 A clinical photograph of a patient with cortical cataract present in the nasal/inferonasal quadrants of the crystalline lens, present bilaterally.

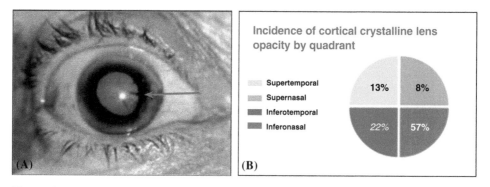

Figure 10 (**A, B**) The inferonasal localization of cortical cataract.

The inferonasal localization of cortical cataract has been reported as far back as 1889 (48). Since then there have been many studies confirming this finding (49–55). It was well known in clinical ophthalmic practice (Figs. 9 and 10A, B). There was a rekindled interest in this observation (12,56,57) following the initial observations of PLF phenomena in the anterior eye in 1982. These transcameral/translenticular pathways were confirmed by ray-tracing experiments (57,17). More recently, large epidemiological (58–67) and morphological (68) studies clearly demonstrated that most cortical cataracts form initially or are prevalent in the inferonasal area of the lens. The germinative zone of the crystalline lens is located equatorially (Fig. 11). This region may be more sensitive to focused UV radiation than other parts of the crystalline lens (69).

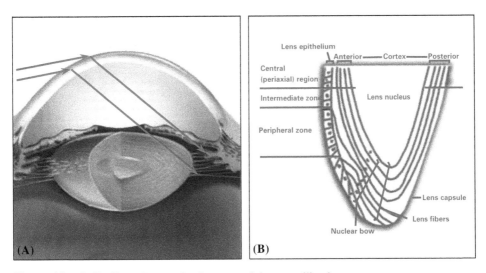

Figure 11 (**A, B**) Show the germinative zone of the crystalline lens.

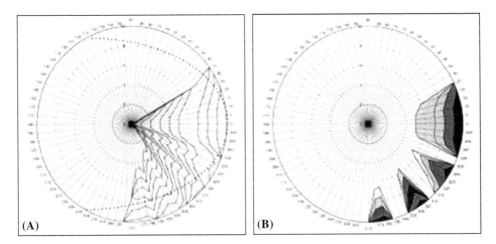

Figure 12 (**A, B**) Fiber growth for one sector in the anterior surface of the adult human lens. A representative light envelope (*broken line*) of standard PLF concentrates light at the equatorial 0° area, consistent with 3 o'clock position (**B**). Cataractous lesions in anterior fibers of the adult lens. Lesion at 0° represents localized damage of Figure 12**A**, but the actual shape depends on the extent of the cellular damage and the initial site of injury. *Abbreviation*: PLF, peripheral light focusing.

A computational model was employed to examine the growth of the normal human lens and the induction of spoke-like cortical cataract (Fig. 12A, B). It was demonstrated that if clusters of germinative cells are caused to opacify, the resultant opacities are predominantly spoke-shaped (70).

Intraocular Lens and Pseudophakic Dysphotopsia

With the development of modern intraocular lenses (IOLs) an unexpected symptom was recognized with particular types of IOLs, known as pseudophakic dysphotopsia; the visual disturbances include glare, streaks, and dark shadows in the temporal visual field and can affect a significant number of pseudophakic patients (71). Pseudophakic dysphotopsia is

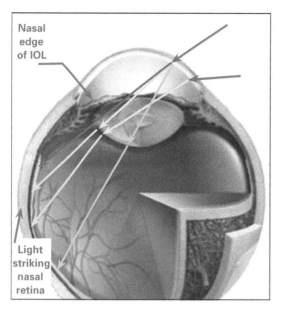

Figure 13 Oblique light incident at the temporal limbus (*right*) is concentrated at the nasal edge of the IOL and reflects to the nasal retina. *Abbreviation*: IOL, intraocular lens.

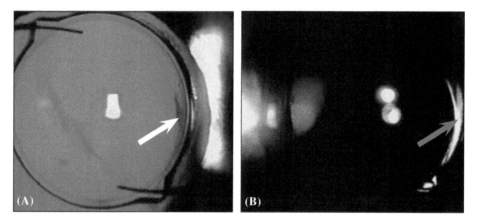

Figure 14 (**A, B**) Clinical photos of a patient with pseudophakic dysphotopsia. Square-edged IOL had been implanted in the right eye of a 47-year-old man (*left panel*). Off-axis lighting from the temporal field elicited foci of intense light on the nasal aspect of the IOL, which resulted in the replication of the visual phenomena noted by the patient. The focusing gain was 2.56 times the incident intensity, and the critical incidence window at the temporal cornea was between 71° and 89° to the sagittal plane. *Abbreviation*: IOL, intraocular lens.

more prevalent than is realized, being reported in 7% to 90% of cases (72). It has been associated, although not exclusively, with square-edged acrylic IOLs designed to reduce capsule opacity (71). Thus, in resolving one problem, a second problem, dysphotopsia, has emerged. Unfortunately, some IOL models also reduce likelihood of an intrinsic solution to the problem, as they inhibit the development of peripheral capsular opacity. Interestingly, dysphotopsia does not appear to have been described in the phakic state, suggesting that the design of the crystalline lens overcomes this problem. It seems that PLF is responsible for these symptoms (Figs. 13 and 14A, B). Oblique light incident at the

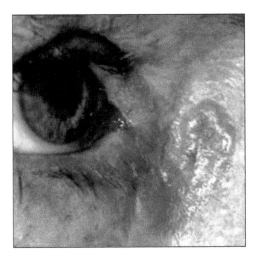

Figure 15 A basal cell carcinoma (BCC) that has commenced in the medial aspect of the eyelids and has grown onto the side of the nose.

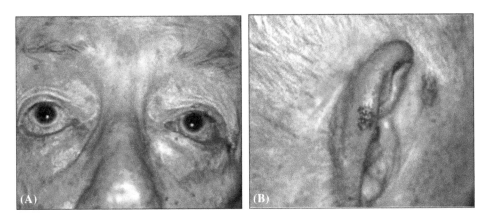

Figure 16 (**A, B**) The weather-beaten facial appearance is not uncommon in outback Australia. This patient suffered from skin malignancies of the ear, face, and eyelids, cicatricial ectropion, pterygium, and cataract. The preponderance of skin malignancy in the postauricular and retroauricular sites and on the posterior aspect of the helix, as compared to the superior aspect of the ear, has been noted (1). This may coincide with the direction of albedo, from below and from behind. These are the directions from which albedo concentration in the anterior eye is best demonstrated.

temporal limbus (right) is concentrated at the nasal edge of the IOL. Light rays continue posteronasally to strike the nasal retina at different areas depending on the angle of incidence. Some light rays may pass between the anterior lens surface and the posterior iris. Another pathway is via the periphery of the IOL (as opposed to the lens edge).

The Eyelids and Peripheral Light-Focusing Effect

A third type of PLF effect is on the eyelid margin. Again the site of a stem cell population, it is postulated (12) that this may account for the nasal predilection for eyelid skin malignancy (73,74).

In some series, basal cell carcinomas (BCC) represent 20% of eyelid tumors and 90% of eyelid malignancies (Figs. 15 and 16A, B). BCC of the eyelids also have a high risk of recurrence. BCC is the most common cause leading to eyelid reconstructive surgery—eyelid reconstructions can entail use of complex methods and require tumor removal, functionality, and an aesthetic outcome (75). This surgery represents a major surgical workload in certain countries.

Sliney recognized early that these phenomena tied together many pieces of a puzzle relating ocular sun exposure and a number of diseases with distinctive locations and features (76). He and others (2,76–86) have called these phenomena the "Coroneo Effect."

Prevention of the Ophthalmohelioses

Hollows, who had a long-term interest in the ophthalmohelioses, after many years of work in outback Australia, set out sensible guidelines for preventing these diseases (87). While on the one hand housing provides shelter from the elements, on the other, modern architecture may allow increased sunlight indoors.

In fact, indoor glare can be problematic (87). Certain materials may also be conducive to high UV reflectance. Thus, it was known in Kenya that hats should be worn indoors in houses with corrugated iron roofs and no ceilings, as "galvanized sheets did not repel all the sun's rays" (87), or more likely, result in high levels of scattered UV light indoors. Corrugated galvanized iron, invented in the 1840s, is a strong, light-weight, corrosion-resistant, inexpensive, easily transported material and has been widely used in buildings, but it seems that it is highly reflective of UV light. Modern paints resist the elements and may also be highly reflective of UV light, potentially increasing our exposure close to, if not in, our shelters.

Sunglasses

Conventional sunglasses are often worn for stylistic reasons, and until recent times, there has been less regard for sunglasses as protective devices. Sunglasses have a number of added disadvantages:

1. They reduce glare from direct, visible light and may allow wearers to increase their exposure to UV albedo (14). It has been pointed out that the eye is the natural and most efficient light warning system and represents the only means to caution a person adequately against the dangers of sunlight, since the skin itself is not able to announce overexposure rapidly enough to force its owner to get out of the sun in time. Modern man has invented remedies for the light sensitivity of the eye to be able to spend more time in the sun without feeling uncomfortable (88). In one study, people wearing sunglasses were less likely to wear hats and protective clothing (89). A possible connection between the use of sunglasses and the risk of developing skin cancer, especially malignant melanoma, has been suggested (88). The development of UV-safe sunglasses that transmit visible light was raised (88).
2. Wearing conventional sunglasses under conditions of extreme albedo (as in the Antarctic) can be associated with the development of photokeratoconjunctivitis ("snow blindness") (11). This may be as a result of inactivation of the natural protective mechanism of squinting (90).
3. As the pupil response is most sensitive to visible light, conventional sunglasses may allow pupil dilation in proportion to the darkness of the sunglasses (91) and increased intraocular insolation.
4. Potential decrease in low-contrast visual acuity (92).

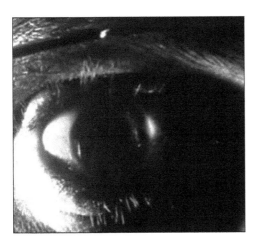

Figure 17 In this image, conventional sunglasses have no effect on PLF at the limbus. *Abbreviation*: PLF, peripheral light focusing.

   5. Reduced visual field attributable to spectacle frame (93).
   6. Inconvenience—discomfort from frame, scratched lenses, fogging, and expense.

A natural protective mechanism in extremely bright light is squinting (that is, narrowing the palpebral fissure)—in this process, the lateral eyelids, as they close, limit the amount of light striking the lateral aspect of the eye.

Interestingly, in extremely bright light, the nondominant eye is closed, explaining why pterygium initially afflicts the dominant eye (41). Sunglass styles vary considerably, particularly since many standards do not address the issue of side protection. As a consequence, side protection can vary from extremely effective to nonexistent (Fig. 17).

Even with wraparound-style sunglasses, side exposure can still be considerable. Thus, in one study, movement of the sunglass frame 6 mm from the forehead resulted in variation of the percentage of UV reaching the eyes ranging from 3.7% to 44.8% (94). It was found that the amount of attenuation is highly variable and depends mainly on their size, shape, and wearing position of the spectacles. One style of sunglasses, popular among surfers and mountaineers, has leather "blinkers." While very effective at reducing glare, these sunglasses greatly reduce peripheral field of vision, which can be dangerous. The effect of spectacle frames on field of vision is well recognized (93,95).

A significant problem, however, is that sunglasses remain inconvenient as protective devices, particularly in certain sports such as surfing in which participants are known to have a high prevalence of pterygium, or sailboard riding in which participants are known to have a potentially high prevalence of pterygium. A range of sunglasses, some of which float, as well as caps have been developed; however, a casual survey on any surfing beach in Sydney, Australia would suggest that these devices are not widely used. Furthermore, there are other sports such as tennis or cricket where sun exposure may be substantial, and sunglasses are inconvenient because of rapid, sudden movements or perspiration resulting in fogging or lens grime. Participants of these sports often play unprotected and would benefit from a more sophisticated protective strategy.

Contact Lenses

UV-blocking contact lenses may play a significant role in solar protection. Incidentally, contact lenses may cause discomfort in patients with pterygium, and this may be an

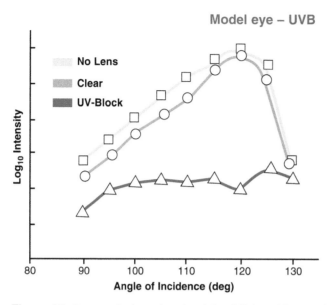

Figure 18 Presents the intensity of peripheral light (arbitrary units) focused at the distal limbus, measured with a UVB detector (□). A conventional 1.50 D contact lens had a slight effect (○). A contact lens of the same 1.50 D optical power and material but with a UV-blocking additive (△) caused a significant reduction in the intensity, but did not show a peak (16).

indication for surgery. An extremely useful role for contact lenses is following pterygium surgery, as a bandage lens—greatly alleviating pain. There is a report of an association of intense UV and contact lens wear, and the development of corneal (limbal) intraepithelial neoplasia (96).

UV-blocking contact lenses have been available for many years (97), but have not been widely adopted (97,98). It has been suggested (99) that this may be due to the longtime lag between UV exposure and disease manifestation, while attitudes to sun exposure may play a role, as for skin protection (100,101).

It may also be that there is a lack of understanding of the light pathways and pathophysiology central to the development of the ophthalmohelioses, since use of UV-blocking contact lenses appears to have no disadvantage yet offers the best ocular protection possible from UV radiation. In recent years, there has however been a resurgence of interest with the development of better contact lenses (102–105) as well as a better understanding of the advantages they offer in relation to the specific ocular advantage of shielding the limbus to prevent PLF (16,17).

Experiments have been carried out confirming that PLF effects are greatly attenuated by the use of UV-absorbing contact lenses (16). UVA and UVB sensors were placed on the nasal limbus of an anatomically based model eye. The temporal limbus was exposed to a UV light source placed at various angles behind the frontal plane. Peripheral light focusing was quantified with the sensor output. The ensemble was mounted in the orbit of a mannequin head and exposed to sunlight in three insolation environments within the region of Sydney, Australia. Peripheral light focusing for UVA and UVB was determined with no eyewear or with sunglasses and commercially available soft contact lenses, with and without UV-blocking capability (Figs. 18–21).

We (16) demonstrated that the intensity of UVA peaked at approximately 120° incidence, the level at which the UVB response was also at its maximum. The

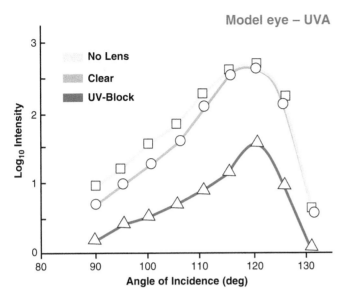

Figure 19 Presents the intensity of peripheral light (arbitrary units) focused at the distal limbus of the aspheric model cornea, measured with a UVA detector (□). A conventional 1.50 D contact lens had a slight effect at lower angles (○). The intensity was significantly reduced in the presence of a contact lens of the same 1.50 D optical power and material, but with a UV-blocking additive (△) (16).

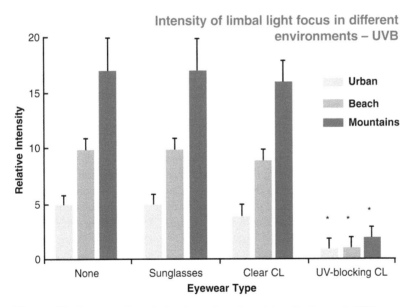

Figure 20 Presents the relative intensity of peripherally focused UVB measured using the mannequin head model in three insolation conditions. In all environments, the UV-blocking contact lens produced significantly lower intensities than no eyewear (*$p < 0.056$) (16).

intensification of UVA was up to 18.3×. The intensity of PLF for UVA and UVB was reduced by an order of magnitude by a UV-blocking contact lens, whereas clear contact lenses had a much lesser effect. Only the UV-blocking contact lens achieved a significant effect on UVA and UVB irradiance in urban, beach, and mountain locales ($p < 0.056$).

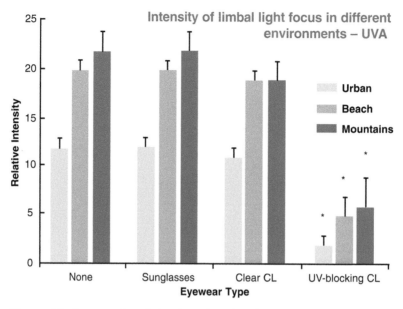

Figure 21 Presents the relative intensity of peripherally focused UVA measured using the mannequin head model in three insolation conditions. In all environments, the UV-blocking contact lens produced significantly lower intensities than no eyewear ($*p < 0.02$) (16).

Experiments have been also carried out demonstrating the PLF of a UV light source in eyes with non-UV-blocking and class 1 and class 2 UV-blocking contact lenses.

A number of studies have clearly identified another type of sunlight hazard: the peripheral focusing of obliquely incident light. UV radiation from albedo (reflected ambient light) is capable of establishing PLF in the anterior segment, but this can be shielded by UV-blocking soft contact lenses. Sunglasses may be unable to shield oblique rays, unless side protection is incorporated. Contact lenses can offer UV protection against all angles of incidence, including the peak-response angle. They can also protect the eye in settings in which the wearing of sunglasses is not feasible or convenient.

However, the external structures of the eye, such as the conjunctiva and the eyelids, remained at risk and would continue to benefit from the use of UV-blocking sunglasses or spectacle lenses.

CONCLUSIONS

Current literature provides strong evidence that the eyes are subject to an increasing risk of damage by UV radiation exposure. It is therefore prudent to consider eye protection against UV radiation, especially those persons who participate in work and leisure activities that expose them to high levels of UV radiation. More recent studies have demonstrated some of the limitations of UV-absorbing spectacle lenses and sunglasses. Contact lenses with UV-blocking characteristics can reduce ocular exposure to the UV radiation implicated in most sun-related disease.

This chapter reviewed the effects of UV radiation on the ocular structures (the limbus, the nasal crystalline lens equator, and the eyelid margin) and discussed the options available to reduce or eliminate the risk of eye damage.

ACKNOWLEDGMENTS

Much of the work described here has been carried out in collaboration with colleagues who have coauthored many of the papers we have published.

I have had collaborations with Professor Denis Wakefield, Dr. Nick Di Girolamo, Dr. Arthur Ho, and Dr. S. Kwok. Funding has been obtained from the National Health and Medical Research Council, the Ophthalmic Research Institute of Australia, and the Rebecca L. Cooper Foundation and from a grant from Johnson & Johnson to specifically study UV-blocking contact lenses. I have no financial interest in any matter discussed here.

REFERENCES

1. Urbach F. Geographic pathology of skin cancer. In: Urbach F, ed. The Biologic Effects of Ultraviolet Radiation. Oxford: Pergamon, 1969:635–650.
2. Sasaki K. International Symposium on the Measurement of Optical Radiation Hazards (MORH) 7 September 1998.
3. Favilla I. Ocular effects of ultraviolet radiation. In Health Effects of Ozone Layer Depletion. Canberra, Australia: Australian Government Publishing Service, 1989:96–113.
4. Davinger M, Evensen A. Role of pericorneal papillary structure in renewal of corneal epithelium. Nature 1971; 229:560–561.
5. Wlodarczyk J, Whyte P, Cockrum P, et al. Pterygium in Australia: a cost of illness study. Clin Experiment Ophthalmol 2001; 29(6):370–375.
6. Javitt JC, Taylor H. Chapter 55: Ocular protection from solar radiation.Duane's Clinical Ophthalmology. Philadelphia: JB Lippincott Co, 1991:1–13.
7. Taylor HR, Hollows FC. Pterygium leading to blindness: a case report. Aust J Ophthalmol 1978; 6:155–156.
8. Fritz MH. Blindness from multiple pterygiums in an Alaskan native. Am J Ophthalmol 1955; 39(4, part 1):572.
9. Sliney DH. The ambient light environment and ocular hazards. In: Landers MB, Wolbarsht ML, Dowling JE, et al. (eds). Retinitis Pigmentosa. New York: Plenum Press, 1977:211–221.
10. Sliney DH. Physical factors in cataractogenesis: ambient ultraviolet radiation and temperature. Invest Ophthalmol Vis Sci 1986; 27(5):781–790.
11. Hedblom EE. Snowscape eye protection. Development of a sunglass for useful vision with comfort from antarctic snowblindness, glare, and calorophthalgia. Arch Environ Health 1961; 2: 685–704.
12. Coroneo MT. Albedo concentration in the anterior eye: a phenomenon that locates some solar diseases. Ophthalmic Surg 1990; 21(1):60–66.
13. Coroneo MT, Muller-Stolzenburg NW, Ho A. Peripheral light focusing by the anterior eye and the ophthalmohelioses. Ophthalmic Surg 1991; 22(12):705–711.
14. Coroneo MT. Pterygium as an early indicator of ultraviolet insolation: a hypothesis. Br J Ophthalmol 1993; 77(11):734–739.
15. Maloof AJ, Ho A, Coroneo MT. Influence of corneal shape on limbal light focusing. Invest Ophthalmol Vis Sci 1994; 35(5):2592–2598.
16. Kwok LS, Kuznetsov VA, Ho A, et al. Prevention of the adverse photic effects of peripheral light-focusing using UV-blocking contact lenses. Invest Ophthalmol Vis Sci 2003; 44(4): 1501–1507.

17. Kwok LS, Daszynski DC, Kuznetsov VA, et al. Peripheral light focusing as a potential mechanism for phakic dysphotopsia and lens phototoxicity. Ophthalmic Physiol Opt 2004; 24: 119–129.

18. von Helmoltz H. Treatise on physiological optics, From the third German edition. In: Southall JPC, ed. Vols 1 and 12. Mechanism of Accommodation. New York: Dover Publications, 1962:143–172.

19. Graves B. Diseases of the cornea. In: Berens C, ed. The Eye and its Diseases. Philadelphia: WB Saunders, 1936:443–557.

20. Mackevicius L. Pterygium. Probable etiology due to persistent photothermal microtrauma. Arch Oftalmol B Aires 1968; 43(5):126–130.

21. Rizzuti AB. Diagnostic illumination test for keratoconus. Am J Ophthalmol 1970; 70(1):141–143.

22. Taylor RL, Hanks MA. Developmental changes in precursor lesions of bovine ocular carcinoma. Vet Med Small Anim Clin 1972; 67(6):669–671.

23. Arenas E. Etiopatologia de la pinguecula y el pterigio. Pal Oftalmol Panam 1978; 2:28–31.

24. Coroneo MT, Di Girolamo N, Wakefield D. The pathogenesis of pterygia. Curr Opin Ophthalmol 1999; 10(4):282–288.

25. Di Girolamo N, Chui J, Coroneo MT, et al. Pathogenesis of pterygia: role of cytokines, growth factors, and matrix metalloproteinases. Prog Retin Eye Res 2004; 23:195–228.

26. Figuera E, Wakefield D, Coroneo MT. Ocular Stem Cells. (In preparation)

27. Tseng SC, Tsubota K. Important concepts for treating ocular surface and tear disorders. Am J Ophthalmol 1997; 124(6):825–835.

28. Hoover HL. Solar ultraviolet radiation—irradiation of the human cornea, lens, and retina—equations of ocular irradiation. Appl Opt 1986; 25:359–368.

29. Podskochy A. Protective role of corneal pithelium against ultraviolet radiation damage. Acta Ophthalmol Scand 2004; 82(6):714–717.

30. Mootha VV, Pingree M, Jaramillo J. Pterygia with deep corneal changes. Cornea 2004; 23(6): 635–638.

31. Bron AJ. Vortex patterns of the corneal epithelium. Trans Ophthalmol Soc U K. 1973; 93(0): 455–472.

32. Every SG, Leader JP, Molteno AC, et al. Ultraviolet photography of the in vivo human cornea unmasks the hudson-stahli line and physiologic vortex patterns. Invest Ophthalmol Vis Sci 2005; 46(10):3616–3612.

33. Sharma A, Coles WH. Kinetics of corneal epithelial maintenance and graft loss. A population balance model. Invest Ophthalmol Vis Sci 1989; 30(9):1962–1971.

34. Kwok LS, Coroneo MT. A model for pterygium formation. Cornea 1994; 13(3):219–224.

35. Vajdic CM, Kricker A, Giblin M, et al. Incidence of ocular melanoma in Australia from 1990 to 1998. Int J Cancer 2003; 105(1):117–122.

36. Detels R, Dhir SP. Pterygium: a geographical study. Arch Ophthalmol 1967; 78(4):485–491.

37. Wu K, He M, Xu J, et al. Pterygium in aged population in Doumen County, China. Yan Ke Xue Bao 2002; 18(3):181–184.

38. Handmann M. Ueber den Beginn des Altersstares in der unteren Linsenhälfte. Klinisch-statistische Studien an 845 Augen mit Cataracta senilis incipiens nebst Bemerkungen über die Cataracta glaukomatosa und diabetica. Klin Montsbl Augenheilkd 1909; 47:692–720.

39. Saad R. Pterygium, pinguecula and visual acuity. Aust J Ophthalmol 1977; 5:52–66.

40. Woodcock M, Huntbach J, Scott R. A case of a uniocular pterygium related to an unusual occupation. J R Army Med Corps 2003; 149(1):56–57.

41. Jensen OL. Pterygium, the dominant eye and the habit of closing one eye in sunlight. Acta Ophthalmol (Copenh) 1982; 60(4):568–574.

42. Ooi JL, Sharma NS, Papalkar D, et al. Ultraviolet fluorescence photography to detect early sun damage in the eyes of school-aged children. Am J Ophthalmol 2006; 141:294–298.

43. Ooi JL, Sharma NS, Sharma S, et al. Ultraviolet fluorescence photography: patterns in established pterygia. Am J Ophthalmol 2007; 143:97–101.

44. Mackenzie FD, Hirst LW, Battistutta D, et al. Risk analysis in the development of pterygia. Ophthalmology 1992; 99:1056–1061.

45. Lee GA, Hirst LW, Sheehan M. Knowledge of sunlight effects on the eyes and protective behaviors in adolescents. Ophthalmic Epidemiol 1999; 6:171–180.

46. Cokkinides VE, Johnston-Davis K, Weinstock M, et al. Sun exposure and sun-protection behaviors and attitudes among U.S. youth, 11 to 18 years of age. Prev Med 2001; 33:141–151.

47. Livingston PM, White V, Hayman J, et al. Australian adolescents' sun protection behavior: who are we kidding? Prev Med 2007; 44:508–512.

48. Duke-Elder S, MacFaul PA. Chapter X. Radiational injuries. In: Duke-Elder S, ed. System of Ophthalmology. Vol XIV, Injuries, Part 2, Non-Mechanical Injuries. London: Henry Kimpton, 1972:912–933.

49. Brailey WA. On some points in the development of cataract. Trans Ophthalmol Soc U K 1891; 11: 66–69.

50. Jackson E. A Manual of the Diagnosis and Treatment of the Diseases of the Eye. Philadelphia: WB Saunders, 1900:412.

51. Greene DW. The association of age and incipient cataract with normal and pathologic blood pressure. J Am Med Assoc 1908; 51:400–405.

52. Schild H. Untersuchungen über die Häufigkeit der lamellaren Zerkluftung, ihre Lage und Verlaufsrichtung in der vorderen und hinteren Linsenrinde an 218 Augen sonst gesunder Personen. Arch Ophthalmol 1922; 107:49–60.

53. Clapp CA. Senile Cataract. Cataract: Its Etiology and Treatment. Philadelphia: Lea & Febiger, 1934:127–134.

54. Berlyne ML. Presenile and senile cataract. Biomicroscopy of the Eye: Slit Lamp Microscopy of the Living Eye, Vol II. New York: Hafner, 1949 (reprinted 1966):1121.

55. Kirby DB. Basic science applied to cataract surgery. Surgery of Cataract. Philadelphia, JB: Lippincott, 1950:75.

56. Coroneo MT. Albedo concentration and eye disease. 18th Annual Scientific Congress, The Royal Australian College of Ophthalmologists, 1986:85.

57. Maloof AJ, Ho A, Coroneo MT. Anterior segment peripheral light concentration and the crystalline lens. Invest Ophthalmol Vis Sci 35:1327 (abstr. 332).

58. Klein BE, Klein R, Linton KL. Prevalence of age-related lens opacities in a population. The Beaver Dam Eye Study. Ophthalmology 1992; 99(4):546–552.

59. Sample PA, Quirante JS, Weinreb RN. Age-related changes in the human lens. Clinical assessment of age-related changes in the human lens. Acta Ophthalmol (Copenh) 1991; 69(3): 310–314.

60. Adamsons I, Munoz B, Enger C, et al. Prevalence of lens opacities in surgical and general populations. Arch Ophthalmol 1991; 109(7):993–997.

61. Schein OD, West S, Munoz B, et al. Cortical lenticular opacification: distribution and location in a longitudinal study. Invest Ophthalmol Vis Sci 1994; 35(2):363–366.

62. Sharma YR, Vajpayee RB, Honavar SG. Sunlight and cortical cataract. Arch Environ Health 1994; 49(5):414–417.

63. Graziosi P, Rosmini F, Bonacini M, et al. Location and severity of cortical opacities in different regions of the lens in age-related cataract. Invest Ophthalmol Vis Sci 1996; 37(8):1698–1703.

64. Mitchell P, Cumming RG, Attebo K, et al. Prevalence of cataract in Australia: the Blue Mountains eye study. Ophthalmology 1997; 104(4):581–588.

65. Rochtchina E, Mitchell P, Coroneo M, et al. Lower nasal distribution of cortical cataract: the Blue Mountains Eye Study. Clin Experiment Ophthalmol 2001; 29(3):111–115.

66. Kawakami Y, Sasaki H, Jonasson F, et al. Reykjavik Eye Study Group. Characteristics and frequency of cortical cataracts at an early stage (Reykjavik Eye Study in Iceland). Klin Monatsbl Augenheilkd 2001; 218(2):78–84.

67. Sasaki H, Kawakami Y, Ono M, et al. Localization of cortical cataract in subjects of diverse races and latitude. Invest Ophthalmol Vis Sci 2003; 44(10):4210–4214.

68. Brown NP, Harris ML, Shun-Shin GA, et al. Is cortical spoke cataract due to lens fibre breaks? The relationship between fibre folds, fibre breaks, waterclefts and spoke cataract. Eye 1993; 7(pt 5): 672–679.

69. Lofgren S, Ayala M, Kakar M, et al. UVR cataract after regional in vitro lens exposure. Invest Ophthalmol Vis Sci 2002; 43:E-Abstract 3577.

70. Kwok LS, Coroneo MT. Temporal and spatial growth patterns in the normal and cataractous human lens. Exp Eye Res 2000; 71(3):317–322.

71. Coroneo MT, Pham T, Kwok LS. Off-axis edge glare in pseudophakic dysphotopsia. J Cataract Refract Surg 2003; 29(10):1969–1973.

72. Davison JA. Positive and negative dysphotopsia in patients with acrylic intraocular lenses. J Cataract Refract Surg 2000; 26:1346–1355.

73. Reifler DM, Hornblass A. Squamous cell carcinoma of the eyelid. Surv Ophthalmol 1986; 30(6): 349–365.

74. Lindgren G, Diffey BL, Larko O. Basal cell carcinoma of the eyelids and solar ultraviolet radiation exposure. Br J Ophthalmol 1998; 82(12):1412–1415.

75. Allali J, D'Hermies F, Renard G. Basal cell carcinomas of the eyelids. Ophthalmologica 2005; 219(2):57–71.

76. Sliney DH. Epidemiological studies of sunlight and cataract: the critical factor of ultraviolet exposure geometry. Ophthalmic Epidemiol 1994; 1(2):107–119.

77. Sliney DH. UV radiation ocular exposure dosimetry. Doc Ophthalmol 1994–1995; 88(3–4): 243–254.

78. Sliney DH. UV radiation ocular exposure dosimetry. J Photochem Photobiol B. 1995; 31(1–2): 69–77.

79. Sliney DH. Ocular exposure to environmental light and ultraviolet—the impact of lid opening and sky conditions. Dev Ophthalmol 1997; 27:63–75.

80. Sliney DH. Geometrical assessment of ocular exposure to environmental UV radiation—implications for ophthalmic epidemiology. J Epidemiol 1999; 9(6 suppl):S22–S32.

81. Sliney DH. The focusing of ultraviolet radiation in the eye and ocular exposure. In: Taylor HR, ed. Pterygium. The Hague: Kugler, 2000:29–40.

82. Sliney DH. Geometrical gradients in the distribution of temperature and absorbed ultraviolet radiation in ocular tissues. Dev Ophthalmol 2002; 35:40–59.

83. Sliney DH. How light reaches the eye and its components. Int J Toxicol 2002; 21(6):501–509.

84. Sliney DH. Exposure geometry and spectral environment determine photobiological effects on the human eye. Photochem Photobiol 2005; 81(3):483–489.

85. Cullen A. International Symposium on the Measurement of Optical Radiation Hazards (MORH) 7 September 1998.

86. Dain SJ. Sunglasses and sunglass standards. Clin Exp Optom 2003; 86(2):77–90.

87. Hollows FC. Ultraviolet radiation and eye diseases. Trans Menzies Foundation 1989; 15: 113–117.

88. Krengel S. Wearing sunglasses a risk factor for the development of cutaneous malignant melanoma? Int J Dermatol 2002; 41(3):191–192.

89. Threlfall TJ. Sunglasses and clothing—an unhealthy correlation? Aust J Public Health 1992; 16: 92–196.

90. Deaver DM, Davis J, Sliney DH. Vertical visual fields-of-view in outdoor daylight. Lasers Light Ophthalmol 1996; 7(2/3):121–125.

91. Sliney DH. Photoprotection of the eye—UV radiation and sunglasses. J Photochem Photobiol B. 2001 Nov 15; 64(2–3):166–75.

92. Morris A, Temme LA, Hamilton PV. Visual acuity of the U.S. Navy jet pilot and the use of the helmet sun visor. Aviat Space Environ Med 1991; 62(8):715–721.

93. Dille JR, Marano JA. The effects of spectacle frames on field of vision. Aviat Space Environ Med 1984; 55(10):957–959.

94. Rosenthal FS, Bakalian AE, Lou CQ, et al. The effect of sunglasses on ocular exposure to ultraviolet radiation. Am J Public Health 1988; 78(1):72–74.

95. Steel SE, Mackie SW, Walsh G. Visual field defects due to spectacle frames: their prediction and relationship to UK driving standards. Ophthalmic Physiol Opt 1996; 16(2):95–100.

96. Guex-Crosier Y, Herbort CP. Presumed corneal intraepithelial neoplasia associated with contact lens wear and intense ultraviolet light exposure. Br J Ophthalmol 1993; 77(3):191–192.

97. Bergmanson JP, Pitts DG, Chu LW. The efficacy of a UV-blocking soft contact lens in protecting cornea against UV radiation. Acta Ophthalmol (Copenh) 1987; 65(3):279–286.

98. Bergmanson JP, Pitts DG, Chu LW. Protection from harmful UV radiation by contact lenses. J Am Optom Assoc 1988; 59(3):178–182.

99. Bergmanson JP, Walsh JE, Harmey J. UV overdose vs hyperoxia. Eye Contact Lens 2005; 31 (3):95.

100. Hillhouse J, Turrisi R. Skin cancer risk behaviors: a conceptual framework for complex behavioral change. Arch Dermatol 2005; 141(8):1028–1031.

101. Naylor M, Robinson JK. Sunscreen, sun protection, and our many failures. Arch Dermatol 2005; 141(8):1025–1027.

102. Hickson-Curran SB, Nason RJ, Becherer PD, et al. Clinical evaluation of ACUVUE contact lenses with UV blocking characteristics. Optom Vis Sci 1997; 74(8):632–638.

103. Giasson CJ, Quesnel NM, Boisjoly H. The ABCs of ultraviolet-blocking contact lenses: an ocular panacea for ozone loss? Int Ophthalmol Clin 2005; 45(1):117–139.

104. Walsh JE, Bergmanson JP, Saldana G Jr., et al. Can UV radiation-blocking soft contact lenses attenuate UV radiation to safe levels during summer months in the southern United States? Eye Contact Lens 2003; 29(1 suppl):S174–S179; (discussion S190–S191, S192–S194. Erratum in: Eye Contact Lens 2003; 29(2):135).

105. Walsh JE, Bergmanson JP, Wallace D, et al. Quantification of the ultraviolet radiation (UVR) field in the human eye in vivo using novel instrumentation and the potential benefits of UVR blocking hydrogel contact lens. Br J Ophthalmol 2001; 85(9):1080–1085.

20
Public Education in Photoprotection

Steven Q. Wang and Allan C. Halpern
Memorial Sloan-Kettering Cancer Center, Dermatology Division, New York, New York, U.S.A.

SYNOPSIS

- A successful public health message must be consistent and straightforward, easy to understand, and simple to repeat.
- There are two major motivating factors in photoprotection campaign: health based (focusing on skin cancers) and appearance based (focusing on photoaging); each appeals to different demographics.
- Message for photoprotection is as follows: sun avoidance; seeking shade; and the use of protective clothing, hat, and sunscreens.
- National and state governments should play a more active role in creating favorable legislative policies, while fashion and beauty industries should be recruited to change public perception on the perceived attractiveness associated with tanned skin.

INTRODUCTION

Skin cancer is the most common type of cancer in the United States. There are more than one million new cases diagnosed each year (1). Basal cell carcinoma (BCC) accounts for more than 75% of the total number of skin cancers and squamous cell carcinoma (SCC) constitutes 15%. Although both skin cancers can be treated effectively with topical medication, radiation, or surgery, unchecked growth of BCC and SCC can lead to local destruction and functional impairment. Advanced stages of SCC can spread and metastasize. Melanoma (MM) only constitutes 5% of the skin cancers but is more deadly. Over the last few decades, the incidence of MM has been increasing steadily. In 2008, it is estimated that there will be 62,480 newly diagnosed MMs, and 8420 deaths from this cancer (1). Currently, there is no effective cure for advanced disease; only early diagnosis followed by prompt excision ensures a good prognosis.

Ultraviolet (UV) exposure from the sun has been attributed as a major culprit for causing skin cancer (2–5). UVB (290–320 nm) is the major wavelength for causing sunburn, and it directly damages the cellular DNA leading to the formation of the 6-4 cyclobutane pyrimidine dimers. UVA (320–400 nm) has longer wavelengths, and there are more UVA rays reaching the earth's surface. Compared with UVB, UVA penetrates deeper into the skin tissue (6). It interacts with endogenous and exogenous photo-sensitizers and generates reactive oxygen species (ROS) that damage the DNA bases and cause cellular mutations (7–11). Chronic UV exposure leads to the formation of actinic keratosis and SCC, while intermittent exposure has been associated with the development of MM and BCC.

The heavy burden of disease and rising incidence of skin cancers are among the major reasons for the introduction of public campaigns focused on primary prevention. The campaigns educate the public about the harmful effects of excessive UV exposure and various photoprotective measures. Hopefully, this knowledge and insight can motivate the public to change behaviors accordingly, and eventually lead to a decreasing incidence of skin cancers. In this review, we will discuss the message regarding photoprotection, outline the challenges encountered, and highlight a number of solutions ranging from new ideas to those proven to be successful.

THE MESSAGE

In general, there are two components of the message of any public health campaign aimed to change beliefs and behaviors of a large group—the motivating factors and the instructions. The motivating factors should be tailored to target different demographic groups, while the instruction should be easy to comply. A successful message must be consistent and straightforward, while at the same time easy to understand and simple to repeat. Lastly, a successful message should appeal to an individual's intellectual and emotional receptivity.

Motivating Factors

There are two major motivating factors in the campaign for promoting photoprotection—health based and appearance based. The rising incidence and burden of disease associated with skin cancer remain the major reasons compelling the launch of various public education programs for photoprotection. The health-based factor emphasizes the risk of skin cancer associated with UV exposure. It focuses on morbidity and mortality. Health care providers, e.g., dermatologists, have long emphasized the need for photoprotection to patients with histories or risks of skin cancers. Nonprofit organizations, such as the American Academy of Dermatology (AAD), the Skin Cancer Foundation, and the American Cancer Society have launched various programs to highlight the danger of skin cancers. For the most part, the health-based approach has received the most attention for it is more relevant and direct to serve the ultimate goal of the campaign, i.e., reducing skin cancer. This approach typically works well with individuals who have personal or family histories of skin cancers. It may not, however, be effective for other segments of the population, such as elderly men and young adults. Older men tend to be generally resistant to health promotion messages. For young adults, the harmful impact of skin cancer may be too distant in their minds to have an immediate effect that would change their current behavior.

In addition to the health-based approach, the appearance-based approach has gained more traction in the recent years, along with a general growing acceptance and interest in cosmetic procedures and antiaging products. This approach highlights all the harmful effects of photoaging, ranging from the formation of dyspigmentation to the appearance of skin wrinkles. It also stresses on the importance of photoprotection as the basis for slowing the process of photoaging. This approach is very effective in reaching the segments of the population that are neither influenced by nor convinced of the risk of skin cancers. A number of studies (12–18) have demonstrated that interventions based on this approach may be more effective than health warnings alone.

In sum, the two sets of different but complementary motives are powerful incentives to change the public's behavior and interaction with the sun. These influences can be used to target different segments of the population.

The Instructions

In the United States, the instructional component of the message for photoprotection involves a series of actions in the following order of importance: sun avoidance; seeking shade; and the use of protective clothing, hat, and sunscreens (Table 1). On a casual glance, the instructions seem straightforward. It can quickly be conveyed by health care providers to their patients or disseminated by the media to the public. On careful review, however, these instructions face a number of challenges in achieving public compliance.

Sun avoidance by definition is the best means to reduce UV exposure, but compliance for most individuals is not easy. There are a number of health benefits associated with sunshine, and active lifestyles involving outdoor activities improve physiologic and emotional state of well being. Furthermore, daily sunlight exposure helps to generate adequate vitamin D. Aside from the health benefit, our current beauty perception identifies tan skin as attractive. This misguided perception is a powerful incentive for individuals to be tanned, let alone practicing sun avoidance. Realizing that total abstinence from sun exposure is not an achievable goal nor desirable for most people, the public has been instructed to limit or minimize UV exposure from the sun during the peak hours (i.e., 10 a.m.–4 p.m.), because the UV rays are most intense during this time period.

Table 1 **Simple Guideline for Photoprotection**

1. Minimize sun exposure and seek shade during 10 a.m.–4 p.m. when the sun is the strongest. Plan outdoor activities for the early morning or late afternoon.
2. Wear a wide-brim hat, long sleeved shirt, and long pants when out in the sun. Tightly woven materials with dark colors offer greater sun protection.
3. Apply sunscreen 20–30 min before going outdoor. Reapply at least every 2 h as long as you stay in the sun. Remember to use sunscreen even on overcast days.
4. Beware of reflective surfaces, such as sand, snow, concrete, and water.
5. Beware of high altitude places, because there is less atmosphere to absorb the UV rays.
6. Avoid tanning salons.
7. Keep infants out of the sun.
8. Teach children sun protection early. Sun damage occurs with each unprotected sun exposure and accumulates over the course of a lifetime.
9. Protect your eyes and your skin. Do not forget to wear UV-filtered sunglasses.
10. Watch for the UV index.

Abbreviation: UV, ultraviolet.

Seeking shade is the next best option for individuals who enjoy the outdoors, while still having a sufficient amount of photoprotection. In Australia, where incidence of skin cancer is higher, shade structures are installed over playgrounds, over pools, and in community centers. Shade trees are planted to block UV exposure from the sun. In the United States, however, such measures only take place in few local communities championed by private citizens and nonprofit organizations, but are not adequately funded by local or national government agencies.

Protective clothing and hats are very effective in blocking UV rays. Tightly weaved clothing with particular fabrics offer excellent UV protection. A number of manufacturers in the United States are producing comfortable and breezy clothing articles that offer high UV protection factor. Wide-brim hats are also important as they can extend coverage over the scalp, forehead, cheek, nose, ears, and neck, all the anatomic sites predisposed to skin cancers. The use of clothing articles for protection has been widely accepted in Australia. Schools have "no hat—no play" policies restricting children without hats from playing outdoors. In the United States, the public has begun to use these articles for protection, especially for kids. Compared with sunscreens, clothing provides a more uniformed blockage of both UVB and UVA rays. In addition, there is no need for reapplication.

Although sunscreen is less effective in preventing UV exposure compared with the above-mentioned strategies, it is the most employed action by the public for photoprotection. A frequent question from patients with histories of skin cancer is "Doctor, so what sunscreens should I use?" This often is the first and only question on their minds when they think about photoprotection. While sunscreen use is important, one should not ignore the need for sun avoidance, seeking shade, and using clothing and hats. This perception of the dominant importance of sunscreen may be the result of market force. Sunscreen sales command an annual revenue of more than one billion dollars in the United States. The sunscreen and cosmetic companies actively promote their products to the public. In contrast, there is little commercial interest in lobbying for sun avoidance, seeking shade, or wearing hats and clothing. Aside from the market force, educators and health care providers also tend to highlight the importance of sunscreen use to their patients on the basis of the observation that it is most likely to be adopted into daily practice. Survey studies examining skin cancer prevention education by pediatricians showed that more pediatricians recommend using sunscreen than wearing clothing and seeking shade (19–21). In sum, the preferred sequence of photoprotection action may be distorted when the message reaches the public. Many individuals use sunscreens as their first line of defense for photoprotection while ignoring sun avoidance practices and using protective clothing.

There are two major hazards in singling out sunscreens as the most important element in photoprotection. First, people do not apply an adequate amount of sunscreen to achieve the desired protection. In the laboratory setting for testing the sun protection factor (SPF) value of sunscreen products, a 2-mg/cm^2 concentration of sunscreen is applied to the subject. However, in real life, most people use much less, i.e., 0.5 to 1 mg/cm^2 (22). To achieve adequate and consistent protection, sunscreens need to be applied 20 to 30 minutes prior to outdoor exposure, and with outdoor activity, reapplied every two hours. Most people do not follow these guidelines. Hence, consumers who use a product with an SPF of 30 may only receive an SPF 15 or less (22). Second, in the United States, the only numerical efficacy rating for sunscreen is the SPF. It is measured on the basis of an in vivo test that assesses protection against sunburn or erythema, a biological response produced mainly by UVB. The SPF value offers no clear indication on the degree of protection against UVA. Although most sunscreen products sold in the United States claim to have broad-spectrum UVA coverage, the extent and magnitude of UVA protection is neither measured nor assessed. Until recently, many products in the United States only offered limited UVA protection (23). Hence, while consumers wearing sunscreen with high SPF can stay out in the sun longer, they may inadvertently receive a large dose of UVA exposure that can induce reactive oxygen-mediated damage to cells and tissues.

THE MESSENGERS

Health Care Providers

Efforts to disseminate photoprotection knowledge and change public behavior are carried out by a host of participants, each with his/her own strengths and limitations. Physicians are the most obvious candidates because of their authoritative status and medical knowledge. Among the different specialties, dermatologists are the most qualified and experienced in delivering the message (24), and the majority of dermatologists believe that counseling their patients about photoprotection is important. Furthermore, as skin specialists, dermatologists can influence their patients using both health-based and appearance-based motives. An annual examination for skin cancer or laser treatment for removal of solar lentigines would be ideal situations to emphasize the need for adequate photoprotection. Unfortunately, in actual practice, not all patients receive such counsel from their dermatologists. In a study by Polster et al. (25), only 27% of the surveyed patients reported that their dermatologists counseled them about the risk of sun exposure. Feldman et al. (24) found that dermatologists only provided counseling 41% of time for high-risk skin cancer patients. The frequency of counseling was much lower, 22%, for all patients' visit.

Pediatricians are another important group engaged in the effort to disseminate photoprotection knowledge and change public behavior because of their interaction with kids and teenagers. Childhood exposure to UV radiation increases the risk for skin cancer as an adult, and childhood education determines lifelong habits regarding sun protection. Therefore, sun prevention in childhood is very important to prevent skin cancer later in life. Yet despite increased public education, studies (26) show that nearly 43% of children aged less than 11 years had experienced a sunburn within the past year of the survey. To reach this segment of the public, pediatricians are the ideal candidates. Approximately 60% of surveyed pediatricians have reported that they usually or always counsel about sun protection (19,27). Most, however, recommend sunscreen use over sun avoidance, shade seeking, and protective clothing.

Family practice (FP) and general practice (GP) physicians provide comprehensive care for patients. Ideally, they can provide primary and secondary prevention efforts (i.e., education and self-examination) for patients who may not have access to dermatologists. Annual examinations would be a timely opportunity to deliver the message regarding the harms associated with excessive UV exposure. Very few patients, however, report that such counsel was given by their GPs. Feldman et al. (24) showed an approximate 1% instance of counseling in office visits by GPs and FPs.

In general, physicians of nearly all specialties agree that counseling on photoprotection is a good idea, but a very small percentage of them actually provide the education in practice. A number of explanations are offered for the gap between perceived good care and actual practice, those ranging from simply not remembering to lack of knowledge. The crucial barrier, however, is lack of time and incentive (28,29). These obstacles are especially evident for GPs and pediatricians who are additionally pushed to perform other screenings to address urgent health issues. Some approaches to resolve these hurdles include using nurses or other health care extenders to perform the education. Although these are reasonable substitutions, direct verbal communication, and education from physicians remain more influential in changing patients' actual behaviors (27,30).

Media and Organizations

The role of media and organizations in this health campaign cannot be underestimated. The public receives most of its knowledge regarding the risk of UV exposure and the need for photoprotection from the media through television, radio, newspaper, posters, magazines, and the Internet. Polster et al. (25) have shown that more patients obtained sun protection knowledge from the media than from their dermatologists. Since media is yet to achieve the desired results, messages need be broadcasted repeatedly over an extended duration, a practice requiring sustained effort and funding.

The major supporters for this effort are government agencies, the sunscreen industry, and nonprofit organizations such as the AAD, the Skin Cancer Foundation, and the American Cancer Society. In contrast to antismoking campaigns, there are no paid advertisements condemning the harm of excessive UV exposure from sun or tanning salons. Advertisements from the sunscreen industry and clothing companies can be seen in printed media or on the Internet, but they lack the sensational effects seen in antismoking advertisements.

The government and various nonprofit organizations have created a number of successful programs and curricula to promote healthy sun behaviors. The SunWise School Program, developed by the U.S. Environmental Protection Agency (EPA) is the first national educational program for sun safety of children in elementary and middle schools (31). The overall goal was to provide sun protection education to at least 20% of the nation's school children. The program uses classroom-based, school-based, and community-based approaches to educate children. Other projects involved the collaboration of a number of governmental agencies. For example, the EPA has partnered with the National Weather Service to include UV index forecasts for large U.S. cities. The UV index information has become widely available to the public. Other efforts have led to the designation of the first Monday in May as "Melanoma Monday" and May as skin cancer awareness month. This has created a recurring opportunity to reach out and educate the public at the beginning of every summer. In addition, each May, the AAD and various other dermatologic organizations combine their efforts to provide free skin cancer screening for the public. These screening sessions have also been the venues for pubic education on photoprotection.

In summary, the messengers in this public campaign include health care providers, media, government agencies, and nonprofit organizations. Each has an important and complementary role in educating the public.

CHALLENGES

Over the past decades, knowledge about the risks of sun exposure and behaviors for photoprotection, specifically sunscreen use, has improved (32–34). There are, however, several areas where additional improvement is needed. A number of studies showed that 50% of children and adults do not protect themselves adequately from UV exposure (35–42). Children and teenagers have become the most difficult demographic group to reach because they do not adopt healthy sun-protective behaviors. In a cross-sectional survey of 10,000 U.S. teenagers, 83% of the responders had at a least one sunburn during the past summer, and 36% had three or more sunburns (43). Less then 40% used sunscreens. More alarmingly, 25% of girls aged 15 to 18 years had used a tanning bed.

The poor protection behavior in teenagers and certain segments of the adult population can be attributed to a number of factors. Some of these have already been discussed in the above sections. The major reason, however, is the disconnect between knowledge and behavior (44,45). In general, the public has comprehended the message about the harmful effects of excessive UV exposure. The beneficial relationship between practicing sun-safe behavior and reducing the risks of skin cancer is sensible and easy to accept. The difficulty lies in adopting these behaviors accordingly. As Jones et al. (46) demonstrated in their study, 90% of surveyed participants knew sun exposure was a major risk factor for skin cancer, and 95% knew that sun beds were not a safe way to tan. Despite the knowledge, less than 20% used sunscreen on regular basis, and 30% had used or were currently using sun beds.

This disconnect between knowledge and behavior exists in other health prevention programs, such as antismoking and blood pressure control education. Why does such a gap exist? Better yet, what are the barriers that impede individuals from changing their behaviors after gaining the insight? Answers to these questions need to be placed within the context and understanding of behavior modification (47). In the first stage of behavior modification (i.e., pre-contemplation), individuals have not identified the need to change. These can be corrected with education and knowledge. In most behavior modification programs, this, perhaps, is the easiest step. Photoprotection education over the past decades should be viewed as effective in this regard.

Moving beyond this step, individuals proceed to the next three stages: contemplation, action, and maintenance. At each of these stages, unique barriers to altering behaviors may exist for different segments of the public. Individuals at the contemplation stage have already understood the potential harms associated with UV, but they may feel that these risks are not applicable to them. This "won't happen to me" attitude is especially prevalent in teenagers who are healthy, energetic, and feel invincible, a combination making most of them more risk prone. Furthermore, the thought of skin cancer and its associated morbidity are too distant to influence these young people.

Individuals moving beyond the contemplation stage into the action and maintenance phases face different challenges. In photoprotection, the return on behavior modification is not immediate or easily noticeable. Daily use of sunscreens by middle-aged men with a long history of sun exposure may not dramatically reduce new cases of actinic keratoses or skin cancers in a short period. Similarly, daily photoprotection practice may not reverse signs of photoaging for appearance-conscious women. Lack of immediate "rewards" or noticeable results can decrease the motivation needed to maintain lifelong practice. In sum, effort, time, discipline, and repeat motivations are needed to sustain continued behavior modification. Hence, it is difficult for individuals to practice a healthy photoprotection lifestyle even though they understand the risks and benefit of these lifestyle modifications.

SOLUTIONS

Ongoing public education on photoprotection is needed as the primary prevention measure to reduce the incidence of skin cancer. To effectively improve behavior changes, we need alternative strategies and programs beyond current public education campaigns. New government policies and legislations can play a major role in promoting photoprotection behavior. Educational departments at the state level, especially in the sunny southern states in the United States, should adopt the Australian "no hat—no play" policy. By restricting children who do not have hats from playing outdoors, this simple rule will be far more effective than any educational message in keeping kids from receiving excessive UV exposure during the peak hours. Tax incentives can be another area of exploration. The government can reduce or remove all taxations on sunscreens or protective clothing, which will in turn remove price as a potential barrier for healthy photoprotective behavior. In contrast, the government should increase tax on all tanning salons, like the tax hikes imposed on the cigarette industry. The increased tax revenue can possibly be used to fund sun safety education and shade structures in public venues. Last, legislations on restricting teenagers from using tanning salons without parental consent can be adopted on a nationwide basis. Currently, only a selective number of states have this requirement. Although these policies are difficult to implement, success in any of the above proposals can have a profound impact on behavior modifications for millions of individuals.

While we wait for sweeping policy changes, we need to develop and focus on interventions that facilitate both education and behavioral changes at the same time. Education messages alone are not adequate in bringing changes to behavior. Furthermore, the interventions need to have multiple components to be more effective in changing behaviors. Adopting such an intervention strategy has proven to be effective in primary school and recreational settings (48). In the primary school setting, children received interactive didactic sessions and take-home activities about sun protection. In addition, parents were given brochures and involved in sessions to develop sun protection plans. These interventions improved behaviors (48,49). In tourism and pool settings, interventions included sun safety training, interactive activities, programs for parents, and providing shaded areas and sunscreen for the participants. Collectively, these actions improved covering-up behavior (48,50,51). The successes of these interventions are based on the principles of social cognitive theory, role modeling, and environmental support.

Apart from multicomponent interventions, actions and messages relying on appearance-based motives should also be emphasized. In comparison to health-based messages, appearance-based messages may have far more reaching impact (12–18). Visual components, such as UV photographs (15,52), can be used to reveal the underlying photodamages that may not be visible on casual glance. Seeing those images can potentially provide an inducement for individuals to modify behaviors. More importantly, a paradigm shift is needed in our society's characterization of beauty. There is a pervasive feeling in our popular culture today that a baseline tan connotes a sense of health, beauty, and even affluence. This must be changed. The fashion and entertainment industries need to lead this effort, because they invariably set the trend in defining beauty. Although the change will not be an overnight process, a number of fashion editors have endorsed the concepts in the Skin Cancer Foundation's campaign—"Go with your own glow." As hinted in the name of the campaign, it attempts to promote the message that one does not need to tan to feel or look attractive. To the skeptics of such campaigns, it is important to mention that it was not too long ago that individuals with fair skin were considered attractive and affluent. It was only at the beginning of the 20th century that this fashion sense changed in the Western world. In Asia, however, fair-skinned complexion is still preferred, and women use sunscreens and even carry umbrellas to protect themselves from the sun. We need this pivotal shift in our collective thinking process. The rejection of tanned skin as an attractive quality will be a powerful incentive for a large portion of the public to practice sun-safe behaviors.

Last, the current instructional portion of the photoprotection message is lacking a crucial component—a discussion on the use of antioxidants for protection and repair. The current instruction focuses only on sun avoidance, seeking shade, protective clothing, and the application of sunscreens. Even in best-case scenarios, individuals practicing all of the above behaviors may experience damage from solar exposure. For most individuals who only use sunscreens for protection, the damage will be more substantial because sunscreens do not block or absorb 100% of the UV rays. To preserve the genetic integrity, the resulting DNA mutations need to be repaired almost on a constant basis. A number of natural antioxidants (53–58) exhibit protective and reparative effects against different oxidative stresses. Of course, additional research, especially in vivo studies, are needed to further characterize the topical and oral antioxidant regimens that can provide an extra degree of protection against UV.

CONCLUSIONS

Photoprotection is an important strategy to reduce skin cancers and prevent photoaging. Looking back over the past few decades, the work by health care providers, government agencies, and nonprofit organizations has raised public awareness on the harms associated with excessive UV exposure. The effort and commitment by all players in this public campaign need to be applauded. There is still, however, a long road ahead. By and large, the public understands that healthy photoprotective behaviors involve sun avoidance, seeking shade, protective clothing, and using sunscreens, but a large segment of the population still does not translate this insight into actual behavior modifications. The disconnect between knowledge and behavior is a real challenge. To improve compliance, sustained effort from all parties is needed to continue this public-health campaign. More importantly, national and state governments should play a more active role in creating favorable legislative policies, while fashion and beauty industries should be recruited to change public perception on the perceived attractiveness associated with tanned skin. Successful effort by these two groups has the potential to change behavior patterns in millions of Americans.

REFERENCES

1. Jemal A, Siegel R, Ward E, et al. Cancer statistics. CA Cancer J Clin 2008; 58(2):71–96.
2. Armstrong BK, Kricker A. How much melanoma is caused by sun exposure? Melanoma Res 1993; 3(6):395–401.
3. Gallagher RP, Hill GB, Bajdik CD, et al. Sunlight exposure, pigmentation factors, and risk of nonmelanocytic skin cancer. II. Squamous cell carcinoma. Arch Dermatol 1995; 131(2): 164–169.
4. Gallagher RP, Hill GB, Bajdik CD, et al. Sunlight exposure, pigmentary factors, and risk of nonmelanocytic skin cancer. I. Basal cell carcinoma. Arch Dermatol 1995; 131(2):157–163.
5. Kricker A, Armstrong BK, English DR. Sun exposure and non-melanocytic skin cancer. Cancer Causes Control 1994; 5(4):367–392.
6. Kochevar I, Taylor, CR, Krutmann, J. Fundamentals of cutaneous photobiology and photoimmunology. In: Wolff K, Goldsmith LA, Katz KI, et al., eds. Fitzpatrick's Dermatology in General Medicine. 7th ed. New York: McGraw-Hill, 2008:797–815.
7. Drobetsky EA, Turcotte J, Chateauneuf A. A role for ultraviolet A in solar mutagenesis. Proc Natl Acad Sci U S A 1995; 92(6):2350–2354.
8. Kvam E, Tyrrell RM. Induction of oxidative DNA base damage in human skin cells by UV and near visible radiation. Carcinogenesis 1997; 18(12):2379–2384.
9. Ley RD. Ultraviolet radiation A-induced precursors of cutaneous melanoma in Monodelphis domestica. Cancer Res 1997; 57(17):3682–3684.

10. Setlow RB, Grist E, Thompson K, et al. Wavelengths effective in induction of malignant melanoma. Proc Natl Acad Sci U S A 1993; 90(14):6666–6670.

11. Staberg B, Wulf H, Klemp P, et al. The carcinogenic effect of UVA irradiation. J Invest Dermatol 1983; 81:517–519.

12. Jones JL, Leary MR. Effects of appearance-based admonitions against sun exposure on tanning intentions in young adults. Health Psychol 1994; 13(1):86–90.

13. Keesling B, Friedman HS. Psychosocial factors in sunbathing and sunscreen use. Health Psychol 1987; 6(5):477–493.

14. Mahler HI, Fitzpatrick B, Parker P, et al. The relative effects of a health-based versus an appearance-based intervention designed to increase sunscreen use. Am J Health Promot 1997; 11(6):426–429.

15. Mahler HI, Kulik JA, Gibbons FX, et al. Effects of appearance-based interventions on sun protection intentions and self-reported behaviors. Health Psychol 2003; 22(2):199–209.

16. Miller AG, Ashton WA, McHoskey JW, et al. What price attractiveness? stereotype and risk factors in suntanning behavior. J Appl Soc Psychol 1990; 20:1272–1300.

17. Novick M. To burn or not to burn: use of computer-enhanced stimuli to encourage application of sunscreens. Cutis 1997; 60(2):105–108.

18. Rossi JS, Blais LM, Weinstock MA. The Rhode Island Sun Smart Project: skin cancer prevention reaches the beaches. Am J Public Health 1994; 84(4):672–674.

19. Easton AN, Price JH, Boehm K, et al. Sun protection counseling by pediatricians. Arch Pediatr Adolesc Med 1997; 151(11):1133–1138.

20. Geller AC, Robinson J, Silverman S, et al. Do pediatricians counsel families about sun protection?: a Massachusetts survey. Arch Pediatr Adolesc Med 1998; 152(4):372–376.

21. Gritz ER, Tripp MK, de Moor CA, et al. Skin cancer prevention counseling and clinical practices of pediatricians. Pediatr Dermatol 2003; 20(1):16–24.

22. Faurschou A, Wulf HC. The relation between sun protection factor and amount of suncreen applied in vivo. Br J Dermatol 2007; 156(4):716–719.

23. Diffey BL, Tanner PR, Matts PJ, et al. In vitro assessment of the broad-spectrum ultraviolet protection of sunscreen products. J Am Acad Dermatol 2000; 43(6):1024–1035.

24. Feldman SR, Fleischer AB Jr. Skin examinations and skin cancer prevention counseling by US physicians: a long way to go. J Am Acad Dermatol 2000; 43(2 pt 1):234–237.

25. Polster AM, Lasek RJ, Quinn LM, et al. Reports by patients and dermatologists of skin cancer preventive services provided in dermatology offices. Arch Dermatol 1998; 134(9):1095–1098.

26. Hall HI, McDavid K, Jorgensen CM, et al. Factors associated with sunburn in white children aged 6 months to 11 years. Am J Prev Med 2001; 20(1):9–14.

27. Dietrich AJ, Olson AL, Sox CH, et al. Sun protection counseling for children: primary care practice patterns and effect of an intervention on clinicians. Arch Fam Med 2000; 9(2):155–159.

28. Nutting PA. Health promotion in primary medical care: problems and potential. Prev Med 1986; 15(5):537–548.

29. Wechsler H, Levine S, Idelson RK, et al. The physician's role in health promotion—a survey of primary-care practitioners. N Engl J Med 1983; 308(2):97–100.

30. Dietrich AJ, Olson AL, Sox CH, et al. A community-based randomized trial encouraging sun protection for children. Pediatrics 1998; 102(6):E64.

31. Kyle JW, Hammitt JK, Lim HW, et al. Economic evaluation of the US Environmental Protection Agency's SunWise program: sun protection education for young children. Pediatrics 2008; 121(5):e1074–e1084.

32. Dixon H, Borland R, Hill D. Sun protection and sunburn in primary school children: the influence of age, gender, and coloring. Prev Med 1999; 28(2):119–130.

33. Robinson JK. A 28-year-old fair-skinned woman with multiple moles. JAMA 1997; 278 (20):1693–1699.

34. Centers for Disease Control and Prevention. Sun-protection behaviors used by adults for their children—United States, 1997. MMWR Morb Mortal Wkly Rep 1998; 47(23):480–482.

35. Lovato CY, Shoveller JA, Peters L, et al. Canadian National Survey on Sun Exposure & Protective Behaviours: parents' reports on children. Cancer Prev Control 1998; 2(3):123–128.

36. Lovato CY, Shoveller JA, Peters L, et al. Canadian National Survey on Sun Exposure & Protective Behaviours: youth at leisure. Cancer Prev Control 1998; 2(3):117–122.

37. Lovato CY, Shoveller JA, Peters L, et al. Canadian National Survey on Sun Exposure & Protective Behaviours: methods. Cancer Prev Control 1998; 2(3):105–109.

38. Shoveller JA, Lovato CY, Peters L, et al. Canadian National Survey on Sun Exposure & Protective Behaviours: adults at leisure. Cancer Prev Control 1998; 2(3):111–116.

39. Hall HI, May DS, Lew RA, et al. Sun protection behaviors of the U.S. white population. Prev Med 1997; 26(4):401–407.

40. Buller DB, Andersen PA, Walkosz B. Sun safety behaviours of alpine skiers and snowboarders in the western United States. Cancer Prev Control 1998; 2(3):133–139.

41. Robinson JK, Rademaker AW, Sylvester JA, et al. Summer sun exposure: knowledge, attitudes, and behaviors of Midwest adolescents. Prev Med 1997; 26(3):364–372.

42. Weinstock MA, Rossi JS, Redding CA, et al. Sun protection behaviors and stages of change for the primary prevention of skin cancers among beachgoers in southeastern New England. Ann Behav Med 2000; 22(4):286–293.

43. Geller AC, Colditz G, Oliveria S, et al. Use of sunscreen, sunburning rates, and tanning bed use among more than 10,000 US children and adolescents. Pediatrics 2002; 109(6):1009–1014.

44. Clarke VA, Williams T, Arthey S. Skin type and optimistic bias in relation to the sun protection and suntanning behaviors of young adults. J Behav Med 1997; 20(2):207–222.

45. Arthey S, Clarke VA. Suntanning and sun protection: a review of the psychological literature. Soc Sci Med 1995; 40(2):265–274.

46. Jones B, Oh C, Corkery E, et al. Attitudes and perceptions regarding skin cancer and sun protection behaviour in an Irish population. J Eur Acad Dermatol Venereol 2007; 21(8):1097–1101.

47. Prochaska JO, DiClemente CC. Stages and processes of self-change of smoking: toward an integrative model of change. J Consult Clin Psychol 1983; 51(3):390–395.

48. Glanz K, Halpern AC, Saraiya M. Behavioral and community interventions to prevent skin cancer: what works? Arch Dermatol 2006; 142(3):356–360.

49. Geller AC, Cantor M, Miller DR, et al. The Environmental Protection Agency's National SunWise School Program: sun protection education in US schools (1999–2000). J Am Acad Dermatol 2002; 46(5):683–689.

50. Geller AC, Glanz K, Shigaki D, et al. Impact of skin cancer prevention on outdoor aquatics staff: the Pool Cool program in Hawaii and Massachusetts. Prev Med 2001; 33(3):155–161.

51. Glanz K, Geller AC, Shigaki D, et al. A randomized trial of skin cancer prevention in aquatics settings: the Pool Cool program. Health Psychol 2002; 21(6):579–587.

52. Mahler HI, Kulik JA, Harrell J, et al. Effects of UV photographs, photoaging information, and use of sunless tanning lotion on sun protection behaviors. Arch Dermatol 2005; 141(3):373–380.

53. Fuchs J. Potentials and limitations of the natural antioxidants RRR-alpha-tocopherol, L-ascorbic acid and beta-carotene in cutaneous photoprotection. Free Radic Biol Med 1998; 25(7):848–873.

54. Fuchs J, Kern H. Modulation of UV-light-induced skin inflammation by D-alpha-tocopherol and L-ascorbic acid: a clinical study using solar simulated radiation. Free Radic Biol Med 1998; 25(9):1006–1012.

55. Hoppe U, Bergemann J, Diembeck W, et al. Coenzyme Q10, a cutaneous antioxidant and energizer. Biofactors 1999; 9(2–4):371–378.

56. Lawrence N. New and emerging treatments for photoaging. Dermatol Clin 2000; 18(1):99–112.

57. Poswig A, Wenk J, Brenneisen P, et al. Adaptive antioxidant response of manganese-superoxide dismutase following repetitive UVA irradiation. J Invest Dermatol 1999; 112(1):13–18.

58. Middelkamp-Hup MA, Pathak MA, Parrado C, et al. Oral Polypodium leucotomos extract decreases ultraviolet-induced damage of human skin. J Am Acad Dermatol 2004; 51(6):910–918.

Index

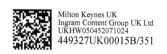

Milton Keynes UK
Ingram Content Group UK Ltd.
UKHW050452071024
449327UK00015B/351